Substance Abuse Treatment

SAGE SOURCEBOOKS FOR THE HUMAN SERVICES SERIES

Series Editors: ARMAND LAUFFER and CHARLES GARVIN

Recent Volumes in This Series

HEALTH PROMOTION AT THE COMMUNITY LEVEL
edited by NEIL BRACHT

ELDER CARE: Family Training and Support
by AMANDA SMITH BARUSCH

SOCIAL WORK PRACTICE WITH ASIAN AMERICANS
edited by SHARLENE MAEDA FURUTO, RENUKA BISWAS, DOUGLAS K.CHUNG, KENJI MURASE, & FARIYAL ROSS-SHERIFF

FAMILY POLICIES AND FAMILY WELL-BEING: The Role of Political Culture
by SHIRLEY L. ZIMMERMAN

FAMILY THERAPY WITH THE ELDERLY
by ELIZABETH R. NEIDHARDT & JO ANN ALLEN

EFFECTIVELY MANAGING HUMAN SERVICE ORGANIZATIONS
by RALPH BRODY

SINGLE-PARENT FAMILIES
by KRIS KISSMAN & JO ANN ALLEN

SUBSTANCE ABUSE TREATMENT: A Family Systems Perspective
edited by EDITH M. FREEMAN

SOCIAL COGNITION AND INDIVIDUAL CHANGE: Current Theory and Counseling Guidelines
by AARON M. BROWER & PAULA S. NURIUS

UNDERSTANDING AND TREATING ADOLESCENT SUBSTANCE ABUSE
by PHILIP P. MUISENER

EFFECTIVE EMPLOYEE ASSISTANCE PROGRAMS: A Guide for EAP Counselors and Managers
by GLORIA CUNNINGHAM

COUNSELING THE ADOLESCENT SUBSTANCE ABUSER: School-Based Intervention and Prevention
by MARLENE MIZIKER GONET

TASK GROUPS IN THE SOCIAL SERVICES
by MARIAN FATOUT & STEVEN R. ROSE

Substance Abuse Treatment

A Family Systems Perspective

Edith M. Freeman

Sage Sourcebooks for
SSHS
the Human Services Series
25

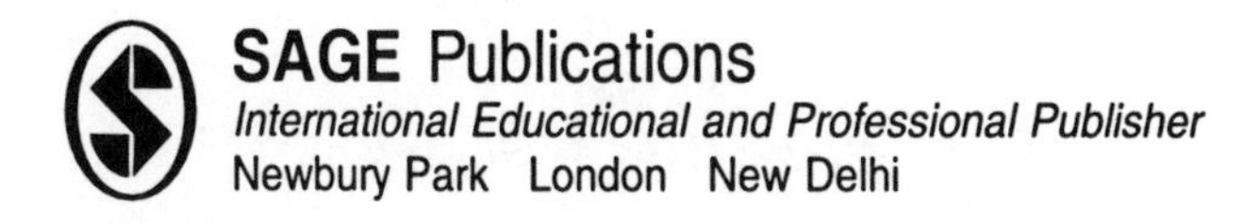

For information address:

SAGE Publications, Inc.
2455 Teller Road
Newbury Park, California 91320

SAGE Publications Ltd.
6 Bonhill Street
London EC2A 4PU
United Kingdom

SAGE Publications India Pvt. Ltd.
M-32 Market
Greater Kailash I
New Delhi 110 048 India

Printed in the United States of America

Library of Congress Cataloging-in-Publication Data

Main entry under title:

Substance abuse treatment: a family systems perspective / edited by
Edith M. Freeman.
p. cm.—(Sage sourcebooks for the human services series; v. 25)
Includes bibliographical references and index.
ISBN 0-8039-4889-1 (cl).—ISBN 0-8039-4890-5 (pbk.)
1. Substance abuse—Treatment. 2. Substance abuse—Patients—Family relationships. 3. Family psychotherapy. I. Freeman, Edith M. II. Series.
[DNLM: 1. Substance Abuse—therapy. 2. Family Therapy—methods. WM 270 S94132 1993]
RC564.S8373 1993
616.86'0651—dc20
DNLM/DLC 93-9209

95 96 10 9 8 7 6 5 4 3 2

Sage Production Editor: Diane S. Foster

When spider
webs unite,
they can tie
up a lion.

African Proverb

CONTENTS

FOREWORD

MAN KEUNG HO

Substance abuse clearly is a major problem in American society today. Substance abuse is not a phenomenon attributable to a single cause or even to a small number of causes. The reasons why a given individual engages in substance abuse are as varied as the range of substances available to abuse; as varied as the social, psychological, and biological makeup of the individual who abuses; and as varied as the families within which abuses develop. Substance abuse is a problem of multiple interactions within and between systems, and the family is the most important part of these systems. Without minimizing the importance of the biological, social, or psychological theoretical explanations of substance abuse, it is the family in which all of these factors are transmitted, reinforced, or modified. It is the family in all of its forms and complexity that must be recognized and addressed in our effort to prevent or intervene in substance abuse problems.

This book, *Substance Abuse Treatment: A Family Systems Perspective,* edited by Edith M. Freeman, represents a pioneering effort to use a family systems perspective as an organizing framework in understanding, treating, and preventing substance abuse. A family systems perspective allows the inclusion of the myriad variables such as family structures, communication and processes, life cycle changes, intergenerational issues, cultural-economic-societal changes, and so on that are needed to provide a richer explanation of any phenomenon pertaining to substance abuse. Consequently a broader range of prevention and treatment approaches can be mounted that have a greater opportunity of showing a significant and positive impact on the problem.

Freeman has capably amassed an outstanding group of practitioners and educators who have produced a thoughtful, challenging, scholarly but practical collection of chapters on substance abuse treatment and prevention adhering to a family systems framework. This book, with its overarching social work person-and-environment perspective and emphasis on "wholeness and wellness," encourages practitioners to empower clients to build on appropriate individual, familial, and environmental strengths. By doing so, this book offers a refreshingly creative, humanistic perspective to the understanding, treatment, and prevention of substance abuse. This book no doubt will be widely read, discussed, and critiqued by both practitioners and scholars. It is a major contribution to the substance abuse and family therapy fields and should be required reading for every substance abuse therapist, program administrator, researcher, and human service professional who works with substance abuse problems.

PREFACE AND ACKNOWLEDGMENTS

EDITH M. FREEMAN

The American family has been described by some authors as the "vanishing family," perhaps an extreme characterization, but most will agree that families have changed in important ways in the past 30-40 years. Both internal and external factors are assumed to be the sources of such changes. As more knowledge of family functioning has been developed through research and the practice experiences of helping professionals, the interdependence between those internal and external factors has become clearer. For example, connections have been clarified between the incidence, patterns, and consequences of substance abuse within a family and a family's internal dynamics, as well as the particular social conditions that are part of its existence. Effective substance abuse treatment must attempt, therefore, to address this broad range of interrelated factors.

The primary purpose of this book is to describe some important aspects of substance abuse treatment within the context of the family—the system most directly affected by the presence of substance abuse problems in one or more of its members. This focus on the treatment of families and on family issues is extremely important, especially when the family is viewed as a system with relationships and norms that may contribute to, as well as help resolve, the addiction problems of a member. Accordingly this book describes various approaches to substance abuse treatment from a family systems perspective. Such a perspective is consistent with the person-in-environment focus of social work that is being emphasized currently in many of the helping professions.

A secondary purpose of the book is to explore some of the common family life span issues that make substance abuse treatment with families a complex and difficult endeavor. Many of these issues are the central focus of various chapters, including identity and coping patterns in the young children of alcoholics across different racial groups, adjustment or launching crises in drug-addicted adolescents, sexual adjustment concerns in adult substance abusers and their partners, and intergenerational role conflicts in families with an elderly member.

The definition of *family* in this book reflects the changing nature of families, these life span issues, and the substance abuse problems that confront the American family today. Definitions are important because they provide guidelines for determining what is normal and what constitutes a problem within a family. Some current definitions focus on the structure of families: for example, on "a group of persons united by ties of marriage, blood, or adoption; constituting a single household; interacting and communicating with each other in their respective social roles of husband and wife, mother and father, son and daughter, brother and sister; and creating and maintaining a common culture" (Burgess, Locke, & Thomas, 1971, p. 6).

Other definitions employ a functional approach to describe what families do or should do, such as "rearing children, meeting affectional needs of adults, and transmitting the values of larger society" (Hartman & Laird, 1983, p. 28). Each definition leaves out all but traditional families by excluding the different family forms that constitute the majority (and yet they too are changing): blended, single parent, cohabiting, intergenerational, same-sex, childless, homeless, foster parent, and matched families. The latter constitute family groups whose members initially do not know each other but who are brought together by a third party to meet the complementary needs of the members (e.g., family-focused independent living homes for adults with dual diagnosis conditions or for recovering adolescents in need of transitional planning for young adulthood).

The definition of a family in this book is inclusive rather than exclusive; it reflects all three dimensions: the continuum of family structures, functions, and forms that represent the varied ethnic and cultural, economic, gender, age, and sexual preference norms that exist in this society. Although those dimensions of the definition are useful to consider in substance abuse treatment, a person's own definitions and perceptions of family are the most important factor to be considered. The conceptual framework of this book emphasizes the importance of building on the perceptions and strengths of families that are in need of substance abuse treatment. This approach supports a belief in the potential for growth and resiliency in individuals and families and in their natural tendency to move toward healing and recovery. The following basic assumptions permeate the discussions about substance abuse treatment throughout this book as the foundation for the conceptual framework:

1. The family is the basic unit of this society in spite of the dramatic changes it is undergoing in structure, function, and form and the related social conditions in which it exists.
2. To be useful, definitions of the family should change consistent with the diversity and changing nature of families, but this change does not diminish the importance or value of the family.
3. Substance abuse attacks and subverts the fabric of a family and the seams of family life, making the addiction its central organizing principle rather than the individual and family life cycle needs and resources.
4. Substance abuse treatment should focus on the manner in which the addiction has subverted the fabric of the family's daily life and the members' connections with each other and with persons external to the family. Effective treatment should address how the family can reorganize itself to manage its central and neglected needs and resources. (Both intergenerational and current family involvement may be helpful, based on the nature of the needs and resources.)
5. All families may not be capable of making this transition. The substance abuse treatment may facilitate the separation of some families during recovery, the members' increased autonomy, and the development of more nurturing relationships in the future.
6. Substance abuse treatment should address the social context in which the addiction, and thus recovery, takes place in order for lasting family systems change to occur.

These assumptions are consistent with the family systems conceptual framework of the book. This framework provides a recurring echo in discussions about (a) individual life span development within the context of the environment (e.g., socialization and positive or negative social conditions), (b) family life cycle development and the system's dual maintenance and growth functions during the addiction and throughout the lifelong recovery process, (c) the organizational dynamics within and between treatment agencies that can affect the quality of assessment and treatment services for and with families, and (d) the linkages between family treatment and related changes that are needed at a policy level in terms of communities and larger social and political institutions. The latter types of large system changes are necessary to support changes in individuals and families as treatment and recovery proceed.

The book's introductory chapter addresses the implications for changes at these different systems levels, along with the significance of substance abuse problems and dynamics within the family system. A family healing and recovery process is conceptualized, as well as the range of appropriate family-focused treatment and prevention services that are needed. The book is organized into two parts that follow this introductory chapter. Part 1 is focused on treatment from the family systems perspective; Part 2 is focused on research related to single system and program evaluation methodology.

The two chapters in Part 2 illustrate how practitioners can apply those respective methodologies and procedures by using case examples from the treatment chapters in Part 1. The case examples included in each chapter were chosen to highlight individual and family life cycle issues relevant to substance abuse treatment. These examples also illustrate the various approaches to family systems treatment at a practical level involving individuals who have family issues to address, subunits of families, family units, and larger systems. The types of addiction discussed in these chapters also are varied, including alcohol addiction, abuse of a variety of other drugs, or both alcohol and drug addiction.

Finally, each of the treatment chapters contains a discussion on the implications for practitioners' roles and the skills needed to implement the recommended family treatment approaches. This fact highlights the value and importance of the range of professional disciplines involved in providing substance abuse treatment to families: addiction counselors, social workers, psychiatrists, nurses, psychologists, sex therapists, mental health therapists, rehabilitation counselors, and physical and occupational therapists.

Therefore this book may be useful as a primary text in family therapy and treatment courses in graduate schools for these various disciplines. It may be appropriate as well for alcohol and drug treatment courses and for family, children, and youth mental health specializations in those same graduate schools. As a supplementary text, the book will be useful for methods or direct practice courses based on the widespread incidence and consequences of addictions, as well as in health, crisis intervention, and criminal justice courses. Experienced clinicians and practitioners from these disciplines may find the book a helpful resource in the range of settings that serve families or address family issues.

Thinking about those complex issues and writing this book over the past several months have provided opportunities for me to "think outside the box": to challenge traditional ways of thinking about families and substance abuse treatment. Being aware of this endeavor has caused friends and colleagues at the University of Kansas to share more of their own family experiences and ideas about family treatment. Their comments, but even more their questions, have helped fuel this creative process. I thank them, along with Man Keung Ho (now deceased) for his enthusiastic comments in the Foreword and Kim Ray for her excellent typing of the manuscript.

The support of my family (Herb, David F., Meredith, Karen, Gloria, Julia, Marvin, David L., and Theo) and the losses we have sustained during this period have renewed my belief in the healing capacity of families.

Edith M. Freeman

REFERENCES

Burgess, E. W., Locke, H. J., & Thomas, M. M. (1971). *The family from traditional to companionship.* New York: Van Nostrand Reinhold.

Hartman, A., & Laird, J. (1983). *Family-centered social work practice.* New York: Free Press.

Chapter 1

SUBSTANCE ABUSE TREATMENT
Continuum of Care in Services to Families

EDITH M. FREEMAN

Each family is unique in the challenging array of needs and resources it has available for responding to problems of daily living and for giving meaning to the lives of its members. Hartman and Laird (1983) call the family the most "intimate environment": a context for the highly individual and often functional adaptations required for coping with a complex environment. Substance misuse and abuse distort and complicate the family's problems of daily living, while draining the unit's creativity and other resources necessary for meeting its basic and developmental needs. Furthermore the chronic nature of addiction gradually diminishes the quality of life and hope among the members.

It is this sense of diminished hope and self-esteem in families with an addicted member that makes substance abuse treatment and recovery extremely complex. Black (1981), Wegscheider-Cruse (1985), and other authors have clarified how the family's shame, dysfunctional roles, and inadequate communication patterns enable not only the addicted member but also the whole unit to remain codependent. Although family issues in treatment have been the focus of recent research and literature, the family treatment approach has not been adopted widely in the substance abuse field. When it has been used, however, as Flanzer and Delany (1992) indicated, the tendency has been to view it "as an adjunct to the primary treatment of medical needs and the recovery process of the individual" (pp. 54-55).

The consequences of keeping treatment focused primarily on the individual can be considerable. From an ecological/systems perspective, the continuous impact of the family in time (intergenerational influences) and the family and peer group in space (influences of the current family and other social relationships) can either impede or enhance the recovery of the addicted member. Even when the addicted member separates from the family and successfully recovers initially, unresolved family issues and the pattern of stressful relationships may cause a relapse in the future. Moreover, if family members are not involved in treatment, they may continue their codependent behavior patterns or become addicted themselves at a later time. In this manner, unfortunately, the addicted and nonaddicted members' dysfunctional experiences with substance abuse can be transmitted to future generations (Bowen, 1974; Pilat & Jones, 1985; Smith, 1988; Steinglass, 1989).

Families need an array of treatment and prevention services in order to eliminate this dysfunctional cycle and the negative impact on future generations. Such an array of services should be theoretically based and grounded in a clear conceptual framework. This introductory chapter summarizes theories and approaches relevant to family treatment for substance abuse problems, emphasizing how families' unique characteristics affect (and are affected by) the process of addiction and treatment. The chapter proposes a range of family-focused services involving many of these approaches along the substance abuse continuum of care. In a final section the implications for the interdisciplinary training of helping professionals are discussed, consistent with the theoretical base and proposed range of services.

A THEORETICAL BASE FOR FAMILY TREATMENT

A number of theories and practice approaches are useful for clarifying the addiction and recovery process in families. The largest group of theories is based on general systems theory and the ecological perspective. Those theories are called the *family systems approaches,* and, when they are combined with theories of alcohol and drug addiction (e.g., the biopsychosocial and stage theories), they provide relevant information about how substance abuse affects the family as a special type of system (Chaudron & Wilkinson, 1988; Freeman, 1992a). Other theories that may be relevant to particular substance abuse issues in addicted families include a focus on cognitive distortion, lack of insight, and value consequences. Those theories are discussed in detail in the literature and are not addressed here (e.g., rational-emotive therapy, psychoanalytic psychotherapy, and reality therapy) (Ellis, McInerney, DiGiuseppe, & Yeager, 1988; Logan, McRoy, & Freeman, 1987; Stream, 1986).

Assumptions: Systems Theories and Substance Abuse

Family systems theories also are called *bridging theories* because they highlight the connections among the life domains of the individual (e.g., the biological, social, and psychological) and connections among the individual, the family, and the larger environment. Bridging theories imply a positive view of human potential and the interactions that take place between these interdependent systems. An underlying assumption is that families do the best they can even when substance abuse and other problems exist. Additional assumptions related to general systems theory and family systems approaches include the following (Hartman & Laird, 1983; Janzen & Harris, 1986; Papp, 1983; Rhodes, 1986; Steinglass, 1989; Usher, Jay, & Glass, 1982):

1. Systems seek to maintain a steady state or the status quo even if the current circumstances are dysfunctional and painful (as when a family has an addicted member).
2. Transitions and milestones represent opportunities for growth and for crises (the latter are threats to the status quo; maintenance of the system becomes associated with maintenance of the addiction/codependency patterns).
3. Open systems are changed by positive feedback; closed systems use negative feedback to correct deviations from the family rules (or the status quo) by the members.
4. Change related to systems is circular rather than linear (the system's circularity indicates that addiction and other problems are both responses to and influences on the family system).
5. A system's "health" is based on its ability to initiate change as needed (to give indications of the need for help in resolving the addiction and other problems, to seek and use help, to use internal and external resources to maintain the necessary changes).
6. Problems develop in boundary areas within and between systems (within the family and between the family and other systems).
7. Problems such as addiction manifest themselves as symptoms that are a response to the system's needs for survival, although they may be contradictory to the members' individual needs.

8. Symptoms or problems such as addiction serve a function for the system and are not viewed as the cause of its problems, based on systems concepts.
9. When the marital subsystem's boundaries become too permeable, generational boundaries (between the parental and child subsystems) may be crossed to stabilize the system (triangulation).
10. A system threatened by intimacy or stressful feelings can stabilize itself in another way—by triangulating an issue such as addiction, financial worries, or sexuality (the issue becomes the focus of the family's energies and is maintained as part of the system while distracting the members from focusing on other more threatening problems).
11. A lack of differentiation occurs in families that are too inflexible, hypersensitive to feelings, and unable to tolerate emotional closeness without anxiety (addicted and other dysfunctional families become fused in their mutual efforts to maintain the system).
12. A lack of differentiation, unresolved family issues, dysfunctional patterns such as addiction, and losses are passed to future generations, often manifested as problems on anniversary dates or stages of the life cycle.

The System Dynamics and Consequences

The assumptions in the previous section identify how systems operate and change under natural circumstances and how problems such as marital conflict or addiction, which are related to the unique properties of systems, can develop. The assumptions indicate also how families are a resource for maintaining the status quo and for precipitating change: They resist change, yet they also provide the initiative that is necessary for change to occur. It is this paradoxical nature that makes the treatment of families with an addicted member both challenging and rewarding (Watzlawick, Weakland, & Fisch, 1974). Usher et al. (1982) commented on this paradoxical maintenance/disruption function of family systems specifically in terms of alcoholism:

> How do families and alcoholism interact? The family is an enduring organized system of related individuals; alcoholism is a chronic psychological and physiological condition. The key to the family-therapy model of alcoholism is found in the examination of that relationship: alcoholismic behavior becomes integrated into the family system and becomes part of the family's life and stability. The maintenance of one becomes the maintenance of the other. (p. 927)

These authors' conceptual framework has implications for the consequences of abuse, as well as what is required for its resolution in families. As an integral part of the structure and daily fabric of the family, the impact of the addiction goes far beyond the effects on individual members. Internally the unit's and the members' needs become secondary to the addicted member's compulsion for alcohol and other drugs and the system's maintenance. Members do not receive the nurturing and support that they require at predictable transitions and milestones: at critical stages of individual and family life cycle development.

At each critical stage of development, the members' potential for becoming self-actualized individuals and for creating healthy, nonaddicted families in the next generation may be stunted (Smith, 1988). This intergenerational addiction pattern is an example of Bowen's (1974) family projection or transmission process. It is not uncommon for other family members to become addicted to the same or different substances or behaviors from this projection process, a behavior resulting in a codependent and coenabling system. Because these dysfunctional patterns serve a function for the unit (they draw attention away from issues that threaten the system's ability to maintain itself), the unit provides powerful feedback to correct any deviations from its rules (efforts by members to end the addiction or to improve relationships) (Flanzer & Delany, 1992; Usher et al., 1982).

Another consequence is that the addiction of a family member can become intertwined with other complex family problems such as incest. Substance abuse is viewed as a contributing rather than a causative factor in sexual abuse because the former decreases inhibitions, blurs generational boundaries, and generally interferes with many functional areas of family life (Mayer, 1985). While these internal consequences are taking their toll on family life, external supports may disintegrate as struggles with the addiction encourage the family to isolate itself more and more. Also, if extended family members or peers call attention to the addiction and its consequences, the family system often will blame those persons by labeling them "mad or bad" (Watzlawick et al., 1974). This process allows the family to maintain its denial that addiction and other problems exist or that they are of consequence.

Often families then become more vulnerable to stress from both "normal" developmental crises and traumatic events. Increased stress leads to less effective responses to crises and family disruptions. Problems that result from the crises and from the family's ineffective responses tend to be manifested in boundary conflicts within the family (triangulation of children or the addiction) and in their external relationships (legal or work problems).

Implications for Family Systems Treatment

The family dynamics and consequences related to general systems theory in the section above can be applied to substance abuse treatment through a variety of family approaches. Goldenberg and Goldenberg (1988) analyzed six of these approaches—the psychodynamic, experiential/humanistic, Bowenian, structural, communication, and behavioral family systems approaches—in terms of specific dimensions. Table 1.1 is an expansion of Goldenberg and Goldenberg's analysis of some of these approaches, with additional approaches and dimensions included. This table highlights the family systems approaches that are illustrated in the case examples throughout Part 1 of this book. Each of the family treatment approaches included in Table 1.1 draws on one or more other theories in addition to family systems theory. For example, the strategic approach draws from cognitive as well as systems theory. Although the strategic and communications family approaches have been combined by some authors, the two approaches have been separated here due to differences in their foci and techniques.

This table presents a number of guidelines for the use of family systems approaches. It also identifies some of the dimensions that indicate how one theory versus another may be more applicable to a particular case situation and how the assumptions are related as well. For instance, the table shows that the intergenerational approach addresses the lack of self-differentiation among family members as part of the addiction problem (which has been transmitted across two or more generations by the family projection process identified in Assumption 11) (Bowen, 1974). If a family's view of its problems, including the addiction, is of members "not being able to think for themselves" or "staying tied to the family," then the intergenerational approach may be useful. In that type of situations and others, it may be appropriate to combine two of these approaches and to use them simultaneously or sequentially as needed (Hartman & Laird, 1983).

These guidelines also help point out certain implications for family treatment, particularly those related to the theories' limitations. One implication is that this range of approaches provides opportunities to use family treatment in a combination of modalities when the total family is not involved in treatment or when other needs must be addressed (in individual, group, couple, and family sessions) (Watzlawick et al., 1974). Examples of various combinations of modalities that can be used to focus on family issues are included in Chapters 2, 6, 7, and 9.

text continued on page 9

Table 1.1

A Comparison of Family Systems Approaches in Substance Abuse Treatment

Dimensions of Each Approach	*Communications*	*Task Centered*	*Structural*	*Problem Solving*
*Focus related to problems in general	Dysfunctional family communication patterns and repetitive games, rigid rules, distractors that determine behavior.	Breakdown in significant family roles, relationships, coping, and problem solving.	Family structure, coalitions, triads, power distribution.	Ineffective patterns in family problem solving (basic and higher needs).
Focus related to substance abuse problems	Role of substance abuse in controlling family rules ("don't feel, don't trust"), double bind messages (denial), repetitive games (victim/rescuer).	Substance abuse viewed as a barrier to mastering the members' psychosocial stages or as ineffective effort to problem-solve.	Triangulation of the addicted member *and* his or her substance, blurring of generational boundaries and parental roles via the addiction (overcompensation).	Efforts to maintain/substance abuse diverts resources from problem solving around higher level needs.
**Goals of treatment	Eliminate dysfunctional behavior/communication sequences in family and rigid rules. Teach family members functional communication.	Completion of shared structured tasks related to significant roles/psychosocial stages to increase family collaboration in effectively meeting needs.	Strengthen permeable boundaries appropriately (cross-generational), individuation of members, restructure family organization (power).	Increase awareness of unmet needs, problem-solving strategies, assertiveness of members.
***Principal treatment strategies	Communication exercises; Analysis of family feedback loop; Message decoding.	Analysis of family in relation to multiple systems (resources/barriers); Task planning/implementation.	Family sculpting; Detriangulation (analysis of triangles); Directives that help realign family alliances and power.	Education in problem-solving steps/strategies; Application of problem-solving exercises by system.
Chapters in which approach is described in this book	2 and 7	3 and 6	4	5

continued

Table 1.1
Continued

	Intergenerational	*Strategic*
Focus related to problems in general	Family-of-origin prescriptions, proscriptions, ghosts, secrets, anniversary dates that affect behavior of current family negatively.	Family resistances to changes, belief systems assumptions, and demands that lead to impasses among the members.
Focus related to substance abuse problems	Family projection process involving addictions in the previous generations, fears of intimacy, and family secrets that enable substance abuse and codependency.	False assumptions of the members about the role/consequences of substance abuse manifested in denial, utopias, demands that members should be responsible for each other's happiness.
Goals of treatment	Address/resolve unfinished family business and cutoffs from previous generations that can prevent recovery.	Resolve family impasses, change family's basic premises/assumptions that enable the addiction, make covert aspects of the family's process overt.
Principle treatment strategies	Construction of the family genogram and analysis; Reenactment; Contacts with family of origin to address unfinished business.	Paradoxical directives or second-order change (reframing, symptom prescription, using resistance); Circular questions; Scaling techniques.
Chapter(s) in which approach is described in this book	8 and 9	9

NOTE: *Culture-specific perspective of these approaches: Most do not focus on this dimension directly (e.g., the intergenerational approach implies that cultural factors related to substance abuse and other family issues may be passed from generation to generation through the family profection process). An attempt has been made in this book to address this omission in the literature on family systems approaches. (See Chapters 2, 4, and 5 for examples of how a culture-specific perspective can be integrated with family systems approaches.)

**Common treatment goals for all family systems approaches, in addition to specific goals for each approach: elimination of substance abuse from the family system, reduction of family stresses that could trigger a relapse, and increase in the system's ability to nurture and support members.

***Common treatment strategies for all family systems approaches: homework assignments, joining, objectifying the family system.

A second implication is that keeping the family unit together may be contraindicated in some cases due to the severity of the addiction and other problems. This task may require that family treatment be focused on helping the members separate, gain closure, and adapt to new family relationships, as illustrated in Chapter 8, where separation and unresolved childhood incest were involved (Janzen & Harris, 1986; Pilat & Boomhower-Kresser, 1992). Often in such situations it is important to combine family systems treatment with other specialized approaches such as loss and grief to address issues not focused on by systems approaches. In other circumstances threats to the system (the need for change) may not signal a breakup of the unit but may indicate the need for support and practitioner-guided family interventions to encourage the addicted member to enter treatment. Thus the need to adapt family approaches to aid in conducting pretreatment interventions is a third implication.

A fourth implication is that systems theory helps predict when natural developmental transitions occur in families and the potential reactions of families according to Erikson (1985). This implication means that such transitions offer opportunities for prevention concurrently with family treatment. Chapter 3, on adolescents, and Chapter 4, on young adults, include examples of this family prevention/treatment process involving the need to apply the approaches to new quasi-family groupings.

A fifth implication is that special adaptations of these approaches may be needed to address the range of diversity among families such as those described in this book. This range includes multiply addicted family systems, ethnic minority families, matched family groups, single-parent families, families living in poverty, and same-sex families. The diverse needs and environmental conditions in which many of these families exist indicate that a range of services and creative applications of family systems and other approaches are required. Moreover, it is clear from Table 1.1 that few of these approaches have been put into operation to address ethnic issues in families, with only a few exceptions (Boyd-Franklin, 1989; McGoldrick, 1982). Creative techniques are needed for involving extended family members and "fictive kin," who are viewed as integral members of the family unit in some ethnic groups. The substance abuse continuum of care provides a useful framework for clarifying which family-focused services are appropriate for supporting the strengths and needs of a range of diverse families.

FAMILIES AND THE SUBSTANCE ABUSE CONTINUUM OF CARE

The limitations of family systems theory identified in the previous section are consistent with gaps in current substance abuse services to families. The lack of conceptual clarity and limited applications of the theory, however, are only two of the reasons why existing services to families are inadequate. Other reasons are the result of general misinformation and biases about families. For example, some helping professionals and program developers assume that most family members will refuse to involve themselves in a member's substance abuse treatment. Other service providers may blame families as the cause of the dysfunctional behavior and unmet needs of the addicted members (Berenson, 1976; Davis, 1987; Treadway, 1989). These and other factors have strongly influenced the nature and range of services that currently are being provided to families.

The Current Service Continuum

Gaps in services to families along the continuum of care tend to be fairly uniform in terms of prevention, intervention, and treatment. The present substance abuse prevention services are geared toward certain high-risk groups. These groups, such as high-risk adolescents, are assumed to be vulnerable to a range of substances, including smokeless tobacco for white youth in rural areas and crack cocaine for some ethnic minority and white inner-city adolescents (Kail, 1992). Other high-risk groups include a growing population of women and elderly who sometimes misuse prescription drugs (see Chapter 9). Some other individuals who have a mental illness are high risk because they combine psychotropic medications with alcohol and other, illegal drugs (see Chapter 6).

The services targeted for these high-risk populations are at a secondary prevention level and typically do not involve family members. *Primary prevention* is focused on the general population of children and youth in schools and on the general public through community education approaches (Office of Substance Abuse Prevention [OSAP], 1991). These services often ignore the natural relationships within families that could be used to strengthen prevention services. Using these relationships as a vehicle for prevention also could strengthen family leadership skills and positive role modeling opportunities. It could prevent the development of dysfunctional roles such as the family hero and mascot that enable addicted systems to maintain their dysfunctional patterns (Freeman & Palmer, 1989; Wegscheider, 1981). Variations may exist in how different ethnic group families function and react to the system characteristics identified in the previous section. However, existing prevention services generally do not address how ethnic and cultural differences among families can make them more vulnerable or resistant to addiction (Freeman & Gordon, 1992).

A similar trend exists in the lack of intervention services for families that are confronted with problems involving addicted members. The growing pattern of multiple family member addictions may have contributed to this situation. The intervention process necessary for moving addicted members into treatment requires the collaboration of family members and other relevant individuals who themselves are not addicted to substances. They must be able to confront the addicted member about the severity of his or her addiction and the consequences that have been experienced by each participant in the intervention. The intervention includes an education and coaching process by a helping professional who then facilitates the addicted member's understanding of what he or she has experienced. The practitioner helps mobilize the internal and external supports that are needed during the transition into treatment and that may have disintegrated due to the addiction (T. Gregoire, personal communication, December 6, 1991).

When more than one family member is addicted, Flanzer and Delany (1992) indicated, the family is a codependent, coenabling system in which all members are engaged in the maintenance of the cycle of chemical dependency. Therefore the collective initiative for change normally found in nonabusing members of a family may not exist, so the members cannot be involved effectively in the type of family intervention described above (Flanzer & Delany, 1992). Thus, currently, interventions may involve significant individuals outside of the immediate family who can help encourage treatment but who are unable to help with resolving family issues that may be central to helping the family address the addiction and other problems. This fact may contribute to higher relapse rates in such families during and after treatment. It also may make helping professionals more resistant to and less convinced about the efficacy of family interventions in moving addicted members into treatment (Berenson, 1976).

Current substance abuse treatment is focused on the general population, with the norm for services having been established with adult, white males. Even with this population, however, the recidivism rates are alarmingly high (ranging from 50%-75%) (Bakeland & Lundewall, 1982). Moreover, families are not included in many conventional treatment programs as a potential resource for decreasing these recidivism rates. In this type of treatment program, family members may be encouraged to attend one of the 12-step programs or to seek treatment in a mental health center (Farris-Kurtz, 1992). Separate treatment for each member may or may not be coordinated between the substance abuse treatment program, the mental health center, the school, child protection services, the probation or parole offices, or other service providers who are involved with the family.

A few recently designed programs were developed as family-centered services and will work only with the total family unit, including its multigenerational members. Family work is considered to be the core service in this second type of program based on the belief that the addiction represents a family system dysfunction, consistent with many of the theoretical assumptions in the previous section (Flanzer & Delany, 1992; Kaufman & Kaufmann, 1979; Steinglass, 1989; Usher et al., 1982).

A third type of treatment program involves work with families as one of a range of services provided to the addicted member. In those circumstances, the family treatment is combined with other services and is viewed as an adjunct to the primary substance abuse and medical treatment for the individual (Davis, 1987; Flanzer & Delany, 1992). In this type of substance abuse treatment program, family dysfunctioning is seen as a consequence of the individual addiction (based on a linear rather than a systems perspective). As a result, in those settings, treatment with the family is focused on the addicted member's recovery based on the assumption that the family functioning will improve automatically once the addicted member has recovered (Steinglass, 1989).

A Proposed Continuum of Care for Families

In light of the resource limitations and problems experienced by families in this current substance abuse service system, additional services are needed that can be provided both singularly and as part of integrated rather than combined services. Summarized in Figure 1.1 are the range and nature of key services needed to make the present continuum of care more integrated, comprehensive, and effective in meeting families' needs. For instance, in terms of *prevention,* services should be developed to supplement the current public awareness/education programs being offered at the community level. Such primary prevention

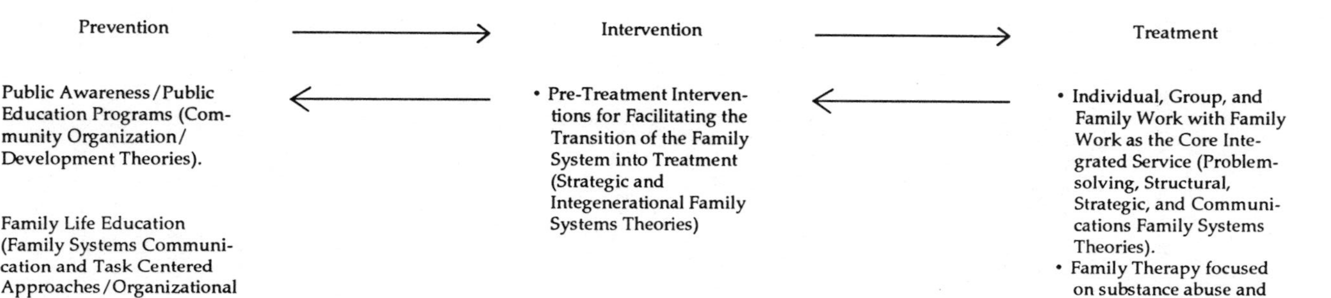

Figure 1.1. Proposed Substance Abuse Continuum of Care: Comprehensive Services to Families (Related Theories/Conceptual Framework)

services do reach members of families, but they do not address family needs directly. Nor do they focus on many of the characteristics of family systems that are evident from the previous assumptions and that influence how prevention messages are interpreted by members and whether they are applied effectively.

The *proposed services* include family life education programs for primary substance abuse prevention that can be provided in sites such as churches, community centers, cultural organizations, and gay or lesbian associations. The use of culture-specific sites and those considered to be supportive of same-sex or low-income families can increase the success of recruitment and outreach efforts. The services might consist of a series of sessions focused on prevention of substance abuse, inadequate individuation/differentiation among family members, dysfunctional communication patterns, low self-esteem, and stress from cultural identity conflicts or discrimination (Hartman & Laird, 1983; Perry & Murray, 1985).

Another type of prevention service could be provided at both primary and secondary levels. A "parents as educators" program could be modeled after the Parents as Teachers program to help parents teach substance prevention to their children. One form of the program could be provided to the general population of families (primary), and a second form could be provided to families in high-risk environments (secondary). Both forms of this program are unique in that they could be provided in the home with year-long, follow-up supportive visits for maintenance of changes after completion of a 2-year program (Freeman, 1991).

Intervention services for families could be useful for the pretreatment period and during treatment. A more comprehensive type of intervention would need to be designed for situations involving multiple family member addictions or addictions in matched families. The use of a team modeled after the Milano strategic family systems approach could be modified for this purpose (Madanes, 1984). The team could help stage a series of family interventions focused on each addicted member. Extended family members and fictive kin (nonblood relations), who are characteristic of matched families and many ethnic minority groups, could be used as supplemental participants. In addition, in treatment programs in which family work is a core service, interventions could be used to move families when they become "stuck" or resistant during treatment. In fact, such barriers often can be predicted to occur after the initial stages of family work in substance abuse treatment, so these interventions could become a regular part of the work (see Figure 1.1) (Black, 1981).

In terms of *treatment,* the range of family services needed is much broader than in prevention and intervention. Family work in various forms is the core integrated service based on the assumptions in the previous section (e.g., the view of addiction as a family system dysfunction). The services include those related to rehabilitation, aftercare, crisis management, respite, 12-step programs, family support groups, and life skills/socialization programs in which religious institutions (churches, synagogues, and mosques) adopt families with recovering members.

Using religious institutions and families that are farther along in the recovery process as sponsors for families entering and continuing in treatment is a unique feature of this continuum of care. This type of peer mentoring of the total family system by an entire church, for example, rather than by individual organizations within a church, could be especially useful and supportive during aftercare. It is at that point, at least initially, when the risk of relapse is high. Families and religious organizations can model spiritual values, cultural traditions, and family leadership skills that are useful for initiating and maintaining recovery. They also can provide both tangible and intangible resources (e.g., employment opportunities and emotional support).

Another unique feature of the proposed continuum of care is the focus on intergenerational and multicultural family issues during sessions with individual families and in groups for multiple families (McRoy, Shorkey, & Garcia, 1985; Pape, 1992; Smith, 1988; Ziter, 1987). Cultural and gender-relevant 12-step programs should be an integral part of the proposed continuum of treatment/support services provided to families (Farris-Kurtz, 1992; Hudson, 1985). These family-focused and culturally relevant services require important knowledge areas and skills for the clinicians, program developers, and evaluators of such programs. The services can be provided most effectively by interdisciplinary teams and individual clinicians who can help families monitor the quality and effectiveness of the services. To meet these requirements, the present focus and structure of training programs for helping professionals will need to be modified and expanded.

IMPLICATIONS FOR PRESERVICE TRAINING AND RECRUITMENT

A number of changes should be proposed and implemented in current preservice programs that prepare helping professionals for substance abuse practice and administration. Many are structural changes that involve large-scale policy and institutional modifications. Some of the recommended changes are in the area of preservice education; others are in the area of recruitment policies and practices for these preservice programs.

Changes in Preservice Education

The complex range of diverse families that need substance abuse services indicates the need to organize and use helping professionals in a more effective and efficient manner. Family diversity includes multiple-member addicted families, culturally diverse families, and family members who are polyaddicted. An approach to addressing this complexity more effectively is to train the different professionals to work in multidisciplinary teams during, rather than after, their preservice education experience. This approach could help institutionalize collaboration and role sharing among these professionals and could lessen turf issues and competition among them. Those types of dysfunctional relationships tend to decrease the field's overall effectiveness in helping families cope with and recover from chemical dependency (Ewan & Whaite, 1982).

The multidisciplinary curricula could be focused on substance abuse practice and administration (U.S. Department of Health and Human Services [DHHS], 1982) as well as the knowledge, skills, and attitudes required for using culturally relevant family treatment approaches (Davis, 1987; Ziter, 1987). The underlying systems theory for these approaches can be applied not only to helping students in preservice programs understand families with an addicted member but also for clarifying the work of the teams and the dynamics within large treatment systems (Kerr, 1982). The content can be provided in an interdisciplinary format through a number of mechanisms, including joint degree programs, jointly sponsored practicums, and interdisciplinary courses. Of course, these changes require structural modifications in training programs from policy, curriculum, and faculty development levels to provide the tangible and intangible supports necessary for lasting changes (Freeman, 1992b).

In addition to the curriculum and faculty development changes identified above, the related and overlapping areas of the service continuum should be emphasized more in substance abuse courses in the various disciplines on policy, research, and practice (Freeman, 1992b). Currently the field is divided into the areas of prevention, intervention, and treatment—an artificial and dysfunctional separation. Often all three service areas are needed within a service program or by one family over the course of its life cycle. The present emphasis on separation decreases the quality and timeliness of services needed by families.

Moreover, current preservice programs should place greater emphasis on training students to integrate research and practice in the field and to involve families more actively in planning and evaluating the services being provided (Weiss & Jacobs, 1988). This type of integration and client family involvement can be empowering to families (Cunningham, 1992), as well as to students and practitioners who will gain a greater understanding of how practice and research complement each other. Family-focused program evaluation and ethnographic single-system evaluation should be an integral part of preservice programs in order to lessen the type of division between practitioners and researchers that students encounter when they enter the field (see Chapters 10 and 11).

Recruitment of Helping Professionals

Just as the above changes can enhance current preservice programs for helping professionals, other changes are necessary in the recruitment practices that are used to encourage individuals to enter the substance abuse field. A more diverse group of students should be recruited in order to address the diverse range of families that currently need prevention, intervention, and treatment services (Freeman, 1992b). Recruitment must take place in a number of forms; for example, it is important not only to continue conventional recruitment within the ranks of recovering individuals but also to target individuals already in the family therapy practice area, the allied health professions, and those practitioners who serve particular population groups in other areas (e.g., families with an elderly member, families with high-risk children and youth, and families in multicultural communities). The emphasis on family-focused substance abuse preservice education will ensure that individuals recruited from these varied practice areas will strengthen their services to families whether the services are related directly or indirectly to substance abuse problems.

CONCLUSION

This chapter has described some of the characteristics of "healthy" and addicted families, along with systems theories that explain the different dynamics and consequences within those families. This knowledge is critical for analyzing and proposing needed services along the substance abuse continuum of care. The current division between prevention, intervention, and treatment in preservice education, practice, and program administration is a barrier to a comprehensive analysis of the continuum. Each area of the field is focused on the services it provides, without a holistic focus on what services are needed by families and in what combination. This division makes the provision of comprehensive and integrated services difficult.

What is required is for practitioners and administrators from a range of professional disciplines to use a more holistic perspective on families by means of the family systems approaches. Although those approaches are limited in terms their cultural relevance and application when the total family unit is not involved in treatment, they currently offer the most useful strategy of treatment in regard to family issues. The use of these approaches should encourage, in the long term, the complementary holistic view and restructuring of the substance abuse continuum of care that has been discussed in this chapter.

REFERENCES

Bakeland, F., & Lundewall, L. (1982). Dropping out of treatment: A critical review. *Psychological Bulletin, 82,* 738-783.

Berenson, D. (1976). Alcohol and family system. In P. J. Guerin (Ed.), *Family therapy: Theory and practice* (pp. 284-297). New York: Gardner.

Black, C. (1981). *It will never happen to me.* Denver: M.A.C.

Bowen, M. (1974). A family systems approach to alcoholism. *Addictions, 21,* 3-4.

Boyd-Franklin, N. (1989). *Black families in therapy.* New York: Guilford.

Chaudron, C. D., & Wilkinson, D. A. (1988). *Theories on alcoholism.* Toronto: Addiction Research Foundation.

Cunningham, M. S. (1992). Multiethnic community empowerment: Affirming diversity, respecting differences, and building common-unity. In State of Washington Division of Substance Abuse, *Planning the future of prevention II in Washington State.* Olympia, WA: Developmental Research and Programs.

Davis, D. I. (1987). *Alcoholism treatment: An integrative family and individual approach.* New York: Gardner.

Ellis, A., McInerney, J. F., DiGiuseppe, R., & Yeager, R. J. (1988). *Rational-emotive therapy with alcoholics and substance abusers.* New York: Pergamon.

Erikson, E. H. (1985). Life cycle. In M. Bloom (Ed.), *Life span development: Bases for preventive and interventive helping* (pp. 35-43). New York: Macmillan.

Ewan, C., & Whaite, A. (1982). Training health professionals in substance abuse: A review. *International Journal of Addictions, 17,* 1211-1229.

Farris-Kurtz, L. F. (1992). Research on alcohol abuse and recovery: From natural helping to formal treatment to mutual aid. In E. M. Freeman (Ed.), *The addiction process: Effective social work approaches* (pp. 13-26). New York: Longman.

Flanzer, J. P., & Delany, P. (1992). Multiple-member substance abuse: Exploring the initiative for change in addicted families. In E. M. Freeman (Ed.), *The addiction process: Effective social work approaches* (pp. 54-64). New York: Longman.

Freeman, E. M. (1991). *Conceptual framework for the Institute on African-American Families* (position paper). Lawrence: University of Kansas School of Social Welfare.

Freeman, E. M. (1992a). Addictive behaviors: State of the art issues in social work treatment. In E. M. Freeman (Ed.), *The addiction process: Effective social work approaches* (pp. 1-9). New York: Longman.

Freeman, E. M. (1992b, April). *Faculty and curriculum development in preservice programs for alcohol and drug professionals in Kansas.* Paper presented at the Faculty Seminar Series on Alcohol and Other Drugs, University of Kansas, Lawrence.

Freeman, E. M., & Gordon, J. T. (1992). *Kansas multicultural substance abuse task force: Training manual.* Lawrence: University of Kansas.

Freeman, E. M., & Palmer, N. (1989). *Reconceptualizing dynamics in the alcoholic family: A preliminary study.* Lawrence: University of Kansas.

Goldenberg, I., & Goldenberg, H. (1988). *Family therapy: An overview.* Belmont, CA: Brooks/Cole.

Hartman, A., & Laird, J. (1983). *Family-centered social work practice.* New York: Free Press.

Hudson, H. L. (1985). How and why Alcoholics Anonymous works for blacks. *Alcoholism Treatment Quarterly, 2,* 11-29.

Janzen, C., & Harris, O. (1986). *Family treatment in social work practice.* Itasca, IL: F. E. Peacock.

Kail, B. L. (1992). Recreational or casual drug use: Opportunities for primary prevention. In E. M. Freeman (Ed.), *The addiction process: Effective social work approaches* (pp. 96-107). New York: Longman.

Kaufman, E., & Kaufmann, P. (1979). *Family therapy and drug and alcohol abuse and addiction.* New York: Gardner.

Kerr, M. E. (1982). Application of family systems theory to a work system. In R. Sagar & K. Wiseman (Eds.), *Understanding organizations* (pp. 121-129). Washington, DC: Georgetown University Family Center.

Logan, S. L., McRoy, R., & Freeman, E. M. (1987). Current practice approaches for treating the alcoholic. *Health and Social Work, 12,* 178-186.

Madanes, C. (1984). *Behind the one-way mirror: Advances in the practice of strategic therapy.* San Francisco: Jossey-Bass.

Mayer, A. (1985). *Sexual abuse: Causes, consequences, and treatment of incestuous and pedophilic acts.* Holmes Beach, FL: Learning Publications.

McGoldrick, M. (1982). *Ethnicity and family therapy.* New York: Guilford.

McRoy, R., Shorkey, C. T., & Garcia, E. (1985). Alcohol use and abuse among Mexican Americans. In E. M. Freeman (Ed.), *Social work practice with clients who have alcohol problems* (pp. 229-241). Springfield, IL: Charles C Thomas.

Office of Substance Abuse Prevention (OSAP). (1991). *Prevention plus III* (DHHS Publication No. ADM 91-1817). Washington, DC: Government Printing Office.

Pape, P. A. (1992). Adult children of alcoholics: Uncovering family scripts and other barriers to recovery. In E. M. Freeman (Ed.), *The addiction process: Effective social work approaches* (pp. 43-53). New York: Longman.

Papp, P. (1983). *The process of change.* New York: Guilford.

Perry, C. L., & Murray, D. M. (1985). Enhancing the transition years: The challenge of adolescent health promotion. In M. Bloom (Ed.), *Life span development: Bases for preventive and interventive helping* (pp. 254-262). New York: Macmillan.

Pilat, J. M., & Boomhower-Kresser, S. (1992). Dynamics of alcoholism and child sexual abuse: Implications for interdisciplinary treatment. In E. M. Freeman (Ed.), *The addiction process: Effective social work approaches* (pp. 65-78). New York: Longman.

Rhodes, S. L. (1986). Family treatment. In F. J. Turner (Ed.), *Social work treatment: Interlocking theoretical approaches* (pp. 432-453). New York: Free Press.

Smith, A. W. (1988). *Grandchildren of alcoholics: Another generation of co-dependency.* Deerfield Beach, FL: Health Communications.

Steinglass, P. (1989). *The alcoholic family.* New York: Basic Books.

Stream, H. S. (1986). Psychoanalytic theory. In F. J. Turner (Ed.), *Social work treatment: Interlocking theoretical approaches* (pp. 19-45). New York: Free Press.

Treadway, D. C. (1989). *Before it's too late: Working with substance abuse in the family.* New York: Norton.

U.S. Department of Health and Human Services (DHHS). (1982). *Planning alcoholism counseling education: A curriculum and instructional resource guide.* Washington, DC: National Institute on Alcohol Abuse and Alcoholism.

Usher, M. L., Jay, J., & Glass, D. R. (1982). Family therapy: A treatment modality for alcoholics. *Journal of Studies on Alcohol, 43,* 927-938.

Watzlawick, P., Weakland, J., & Fisch, R. (1974). *Change: Principles of problem formulation and problem resolution.* New York: Free Press.

Wegscheider, S. (1981). *Another chance: Hope and health for the alcoholic family.* Palo Alto, CA: Science and Behavior Books.

Wegscheider-Cruse, S. (1985). *Choice-making for co-dependents, adult children and spirituality seekers.* Palo Alto, CA: Public Health Communications.

Weiss, H. B., & Jacobs, F. H. (1988). *Evaluating family programs.* Hawthorne, NY: Aldine.

Ziter, M. L. P. (1987). Culturally sensitive treatment of black alcoholic families. *Social Work, 32,* 130-135.

Part I

SUBSTANCE ABUSE TREATMENT ACROSS THE LIFE SPAN

EDITH M. FREEMAN

Involvement of families in substance abuse treatment is both a benefit and a complicating factor in such treatment. Despite the complex nature of family treatment, however, professional ethics, practice wisdom, and the research literature support the need to consider all factors that impinge on the addiction and recovery of family members. The eight chapters in Part 1 of this book attest to this need and to the array of variables that are important in effective assessment and treatment with families. These chapters clarify, as well, the role of multidisciplinary practitioners and administrators in actively involving family members in the work through specific methods for structuring practice and programs. The expected result, as reflected in these chapters, is families actively participating in the planning and implementation of the assessment/treatment process.

Implicit in this process is the importance of building on individual and family system strengths and on an appreciation for the range of family diversity that may be present. The treatment process can be enriched by an appreciation for the diversity in ethnicity and culture (Chapters 2, 4, and 5), gender (Chapters 5 and 8), sexual preference (Chapters 5 and 6), and life span development and age (Chapters 2, 3, 4, and 9). In fact, the chapters in Part 1 are organized to reflect life span family issues that can affect young children, adolescents, adults, and the elderly and that need to be addressed during substance abuse treatment. The treatment for family and life cycle issues is described in a variety of modalities, including individual, couple, group, and family sessions.

Some of these chapters focus on problems within service-providing systems that impact the effectiveness of substance abuse treatment. For example, Chapter 4 contains a summary of how culturally relevant community organizations and informal leaders can be used to recruit and treat addicted young adults from ethnic minority groups and their families, in contrast to the lack of effectiveness in some traditional mental health agencies. Highlighted in Chapter 6 are the barriers within the mental health and substance abuse treatment systems that create conflicts about the treatment of choice for dually diagnosed clients with an addiction and a mental illness. Similarly explored in Chapter 7 is how community-based Vet Centers have resolved some of the VA hospital barriers to family treatment with dually diagnosed clients: with addicted veterans who suffer also from PTSD.

The focus of other chapters is on developmental factors that complicate treatment, as in the case of drug-addicted runaway youth (Chapter 3) and elderly substance abusers involved in intergenerational family dynamics (Chapter 9). In Chapter 3, preparation for adult decision making and emancipation are an integral part of the developmentally focused substance abuse family treatment being described there. The dynamics of family systems treatment for substance abuse with young children, codependent adults, and clients with sexual dysfunction problems are addressed in Chapters 2, 5, and 8, respectively. In these and the other chapters, case studies or vignettes are used to highlight the individual and family life cycle issues that are relevant to substance abuse treatment.

Chapter 2

A CROSS-CULTURAL TREATMENT APPROACH FOR FAMILIES WITH YOUNG CHILDREN

RUTH G. McROY
MARIAN A. AGUILAR
CLAYTON T. SHORKEY

The impact of untreated parental substance abuse on the development and healthy functioning of young children has received increased attention by researchers during the last three decades. Information related to the effects of parental substance abuse on children has been developed from the study of children receiving services from child welfare, medical or psychiatric clinics, or from the study of children whose parents were receiving treatment for chemical dependence. Because most of the research completed in this area has involved parental dependence on alcohol, generalizations that pertain to children whose parents are dependent on other substances remain tentative. A recent study by the National Center for Health Statistics of children's exposure to alcoholism in the family provides the best estimate to date of the percentage of U.S. children affected by this disease (Schoenborn, 1991). Approximately 18% of this national sample of more than 43,000 adults reported living with an alcoholic at some time during their first 18 years of life. Anglo Americans (18.5%) were more likely than African Americans (15.6%) to grow up with an alcoholic. The percentage of Hispanics growing up with an alcoholic in their family (17.4%) was closer to percentages for Anglo Americans than African Americans. These data are consistent with a report by the National Institute on Alcohol Abuse and Alcoholism (NIAAA) (1990b) indicating that overall drinking rates are lower among African Americans, compared with rates for Anglo Americans and Hispanics. Estimates of the percentage of children exposed to parental abuse of drugs other than alcohol are not available. The National Institute on Drug Abuse (NIDA) (1991) reported that 7.3% of the U.S. population, or 14.5 million people, were current users of illicit substances in 1988. The rate of cocaine use by both African Americans and Hispanics was higher than for Anglo Americans, and the rates of heroin use and intravenous drug use was most frequent for African Americans. Current data related to the rates of use and choice of chemicals by various ethnic/racial groups are incomplete and inconsistent (NIDA, 1991). Although specific data on the numbers and impact of illicit drug use on children are not available, it is clear that large numbers of children are affected by the abuse of these chemicals by family members. This chapter reviews research findings on the impact that chemically dependent family members have on young children, reviews specialized treatment approaches used with these children, and introduces a systems-oriented model for work with these families. Specific cultural considerations are explored for work with culturally diverse populations. Case illustrations are included, and useful intervention techniques, based on important age/developmental considerations, as well as cultural factors, are identified.

RESEARCH RELATED TO CHILDREN IN CHEMICALLY DEPENDENT FAMILIES

Research related to the impact of chemical dependence of family members on young children has developed during the past 30 years from the study of children receiving services from child welfare and medical or psychiatric programs rather than through chemical dependency treatment agencies. In *Wednesday's Children,* Leontine Young (1964) reported on her study of child abuse and neglect in 300 families characterized by poverty, poor housing, unemployment, and large numbers of children. Families in her sample were identified by public and private child welfare agencies serving rural, suburban, and inner-city areas. She concluded that the most acute problem, other than poverty, was alcoholism in these families. In the sample, 186 parents were categorized as severe and chronic drinkers, and many others drank heavily. The sample included 237 Anglo-American, 54 African-American, and 9 Native-American or Asian-American families. Young found no relationship between the race of the parents and the incidence or type of abuse or neglect.

In 1969, R. Margaret Cook published *The Forgotten Children,* her study of 115 children with alcoholic parents. The majority of children included in the study were from middle or upper class families receiving services from the Addiction Research Foundation of Ontario. According to Cook's estimates, 106 of these abused and neglected children were fairly or severely emotionally damaged in their alcoholic families. Only nine children were rated as slightly damaged. The accounts that these children gave of their interactions with their parents, siblings, or peers were important in gaining initial insight into the daily stresses these children of alcoholics often endure. The following is a sample of the comments made by these children: "Everybody at our house is angry all the time" (p. 24), "I worry all afternoon at school about how things will be when I get home" (p. 26), "I can take it when one of them [parent] drinks, but I really get scared when they both start" (p. 30), "Mom doesn't look after us. I have to be the mother myself" (p. 31).

Chafetz, Blane, and Hill (1971) compared a sample of 100 children of alcoholic parents to a sample of 100 children whose parents had no alcohol problem. The researchers used information from case records available from the Child Psychiatric Clinic at Massachusetts General Hospital. In the experimental group, 41% of the parents were separated or divorced, compared with 11% of the parents in the control group. The authors found that children of alcoholic parents differed significantly from controls in extended separations of their parents, incidence of serious illnesses or accidents, school problems, and problems with the police or the courts. The authors concluded that children of alcoholic parents were at high risk for developing emotional disorders and emphasized these children's need for special services.

Obuchowska (1974), using responses to a picture projection test that was scored according to verbalized needs, compared 50 children of alcoholic fathers to 12 children of alcoholic mothers *and* fathers. Of the children with alcoholic fathers, 44 were judged to have a positive emotional contact with their mothers. Of the children with alcoholic fathers, those who had positive emotional contact with their nonalcoholic mothers displayed high achievement and affiliation motivation related to their school life. Children whose parents were both alcoholic or whose father was alcoholic and emotional contact with their mother was poor did not display needs for achievement or affiliation motivation at school. These children were characterized by various forms of aggression, isolation, and resignation. Emotional contact with the mothers was identified as an extremely important compensatory factor for children with alcoholic fathers.

In 1977, Mayer and Black reported on a study comparing physical or sexual abuse of children of 19 Anglo-American and 5 African-American alcoholic parents, and 23 Anglo-American and 30 African-American opiate-addicted parents from the Washingtonian Center for Addictions in Boston. Children in ten of these families (13%) were classified as physically or sexually abused. Nine of the abusing families included opiate abusers, and one child was in an alcoholic family. In addition to the findings that physical abuse was significantly more frequent in opiate-addicted families as compared to alcoholic families, it must be noted that the majority (78%) of opiate addicts in the sample were female and that the majority (79%) of alcoholics were male. Therefore it is unclear whether the gender of the chemically dependent parent or the choice of substance accounted for the major difference between the samples.

Also in 1977, Miller and Jang reported on a 20-year longitudinal study of children from lower socioeconomic, multiproblem, urban families. The study included 147 children who had an alcoholic parent and 112 who did not. The researchers traced the social, educational, health, legal, birth, death, and marital records of the subjects from 1956 through 1975. The researchers used a path analysis to trace the linkages of parental alcoholism to problems identified over the course of the child's development. The overall finding of the study was that the greater degree of parental alcoholism, the greater the negative impact on the children both during their developmental years and in their adult social and psychological adaptation. Children of alcoholic families were more likely to have failed in marriage and in their ability to support themselves and their families and were found to have more mental health problems and suicidal acts.

Behling (1979) reported on the incidence of alcoholism in predominantly middle class military families of 51 children referred for abuse or neglect to a naval hospital in California. Alcoholism was a factor in 51% of the 26 physical abuse cases, in 20% of the 20 neglect cases, and in 10% of the sexual abuse cases. Alcoholism or alcohol abuse was present in both parents in 12% of the cases. Ninety-two percent of the children were abused by the alcoholic or alcohol-abusing parent.

Rimmer (1982) reported on a study comparing 180 children of 71 alcoholic patients admitted to a private psychiatric hospital to 51 children of 20 depressed patients and 128 children of patients served by the obstetrics-gynecology division of the hospital. Children were compared on the frequency of health problems, learning problems, and behavior problems. Data were collected through interviews with the parents and children and from questionnaires provided by the children's teachers. No significant difference was found in the frequency of health or learning problems among the children of alcoholics and those of depressed and normal parents. Children of alcoholics, however, had higher frequencies of childhood behavior problems than the other two groups, including lying and stealing at home and school, fighting, skipping school, and discipline problems at school.

Werner (1986) compared the characteristics and family environments of children of alcoholics who exhibited serious coping problems by age 18 to children who did not display these problems. The sample included 22 males and 27 females from a multiracial group of children born on the island of Kauai, Hawaii, in 1955. The children of alcoholic mothers, and male children in general, were found to have larger numbers of psychosocial problems in childhood and adolescence than children of alcoholic fathers and female children. Children with serious coping problems by age 18 scored lower on the Primary Mental Abilities Test and seven subscales of the California Psychological Inventory: sense of well-being, responsibility, socialization, self-control, tolerance, intellectual efficiency, and achievement via conformance.

Bennett, Wolin, and Reiss (1988) studied 82 families in the Washington, DC, area, including 37 families with one or more alcoholic parents and 45 families with nonalcoholic parents. Data were collected by means of a structured interview and two rating instruments of the children's behavior completed by the parents. The children were tested at school with the WISC-R, the Peabody Achievement Test, the Piers-Harris Self-Concept Scale, and the Herjalnic Diagnostic Interview. Children from the alcoholic families were rated as exhibiting significantly greater numbers of behavior and learning problems and psychosomatic and impulsive hyperactive symptoms, as well as lower self-esteem and lower full scale IQ scores than controls.

Tubman (1991) studied the emotional and behavioral characteristics of 26 children of problem-drinking men and 27 children of control subjects. Subjects were recruited through advertisements and newspaper notices in a Northeastern community. The children's mothers rated their children's behavior by means of standardized test instruments. The children of alcoholics were rated significantly higher on measures of anxiety and depression and on the frequency of behavior problems at home and at school. A comparison of alcoholic and nonalcoholic families also using data from the mothers indicated major problems in family functioning, marital conflicts, and availability of social support for the families with alcoholic fathers.

Summarizing the preceding research studies, it appears that children of alcoholics (COAs) are at a substantially higher risk of neglect and physical, emotional, and sexual abuse than children whose parents are not chemically dependent. A broad range of problems may be present in these children, such as anxiety, low self-esteem, isolation, resignation, depression, aggression, and a variety of behavioral disorders at home and at school. Research suggests that children whose mothers are chemically dependent or those with two chemically dependent parents are at highest risk for developing emotional and behavioral problems. A 1990 summary of the literature on children of alcoholics, published by the National Institute on Alcohol Abuse and Alcoholism, warns that "research on COA's is still in its infancy" and that "because of limitations in the methodology and the inadequate number of comprehensive studies, research findings cannot be generalized to all children who grow up with alcoholic parents" (NIAAA, 1990a, p. 3). Individual assessment of cognitive, emotional, and behavioral problems is paramount in individualizing clinical treatment of young children whose parents are addicted to alcohol or illicit chemicals.

SPECIALIZED TREATMENT APPROACHES FOR CHILDREN FROM CHEMICALLY DEPENDENT FAMILIES

The most frequent method for treatment of young children of substance-abusing parents is the group work model. Hawley and Brown (1981) outlined a successful program for working with children in groups, including education about chemical dependence and identification and expression of feelings about life experiences in a chemically dependent family. Reducing self-blame and developing skills for coping effectively with a chemically dependent parent are other important aspects of the program. Techniques used with children in these groups include skits, puppet shows, role playing, and practice of coping skills.

Brown and Sunshine (1982) described the use of group work with children of chemically dependent clients to reduce confusion, helplessness, shame, and guilt and to develop healthy interactions with peers. Robinson (1983) emphasized the need for prevention-oriented group work with children of substance-abusing parents that includes educational, creative, recreational, and therapeutic activities. The author stressed the significance of holding groups at YMCAs or other activity-oriented facilities, rather than in schools or at mental health facilities, to reduce the stigma associated with the children's life situation. Research by Burk and Sher (1990) related to negative stereotyping of children of alcoholics in schools and mental health centers provides support for the importance of avoiding labeling of these children through provision of services that cause them to stand out from their peers.

Pilat and Jones (1984/1985) described a suggested three-phase process for work with children from chemically dependent families in age-appropriate groups, beginning with education, that deals with denial issues, expression of feelings, and problem solving. A wide range of group activities is used, such as chalk and felt-tip marker art work, clay work, story telling, word games, small group exercises, and discussion. The second phase of the process begins when the children become more open about their feelings and the impact that their parents' abuse of chemicals has had on their lives. Group problem solving allows the children to share and develop coping skills for use in their families. Children in this long-term program graduate to the third phase of the program when they are old enough to participate in community Alateen groups, 12-step groups oriented toward adolescents in chemically dependent families.

A broad range of resources is available in general for programming group activities with children from chemically dependent families. Schaefer and Reid (1986) reviewed the use of therapeutic games focused on enhancing communication skills, problem-solving skills, socialization skills, and self-esteem. Dozens of educational and therapeutic games applicable for use in children's groups are available from the Center for Applied Psychology (Center for Applied Psychology, Inc., P.O. Box 1586, King of Prussia, PA 19406, (800) 962-1141). Educational workbooks such as *My Dad Loves Me, My Dad Has a Disease* (Black, 1979) and *Our Secret Feelings* (Molchan, 1989) contain creative exercises that allow children to express their feelings related to life in a chemically dependent family and are useful tools. The use of fiction and nonfiction books as bibliotherapy is recognized as a valuable tool for educating children of chemically dependent parents about the disease of chemical dependence (Manning, 1987).

Brisbane (1985) provided an annotated bibliography of contemporary fiction especially suited for work with African-American children. Play therapy techniques often are incorporated into treatment groups as a vehicle for expressing and working through the anger, fear, guilt, and denial often experienced by children of alcoholics (Hammond, 1985).

WORK WITH CHEMICALLY DEPENDENT FAMILIES

As described by Wegscheider (1981), the disease of chemical dependence affects all members of the family. As the disease progresses, the functioning of the family system and its members gradually deteriorates and emotional, medical, financial, and other problems increase. When possible, the treatment of members of chemically dependent families should focus on the total family system. The ideal treatment model (Wegscheider, 1981, p. 167) includes 4-6 weeks of primary treatment for the chemically dependent family member, with concurrent treatment of all other family members. Initial individual and group treatment is followed by 10-12 weeks of individual family therapy or multifamily therapy. During the 1980s, many private alcohol and drug treatment programs attempted to implement this idealized approach to family treatment. Practical realities associated with treatment of family members other than the chemically dependent client have forced many programs to substitute scaled-down family week or family weekend components to their treatment program. It is a rare occurrence for public or low-cost, nonprofit treatment agencies to include comprehensive family treatment as a part of their programs due to lack of funding to support these efforts. In many cases the chemically dependent family member or others may refuse treatment, parents may separate or divorce, and children may be removed to foster care facilities or are cared for by relatives. Nevertheless the more comprehensive family treatment approach is likely to achieve greater effectiveness, and it should be used with whoever in a family agrees to treatment (even if only one or two members can be involved).

Conceptual Framework for Treatment

In this chapter a systems-oriented framework is proposed for service delivery to chemically dependent families with small children. The framework involves a combined communications and problem-solving family systems approach that can be used with two or more members of a family. Work with chemically dependent families should focus first on the family members requesting services and "should be centered on their own needs and choices" (Deutsch, 1982, p. 159) rather than placing primary emphasis on the alcoholic or addict. Even if the chemically dependent family member refuses treatment, "other family members can change the way in which their lives are affected" (Black, 1979, p. 67).

Basic Services

Basic services focus on the use of community resources to meet the initial needs of family members who request or are referred for assistance. These resources may include emergency assistance for food, utilities, clothing, housing, and shelter, and assistance in obtaining AFDC, Medicaid, or food stamps. Linkage to appropriate community self-help groups is helpful for providing support and education to members of chemically dependent families. These self-help groups include Alcoholics Anonymous, Narcotics Anonymous, Cocaine Anonymous, Families Anonymous, Al-Anon, and Alateen.

Often the initial presenting problem is the need for specialized treatment services for children who are suffering from emotional or behavioral problems associated with chemical dependence of family members. An understanding of the special needs of these children can be facilitated through the use of several assessment tools available to measure attitudes, perceptions, feelings, and behaviors of children, such as the Children of Alcoholics Screening Test (Pilat & Jones, 1984/1985) and the Children of Alcoholics Life-Events Schedule (Roosa, Sandler, Gehring, Beals, & Cappo, 1988). As previously discussed, individualized assessment of problems and needs of children of substance-abusing parents is extremely important in making appropriate referrals for psychoeducational and clinical services.

Ongoing Services

Ongoing services should emphasize support for family members and build on the functional aspects of family life. Assessment of the family system and identification of needs and priorities of its various members are important aspects of the process. Ongoing services may include coordination of a broad range of resources for family members, including (a) alcohol and drug treatment for the parents; (b) women's advocacy programs; (c) educational programs such as literacy, English as a second language, and General Education Development (GED); (d) classes in budgeting and child management; and (e) services of various public and private family agencies, including those operated by churches and nonprofit groups for specific minority populations. An important aspect of these ongoing services is the removal of the chemical from the system as soon as possible (Usher, Jay, & Glass, 1985). Education and training of the family members to intervene with the chemically dependent family member in order to motivate that person to accept initial treatment offers the greatest promise for initiating recovery for the entire family system (Johnson, 1986). Because acceptance of treatment by the chemically dependent family member is viewed generally as a prerequisite for family therapy involving all of the members, success with this goal determines the focus of additional services (Heath & Stanton, 1991). If the alcohol and drug treatment facility does not house a comprehensive family treatment program, the family may need to be referred to local family service agencies that provide family therapy focused on "modification of family relationship patterns" (Bowen, 1974, p. 102). In either circumstance, family therapy or family treatment should be provided only by specially trained family therapists who also have knowledge and experience in the field of chemical dependence (Knott, 1986).

Cultural Factors as Special Considerations in Work With Families With Young Children

In providing ongoing treatment services to chemically dependent ethnic minority families with young children, it is essential to assess these families from a culturally sensitive perspective. Assessment from that perspective provides the guidelines for which areas should be the focus of family therapy or treatment, individual sessions with the child, or group approaches with these children. Five specific factors should be taken into account in all phases of assessment, treatment planning, and service delivery: (a) personal family characteristics and ethnic identity, (b) family structures and informal helping networks, (c) values and beliefs, (d) communication patterns and barriers against help seeking, and (e) environmental and social stressors. As can be seen in Table 2.1, these five factors often are interrelated; for example, on the one hand, cultural roles within the family often affect how involved extended family members are in providing support, while the level of acculturation can affect a child's or other member's attitudes about alcohol use in the family. On the other hand, stress from racism may be

Table 2.1
Cultural Considerations in Assessment and Treatment Planning

1 (a)	Personal/Family characteristics	Socioeconomic status, marital status, educational background, family history, including immigration status; characteristics and/or experiences with oppression and racism; eligibility for social services; personality characteristics such as self-image and coping styles; life cycle issues; cultural experiences of the family in the community
(b)	Ethnic identity	Degree of bi-culturality: traditional, culturally immersed, bicultural, bilingual, or acculturated
2 (a)	Family structure	Marital status and household composition; nuclear family, extended family, augmented family; role of family members, including children and *compadres*
(b)	Informal helping networks	Church, extended family, neighborhood, and community
3	Values and beliefs	Religious beliefs and spirituality; importance of the individual and the family; respect, *personalismo*; attitudes about alcoholism and drinking behavior; communication about alcoholism in the family; attitudes about the use of social services and treatment
4 (a)	Communication patterns	Language fluency; impact of language skills on the ability to secure a job or to broker community systems; patterns of communication within the family and with those external to the family
(b)	Barriers toward help seeking	Lack of trust, cultural paranoia, lack of support systems, sense of powerlessness, denial, resistance, emotional disorders, chemical dependence, access to resources, and economic stability
5	Environmental and social stressors	Homeless or inadequate housing; accessibility to liquor stores and illegal drugs; peer and family influence for drinking and drug use; stress associated with unemployment, underemployment, or current employment situation; racism and discrimination; health problems, parenting issues, poverty, mobility issues, and relationship problems

coped with differently, on the basis of the level of acculturation in the members and the presence of positive role models for informal cultural social supports. It is also important to consider how these factors may affect family members differentially, causing their needs and the type of help required to vary. For instance, some members may have used cultural and social support networks more effectively than other members.

1. Personal and Family Characteristics and Ethnic Identity

It is important to assess the family's socioeconomic status, marital status, educational background, historical background including information on the family's immigration status and/or experiences with oppression and racism, and eligibility for social services and assistance. Personality characteristics, self-image, coping style, life cycle tasks, experiences within the family, the community, as well as cultural influences on the family should be explored in the initial assessment (Logan, Freeman, & McRoy, 1990). This information is also helpful in assessing interpersonal styles or level of acculturation.

Ethnic minority families vary in their level of acculturation, and this difference must be considered in treatment planning. For example, "acculturated" African-American families have adapted to the mainstream Anglo-American culture and may reject their African-American identity as inferior to the dominant culture's norms. "Bicultural" African Americans, however, may be comfortable functioning in the "white world" but also may maintain ties in the African-American community. Bilingual/bicultural Mexican Americans also have a dual perspective and feel comfortable with and have pride in their Mexican-American identity but also seek racial diversity. "Culturally immersed" African Americans may have experienced so much prejudice and discrimination that they may totally reject whites' values, distrust whites, and assume a pro-African-American stance. In addition, there may be different levels of acculturation within a family in this area. For instance, a child in an African-American family may be culturally immersed, while parents and other members are traditional. In assessing or intervening in such families, stress or conflicts about these differences may affect a parent's recovery. These conflicts may increase the difficulties in family treatment: in getting a child to "give up" adult roles that he or she assumed due to the emotional absence/dysfunctioning of the addicted parent. Similar conflicts may occur in Mexican-American families where differences may exist in family members' bilingual skills, as well as their levels of acculturation.

Persons adopting a "traditional" interpersonal style tend to have their survival needs met in the white world, but their human needs are met in the African-American world. They may be accepting of their African-American identity but typically work for whites and often maintain a position of deference to whites (Bell & Evans, 1981; McRoy, 1990; McRoy & Shorkey, 1985). The type of interaction and willingness to be open with counselors may be affected by the individual's interpersonal style. Service providers must employ treatment approaches that take into consideration the interpersonal styles and level of acculturation of individual family members and must be aware of how the helping person is viewed by the client or family members.

2. Family Structures and Informal Helping Networks

Minority family structures may range from simple nuclear families that include only parents and children, to extended families that include other relatives, to augmented families that also may include nonrelatives (Billingsley, 1968; Logan et al., 1990). Families may be characterized as single parent (divorced, never married, or widowed), married, or remarried. The type of family constellation must be considered in assessing stressors. Numerous variations of these basic family forms may exist within minority communities, and they tend to be adaptive responses to contemporary economic realities, as well as to a history of oppression. Although rather unusual, in some crime-involved families, children are considered to be the head of household because of their earnings from selling drugs, especially crack (Staples, 1988). Efforts to change the family's structure and the underlying values should be the focus of family therapy in such circumstances. The parents' prior support of values (selling drugs, for example) that are inconsistent with their current efforts to initiate and maintain recovery has to be discussed with the children in such families, and the conflicts worked through. These interventions are necessary for the parents' recovery, as well as the child's giving up drug sales and abuse when the latter is a factor.

Information on informal helping networks such as the church, extended family members, *compadres,* and other support systems in the neighborhood and community provide much-needed information to the social worker responsible for assessing ethnic minority families. Using an ecomap to depict the family in its relationships with other systems and a genogram to assess how family-of-origin issues may impact current concerns, the worker is able to assess both strengths and weaknesses (Cournoyer, 1991; McGoldrick & Gerson, 1986).

3. Values and Beliefs

Religion and spirituality continue to be dominant values among African Americans (Dillard, 1987). Not only have the church and religious belief systems served as a source of strength, but the church also has been an organizational base for social action (Taylor & Chatters, 1991). Treatment programs that involve collaborative efforts with the church are often more successful in outreach to African-American families. Because drinking is socially acceptable to many Mexican-American Catholics, the recognition of drinking as a problem may be slow (Gilbert & Cervantes, 1987). It is important to assess the Mexican-American client's religious beliefs and values and attitudes. In addition, as the church and other spiritual organizations may be part of the natural helping network, it is important to assess to what extent the family views and uses these institutions as resources (Aguilar, DiNitto, Franklin, & Lopez-Pilkinton, 1991).

Attitudes about alcoholism and drinking behavior may vary by ethnic group. For example, among many Mexican Americans, alcoholism is not discussed openly. Delving into these issues in the presence of children is not acceptable. These factors must be considered in working with Mexican-American families, and the heads of the household need to be educated in the treatment process and alerted to the discussion and context of these issues. This education may involve first acknowledging the cultural pattern with parents that inhibits discussing the issues in the presence of children. Then education about the effects of both the cultural pattern and the substance abuse pattern can pave the way for initiating family treatment that involves the children along with other family members.

The most common cultural values of Mexican Americans discussed in the literature are familialism, respect, sharing, and cooperation. These strengths have contributed to the survival of the Mexican-American family. These values, if used constructively, have a positive impact on treatment. A related concept, *personalismo,* provides the expectation that professionals can interact with family members on a person-to-person level (McRoy, Shorkey, & Garcia, 1985).

Because both the immediate family and the extended family members in minority groups are valued and both play a role in the socialization of the children, the assessment process needs to include the extended family. The extended family may either be a source of support during treatment or create a positive milieu for alcohol and other drug consumption. For example, the extended family often is included in family celebrations where alcoholic beverages may be freely consumed. If the extended family creates a positive milieu for substance abuse, the treatment may be sabotaged unless these members are included. Education also should be a component of the treatment program, as the older members of the household may not perceive alcoholism as a disease.

4. Communication Patterns and Barriers Toward Help Seeking

The communication style of family members provides clues about their acculturation status. For example, in Mexican-American families, initial assessment must include an analysis of each family member's fluency in Spanish and English and his or her level of interaction with the Mexican-American community and wider society. Family members with fluency in both Spanish and English are more likely to be bicultural. In some Mexican-American families, bilingual children are expected to interpret for their Spanish-speaking parents. Inability to speak English can be very stressful and may affect an individual's ability to achieve in school, advance in a job, or use nonsubstance alternatives for coping effectively. Awareness of verbal and nonverbal communication patterns is critical to progress in treatment of Mexican-American and other minority families. Taking time to create an informal atmosphere in order to establish trust is essential (McRoy et al., 1985).

One of the biggest problems that practitioners may encounter in working with ethnic minority populations in a culturally appropriate environment is resistance to, as well as retention in, treatment (Gilbert, 1987; Gonzales-Ramos, 1990). Many families may have developed a strong cultural paranoia due to negative cross-cultural experiences and have become afraid to trust therapists who are of a different race, cultural background, or socioeconomic status (Boyd-Franklin, 1989). Some family members may be uncooperative because of the impact of drug addiction on their personality, temperament, and behavior (Staples, 1988). Families that do seek treatment are also confronted with barriers such as lack of child care, inadequate language skills, or a sense of powerlessness, which may cause some family members to discontinue treatment. Often children are not involved in decisions about whether to continue family treatment. When parents make decisions to discontinue, it is important to help children find other cultural supports and ways to influence parents to at least allow the children to be involved in some other form of treatment and/or self-help group. Providing bilingual therapists and child care services, as well as involving minority families in goal setting, increases the likelihood that such families will continue in treatment. There is a need for more culturally competent or culturally sensitive counselors in social service settings (Dillard, 1987; Wright, Kail, & Creecy, 1990).

5. Environmental and Social Stressors

The extent to which economic factors, as well as other stressors and demands from the external environment, might be influencing the family's substance abuse problem must be explored. For example, many African-American families today are faced with a grim economic picture. Some 31% of African-American families live in poverty (Wilson, 1987). The majority of low-income families live in large, densely populated communities where liquor stores and illegal drugs are highly accessible. Heavy drinking and drug use are a pervasive problem in inner-city areas, especially among low-income populations. The frustration from being unable to obtain the types of jobs needed to fulfill financial responsibilities may cause some African Americans to engage in substance abuse. Middle-class African Americans are also not immune to the problems of everyday life, such as employment-related stress, adjusting to dual career marriages, parenting issues, upward mobility, and identity conflict, as well as racism. All of these factors must be explored in working with African-American impoverished and middle-class families in which drugs and alcohol are used as a "temporary" escape (Coner-Edwards & Edwards, 1988).

Similarly Mexican-American males, particularly young males, suffer disproportionately from alcohol dependence and problems related to abuse (Gilbert & Alcocer, 1988). Alcohol-related arrest rates in this group continue to increase (Caetano, 1987). An increase has occurred in consumption of alcohol by Mexican-American women, and there appears to be a relationship between acculturation and increased substance use by Mexican-American women. Family drinking behavior and peer drinking patterns appear to determine consumption in Mexican Americans (Gilbert & Cervantes, 1987). With increases in drinking rates among Mexican Americans, there has been an increase in the rate of social problems. These factors have implications for the family as a whole, especially when the identified substance abuser loses a job, becomes ill, or physically abuses the children or other family members. For the Mexican-American family, drug dependency is a family problem. Substance abuse is related to increases in the rates of poverty and social problems among the Mexican-American and other minority families (Caetano, 1989). Under these circumstances, even when a parent is involved in alcohol or drug treatment and recovery, these social problems affecting children and other family members are not automatically resolved. For instance, when children in such families have been neglected or abused physically or sexually, more specialized treatment should be provided to address the family patterns that have given rise to and have maintained the abuse. Other environmental and social stressors that are part of the problem, such as employment discrimination or inadequate inner-city housing, need to be resolved as part of the basic services being provided.

CASE STUDIES OF SUBSTANCE ABUSE TREATMENT IN FAMILIES WITH YOUNG CHILDREN

The five major cultural considerations described in the foregoing section can provide the worker with a beginning awareness of the unique issues that must be explored when dealing with African-American and Mexican-American families. The cultural meaning of drinking and the societal inequities that may promote substance-abusing behavior are as significant in family treatment as gaining information on the extent of the substance abuse. To illustrate the significance of these cultural, environmental, and family factors, three case examples of African-American and Mexican-American families are included.

Case Example 1

Jaime, a 10-year-old Mexican-American boy, was referred to the school social worker by his teacher due to difficulty in adjusting to his new school. Jaime has displayed defiant and disruptive behavior in the classroom. The social worker arranged a home visit with the child's 31-year-old mother, Angela. On visiting the home, the worker learned that the family lives in a one-bedroom house behind the home of Angela's oldest sister. Angela has two children by her first husband, Jaime and a 14-year-old daughter. Her first husband maintained close contact with the two children but was killed recently in an alcohol-related accident. The death of her first husband has had a strong impact on Jaime, who had a close relationship with his father. Angela's second marriage ended in divorce, having lasted only 1 year. After her divorce, the family moved into the small house on her sister's property, and the children were required to change schools. The worker learned that the children have limited interaction with the mother and often are left to take care of themselves after school. Since her divorce, Angela has received AFDC and food stamps. She spends much of her time away from home with friends who drink heavily.

During the home visit, the worker discussed Jaime's problems in school and explored the relationship between his anger and hostility, the loss of his father, and current changes in his home and school situations. The worker received permission from the mother to refer Jaime for individual counseling and to an activity-oriented treatment group for children that is conducted by a male, bilingual/bicultural Mexican-American social worker in the community. Although family treatment was suggested for all three members, the mother currently does not see the need for additional services for either herself or her daughter. Angela freely admits drinking and partying frequently but does not consider this to be a problem for herself or her children.

Angela is an attractive and physically healthy woman with good language and social skills and is able to access community resources when needed. When she became pregnant and married her first husband at age 17, her family strongly disapproved of the marriage. After moving from her parents' home, she and her husband developed a close relationship with numerous friends who frequently spent time together drinking and socializing. After her divorce from her first husband, she was increasingly isolated from her family and dependent on friends. Angela could best be described as selectively bicultural. She is bilingual and participates in many aspects of the Mexican-American community with her friends, but she has become estranged from the Catholic Church due to her divorce and does not interact regularly with her family. Because her male and female peers use alcohol as an important part of their life-style, she has rejected many of the traditional attitudes of Mexican-American women associated with abstinence from alcohol. She is emotionally immature and is self-oriented rather than family-oriented in terms of her children. Angela feels hurt and angry about her extended family's disapproval and lack of support. Her continued unconventional life-style has contributed to socioemotional separation from her family.

After 6 weeks of individual and group treatment involving a communications and problem-solving systems approach, Jaime's behavior has improved significantly in school. He has developed a positive relationship with his teacher; with the other children, he is participating in activities in which he now expresses his feelings appropriately. He has been helped to discuss and use activities to problem-solve how to adjust to the school and family changes, including the mother's alcohol use. The worker has helped Jaime identify other social supports, including the mother's sister who lives nearby. The worker has met with the mother on two subsequent occasions to provide progress reports on the child's changing behavior at school and to foster a trusting relationship with Angela. The long-term goal of the worker is to provide Angela with the opportunity to talk about her personal concerns and unfulfilled needs, her possible relationship problems, distance from her family, and dependence on alcohol as a major part of her social life. The worker would like the opportunity to connect

Angela with a local bicultural alcohol and drug treatment program that also provides counseling, education, and job training. The worker's goal is to connect her with social groups for adults in the Mexican-American community that do not emphasize alcohol in their functions.

Case Example 2

Gina, a 4½-year-old African-American female, is the youngest of three children in the Jones family. She has an older brother aged 12 and a sister aged 13. Esther Jones, her mother, is in her late 30s; her father, David, is in his early 40s. Gina was referred by her pediatrician to a community center for counseling due to symptoms of depression. She was having trouble sleeping and was not eating. Her preschool teacher also had informed Gina's mother that the girl was extremely quiet and withdrawn. On meeting with the mother, the community center social worker learned that Gina's father was an alcoholic and was verbally and physically abusive to the mother when he was drinking. The referring physician believed that Gina was depressed because of the fighting and abuse going on at home. On several occasions, when Gina's father was drunk, he threatened to "beat her," according to her mother. However, she did not indicate that this beating had ever happened. Acknowledging that Gina should not be the sole focus of the treatment, the worker began spending more time with Ms. Jones just prior to beginning Gina's therapy each week. This strategy represented the worker's nonthreatening efforts to involve Gina and the mother in family treatment, along with individual treatment for Gina.

Ms. Jones is willing to seek whatever help Gina needs but fears seeking help herself. She believes that if her husband learned that she was talking to a therapist about the problems at home, he would really become abusive. Mr. Jones is extremely concerned that he could lose his job if others learned he was a heavy drinker. He has been careful only to drink on the weekends and after work. Ms. Jones does not plan to tell her husband that Gina is being seen at the center.

Ms. Jones works as a dental assistant, and her husband is a supervisor at a department store. They consider themselves to be middle income and bicultural. Both Mr. and Ms. Jones are members of a neighborhood Baptist church, but Mr. Jones rarely attends services. Ms. Jones's parents live in another state, and she sees them once every 2-3 years. Mr. Jones's mother and stepfather live about 50 miles away and often keep Gina over the weekend and on holidays. The older son has a job mowing lawns in the neighborhood, and his sister baby-sits for neighbors. They try to spend as much time as possible either working, at school, or spending the night with friends. All three children have observed their father cursing or striking their mother when he is drinking, and on several occasions they have tried to stop their father from hitting the mother.

The worker used play therapy with Gina to help her talk about her feelings when the father drinks and is abusive. She clearly loves her father and especially enjoys the attention he gives her when he is sober. However, she fears his outbursts when he is drinking and had experienced nightmares about him smothering her to death. During one session, the worker and Ms. Jones completed an ecomap on the family to begin to identify stressors and supports. She also gave Ms. Jones two books on alcoholism for her and the children to read. This use of bibliotherapy can be helpful in opening closed communication channels in families where the rule has been not to talk due to secrecy about the addiction. The secrecy can extend beyond the nuclear family, as it did in the Jones family.

Ms. Jones noted that Mr. Jones's parents deny his drinking problem even though he has regular contact with them. They are abstainers and extremely religious. They have difficulty believing that Mr. Jones is alcoholic and deal with the issue by spending as little time as possible in the Jones home. Ms. Jones indicated that she is basically noncommunicative with her spouse, as she is exasperated with his drinking problem. She says, "As long as he pays the bills, I'll just ignore how he acts." She often speaks of a "better life in the hereafter."

Slowly, after several weeks of family treatment sessions with the worker, Ms. Jones began to trust the worker enough to state that she had been considering divorcing Mr. Jones. She had discussed this possibility with her minister on several occasions, and he had advised her first to try getting her husband to seek treatment. The worker urged Ms. Jones to use some of the communications skills they had discussed in the sessions to confront her husband and explain how his drinking behavior was affecting the whole family. Ms. Jones was fearful of this confrontation because she still loved her husband. She did give permission for the worker to contact her minister to discuss the situation further.

With the help of the minister, the worker finally was able to get Ms. Jones to begin attending a racially mixed Al-Anon group. She also notified her extended family of the problems she was having and found that she had their emotional support. In fact, they offered to keep all three children during the summer so that Ms. Jones could attend family therapy sessions and find ways to manage in the event she decided to leave Mr. Jones. Her family also offered her financial support.

With this family support and her increased awareness and communication skills, Ms. Jones confronted Mr. Jones about the drinking and the abuse. However, he refused to admit the problem and refused to get treatment.

About 8 months after the initial referral for Gina, Ms. Jones and the children moved out and she filed for divorce. With the support of her family and the church and her new friends at the Al-Anon group, Ms. Jones, as she puts it, has been able "to begin all over again." Gina's older brother and sister attend a support group at school for children of divorce, and Gina is no longer exhibiting signs of depression. Gina's worker has since encouraged Ms. Jones to join a group for battered women sponsored through the center.

Case Example 3

Carlos is a 7-year-old Mexican-American boy who was referred to an at-risk school program for disruptive classroom behavior. The mother's permission was sought to begin therapy with Carlos. On visiting the mother, Carmen Garcia, at the home, the bilingual social worker found that she could not speak English and was undocumented. The household consisted of the mother, Carmen, the father, and two other siblings (a 6-year-old boy and a 12-year-old girl). The mother reported that her husband was a heroin addict and spent money as fast as he made it. Her way of coping with the stress was to drink heavily. She had not sought any help for fear of being deported.

At the time of the initial interview, the mother had only one close friend, her *comadre.* The rest of her family lived in Mexico. She had been a homemaker since her marriage and had not tried to obtain employment in this country because of her undocumented status. She reported feeling very isolated at times. She did go to the Catholic Church in her neighborhood on Sundays but did not make friends. She discouraged anyone from visiting the home for fear that her husband's problem would be discovered. Although Carmen was literate, she had not had the opportunity to learn English except what little her children taught her.

Permission was readily obtained from the mother to place Carlos in a group of boys his age that met weekly. When Carmen realized the impact her husband's addiction was having not only on herself but also on her children, she pleaded with him to seek help but he refused. After much reassurance that going for therapy would not jeopardize her status, she went to Catholic Family Services, where she had been referred by the school social worker. The school social worker continued as Carmen's case manager, using primarily a problem-solving family systems approach.

Eventually Carmen was able to separate from her husband and now participates in an AA group through her church to stop drinking. Her *comadre* offered to baby-sit if Carmen wanted to go to night classes. Consequently Carmen followed up on a referral to a women's center for classes in English and GED. She also took advantage of job readiness skills classes even though she was unable to obtain employment because of her undocumented status. At the women's center, she was assisted in placing an application with the Naturalization Service to begin the process of legalizing her status in the United States. She was able to do this because the youngest child had been born in the United States.

Carlos's acting-out behavior began to improve as a result of the group work and the mother's problem-solving activities to reduce some of the home and environmental stressors. Today Carlos is making straight A's and is a model student. Carmen has since taken parenting classes at AVANCE (a culturally relevant agency serving mothers in developing parenting and other skills). She currently is enrolled at the local junior college. She has become an advocate for other mothers and now is teaching parenting, as well as problem-solving and coping skills, to other mothers at the agency where she was given help and where she later was hired as a paraprofessional. The Garcia family has made great strides during the 2 years they have received family treatment and support. In addition to Carlos, the other siblings are doing well at school. Their environment has changed, and they have seized the opportunity to make the best of the services provided.

CONCLUSION

These cases illustrate how untreated parental substance abuse can adversely affect all members of the family. In each of the three cases, the child was identified initially as the client. Referrals for intervention typically were made by the teacher, physician, or school social worker, and the children were exhibiting problems of depression or disruptive behavior. During the assessment, however, it became apparent that the child was exhibiting problems symptomatic of problems in the home environment. The workers used the two-phase (basic services and ongoing services) family treatment model and cultural framework, discussed earlier, in their work with the client and the family. Play therapy, bibliotherapy, group work, and modified family therapy techniques for reaching children and families proved to be very effective with these cases. The combined problem-solving and communications family therapy strategies were particularly useful for helping the parent involved in treatment assess his or her situation and confront the addicted parent. These strategies were also useful in helping the worker get beyond parental denial in the case where both parents were addicted (the Garcia family). The involvement of parents, as well as the identification of support systems within the community, extended family, and church, was a critical part of the culturally appropriate interventions that were used in work with each of these families.

REFERENCES

Aguilar, M. A., DiNitto, D. M., Franklin, C., & Lopez-Pilkinton, B. (1991). Mexican-American families: A psychoeducational approach for addressing chemical dependency and codependency. *Child and Adolescent Social Work, 8*(4), 309-326.

Behling, D. W. (1979). Alcohol abuse as encountered in 51 instances of reported child abuse. *Clinical Pediatrics, 18*(2), 87-88, 90-91.

Bell, P., & Evans, J. (1981). *Counseling the black client: Alcohol use and abuse in black America.* Center City, MN: Hazelden.

Bennett, L. A., Wolin, S. J., & Reiss, D. (1988). Cognitive, behavioral, and emotional problems among school-age children of alcoholic parents. *American Journal of Psychiatry, 145*(2), 185-190.

Billingsley, A. (1968). *Black families in white America.* Englewood Cliffs, NJ: Prentice-Hall.

Black, C. (1979). *My dad loves me, my dad has a disease.* Newport Beach, CA: ACT.

Bowen, M. (1974). Alcoholism as viewed through family systems theory and family psychotherapy. *Annals of the New York Academy of Sciences, 233,* 115-122.

Boyd-Franklin, N. (1989). *Black families in therapy: A multisystems approach.* New York: Guilford.

Brisbane, F. L. (1985). Using contemporary fiction with black children and adolescents in alcoholism treatment. *Alcoholism Treatment Quarterly, 2*(3/4), 179-197.

Brown, K. A., & Sunshine, J. (1982). Group treatment of children from alcoholic families. *Social Work with Groups, 5*(1), 65-72.

Burk, J. P., & Sher, K. J. (1990). Labeling the child of an alcoholic: Negative stereotyping by mental health professionals and peers. *Journal of Studies on Alcohol, 51*(2), 156-163.

Caetano, R. (1987). Acculturation and attitudes toward appropriate drinking among U.S. Hispanics. *Alcohol and Alcoholism, 22,* 427-433.

Caetano, R. (1989). Concepts of alcoholism among whites, blacks, and Hispanics in the United States. *Journal of Studies on Alcohol, 50*(6), 580-582.

Chafetz, M. E., Blane, H. T., & Hill, M. J. (1971). Children of alcoholics: Observations in a child guidance clinic. *Quarterly Journal of Studies on Alcohol, 32,* 687-698.

Coner-Edwards A. F., & Edwards, H. E. (1988). Relationship issues and treatment dilemmas for black middle-class couples. In A. F. Coner-Edwards & J. Spurlock (Eds.), *Black families in crisis: The middle years* (pp. 227-238). New York: Brunner/Mazel.

Cook, R. M. (1969). *The forgotten children.* Toronto: General Publishing.

Cournoyer, B. (1991). *The social work skills workbook.* Belmont, CA: Wadsworth.

Deutsch, C. (1982). *Broken bottles, broken dreams: Understanding and helping the children of alcoholics.* New York: Teachers College Press.

Dillard, J. M. (1987). *Multicultural counseling: Toward ethnic and cultural relevance in human encounters.* Chicago: Nelson-Hall.

Gilbert, M. (1987). Programmatic approaches to the alcohol-related needs of Mexican Americans. In M. J. Gilbert & R. C. Cervantes, *Mexican-Americans and alcohol* (Monograph No. 11, pp. 95-107). Los Angeles: University of California, Spanish Speaking Mental Health Research Center.

Gilbert, M. J., & Alcocer, A. A. (1988). Alcohol use and Hispanic youth: An overview. *Journal of Drug Issues, 18*(1), 33-48.

Gilbert, M. J., & Cervantes, R. C. (1987). Patterns and practices of alcohol use among Mexican Americans: A comprehensive review. In M. J. Gilbert & R. C. Cervantes, *Mexican-Americans and alcohol* (Monograph No. 11, pp. 1-60). Los Angeles: University of California, Spanish Speaking Mental Health Research Center.

Gonzalez-Ramos, G. (1990). Examining the myth of Hispanic families' resistance to treatment: Using the school as a site for services. *Social Work in Education, 12*(4), 261-273.

Hammond, M. L. (1985). *Children of alcoholics in play therapy.* Deerfield Beach, FL: Health Communications.

Hawley, N. P., & Brown, E. L. (1981). The use of group treatment with children of alcoholics. *Social Casework, 62*(1), 40-46.

Heath, A. W., & Stanton, M. D. (1991). Family therapy. In R. J. Frances & S. I. Miller (Eds.), *Clinical textbook of addictive disorders* (pp. 406-430). New York: Guilford.

Johnson, V. E. (1986). *Intervention: How to help someone who doesn't want help.* Minneapolis: Johnson Institute Books.

Knott, D. H. (1986). *Alcohol problems: Diagnosis and treatment.* New York: Pergamon.

Logan, S. M. L., Freeman, E. M., & McRoy, R. G. (1990). *Social work practice with black families: A culturally specific perspective.* New York: Longman.

Manning, D. T. (1987). Books as therapy for children of alcoholics. *Child Welfare, 66*(1), 35-43.

Mayer, J., & Black, R. (1977). Child abuse and neglect in families with an alcohol or opiate addicted parent. *Child Abuse and Neglect, 1,* 85-98.

McGoldrick, M., & Gerson, R. (1986). *Genograms in family assessment.* New York: Norton.

McRoy, R. G. (1990). Cultural and racial identity in black families. In S. M. L. Logan, E. M. Freeman, & R. G. McRoy (Eds.), *Social work practice with black families: A culturally specific perspective* (pp. 97-111). New York: Longman.

McRoy, R. G., & Shorkey, C. T. (1985). Alcohol use and abuse among blacks. In E. M. Freeman (Ed.), *Social work practice with clients who have alcohol problems* (pp. 202-213). Springfield, IL: Charles C Thomas.

McRoy, R. G., Shorkey, C. T., & Garcia, E. (1985). Alcohol use and abuse among Mexican Americans. In E. M. Freeman (Ed.), *Social work practice with clients who have alcohol problems* (pp. 229-241). Springfield, IL: Charles C Thomas.

Miller, D., & Jang, M. (1977). Children of alcoholics: A 20-year longitudinal study. *Social Work Research and Abstracts, 13*(4), 23-29.

Molchan, D. S. (1989). *Our secret feelings: Group activities for children of alcoholics.* Holmes Beach, FL: Learning Publications.

National Institute on Alcohol Abuse and Alcoholism (NIAAA). (1990a). Children of alcoholics: Are they different? *Alcohol Alert, 9,* 1-3.

National Institute on Alcohol Abuse and Alcoholism (NIAAA). (1990b). *Seventh special report to the U.S. Congress on alcohol and health* (DHHS Publication No. ADM 281-88-0002). Alexandria, VA: Editorial Experts.

National Institute on Drug Abuse (NIDA). (1991). *Drug abuse and drug abuse research: The third triennial report to Congress from the Secretary, Department of Health and Human Services* (DHHS Publication No. ADM 91-1704). Washington, DC: Government Printing Office.

Obuchowska, I. (1974). Emotional contact with the mother as a social compensatory factor in children of alcoholics. *International Mental Health Research Newsletter, 16*(4), 2, 4.

Pilat, J. M., & Jones, J. W. (1984/1985). Identification of children of alcoholics: Two empirical studies. *Alcohol Health and Research World, 9*(2), 27-33.

Rimmer, J. (1982). The children of alcoholics: An exploratory study. *Children and Youth Services Review, 4,* 365-373.

Robinson, G. M. (1983). Children of alcoholics. *Social Casework: The Journal of Contemporary Social Work, 64*(3), 178-181.

Roosa, M. W., Sandler, I. N., Gehring, M., Beals, J., & Cappo, L. (1988). The Children of Alcoholics Life-Events Schedule: A stress scale for children of alcohol-abusing parents. *Journal of Studies on Alcohol, 49*(5), 422-429.

Schaefer, C. E., & Reid, S. E. (Eds.). (1986). *Game play: Therapeutic use of childhood games.* New York: John Wiley.

Schoenborn, C. A. (1991). Exposure to alcoholism in the family: United States, 1988. *Advance Data, 205,* 1-13.

Staples, R. (1988). Substance abuse and the black family crisis: An overview. In R. Staples, *The black family: Essays and studies* (pp. 257-267). Belmont, CA: Brooks/Cole.

Taylor, R. J., & Chatters, L. M. (1991). Religious life. In J. S. Jackson (Ed.), *Life in black America* (pp. 105-123). Newbury Park, CA: Sage.

Tubman, J. G. (1991). A pilot study of family life among school-age children of problem drinking men: Child, mother, and family comparisons. *Family Dynamics of Addiction Quarterly, 1*(4), 10-20.

Usher, M. L., Jay, J., & Glass, D. R., Jr. (1985). Family therapy as a treatment modality for alcoholism. In E. M. Freeman (Ed.), *Social work practice with clients who have alcohol problems* (pp. 106-118). Springfield, IL: Charles C Thomas.

Wegscheider, S. (1981). *Another chance: Hope and health for the alcoholic family.* Palo Alto, CA: Science & Behavior Books.

Werner, E. E. (1986). Resilient offspring of alcoholics: A longitudinal study from birth to age 18. *Journal of Studies on Alcohol, 47*(1), 34-40.

Wilson, W. J. (1987). *The truly disadvantaged: The inner city, the underclass, and public policy.* Chicago: University of Chicago Press.

Wright, R., Jr., Kail, B. L., & Creecy, R. F. (1990). Culturally sensitive social work practice with black alcoholics and their families. In S. M. L. Logan, E. M. Freeman, & R. G. McRoy (Eds.), *Social work practice with black families: A culturally specific perspective* (pp. 203-222). New York: Longman.

Young, L. (1964). *Wednesday's children: A study of child neglect and abuse.* New York: McGraw-Hill.

Chapter 3

DEVELOPING ALTERNATIVE FAMILY STRUCTURES FOR RUNAWAY, DRUG-ADDICTED ADOLESCENTS

EDITH M. FREEMAN

The child welfare system traditionally has focused on the needs of young children in relation to adoption, foster care, and protective custody. Although the needs of adolescents have been acknowledged by the system, services to this population often have been provided in a fragmented manner, along with services from residential treatment facilities, public schools, and the juvenile justice system (Kurtz, Jarvis, & Kurtz, 1991; Nystrom, 1989; Sims, 1988). The problems experienced by youth, in part, have accounted for this pattern of service. For example, emotional and behavioral disorders, school failure, and legal offenses are the most common presenting problems of this group. Another reason may be the assumption that most teenagers' problems will be resolved through maturation. This assumption means by implication that the majority known to the child welfare system will reach emancipation eventually and achieve an acceptable level of independent living (Timberlake, Pasztor, Sheagren, Clarren, & Lammert, 1987; *To Whom Do They Belong,* 1991).

Recent changes in society indicate that this maturational process may be delayed for many youth; some of these changes include adverse economic conditions, high unemployment among youth, increasing school dropout rates, the alcohol and drug epidemic, and a rapidly growing subgroup of runaway and homeless youth (Clayton & Ritter, 1985; Freeman

& McRoy, 1986; Harris, 1983; Segal, 1991). The two latter conditions pose a significant threat to some adolescents and their families. Researchers and policymakers have characterized the communities in which drug use is at epidemic proportions as "war zones" and have indicated that a substantial percentage of runaways are "push-outs" or "throwaways" who have not voluntarily decided to leave their homes or an out-of-home placement (Clayton & Ritter, 1985; Moroz & Segal, 1990; Rothman, 1989). Others have labeled them "children of the night" who are caught "in the middle of the madness" (Dio, 1987) to emphasize their vulnerability to a system that has failed them and to highlight their identity confusion.

Identity confusion can lead to alienation of youth at a point when, paradoxically, they have a strong developmental need to affiliate (Freeman & McRoy, 1986; Harris, 1983). Some unscrupulous adults use this need for affiliation and acceptance, along with drugs, to entice runaways into prostitution. Prostitution and other crimes become both a way to earn money for drugs and a reason to continue the drug abuse for self-medication reasons. The drugs are used to mask emotional pain and the stress inherent in the life-style. There is a growing body of research on adult prostitution, but there is little information about juvenile prostitution among males and females. Nor has the association between that problem, family dysfunctioning, and drug abuse been clarified, even though all of these problems have increased markedly during the past 10 years (Clayton & Ritter, 1985; Schaffer & DeBlassie, 1984).

The purpose of this chapter is to describe the incidence and process of exploiting young people into drug use, prostitution, and other serious crimes. The connection between running away and individual/family developmental issues is explored to lay a foundation for the discussion about drug addiction. Finally treatment strategies are included for social workers, psychologists, community outreach workers, addiction counselors, and other helping professionals with a goal toward effective independent living for youth. The strategies also address ways to correct some of the existing societal conditions that can prevent the development of strengths in this area.

RUNNING AWAY: INDIVIDUAL AND FAMILIAL DEVELOPMENTAL ISSUES

Rothman (1989) noted that "runaway behavior is a complex, multifaceted phenomenon" (p. 14), indicating that a breakdown has occurred in the family's relational system. Moreover, *running away* can be defined as a psychological, physical, and legal act. Often there is an emotional detachment from significant others, a psychological leave-taking by youth prior to the act of physical flight. The psychological leave-taking may be characterized by a rapid escalation of conflict or lack of communication within a family, along with less time being spent with relevant others, whether the youth is physically at home or spending time elsewhere.

The physical running away can occur at the peak of a period of conflict, during a lull in the conflict when all seems well, or from an accumulation of seemingly small frustrations. Clothing and other possessions may be left behind; moreover, the adolescent usually has few financial resources. The plan to run away is often impulsive, and it is frequently shared with a sibling or peer but seldom with an adult (Morgan, 1982). More youth from dysfunctional homes and families run away than from the general population of adolescents, across all racial and socioeconomic groups (D'Angelo, 1987; Nye & Edelbrock, 1980; Palenski & Launer, 1987; Thompson, 1990).

Legally, running away is considered to be a status offense that would not be a criminal act if the runaway were an adult. Usually a youth must be gone for 24-48 hours before police will take action, depending on the state or locality involved (Morgan, 1982). This interval may delay the possibility of locating some teenagers, while in other circumstances the "cooling off" period can provide an opportunity for youth to reconsider the situation and to return home voluntarily. Such concerns about decision making and control are paramount to these adolescents developmentally. Those concerns are useful for understanding both the incidence and the reasons for adolescent runaways.

The Incidence of Runaway Behavior

Most runaway episodes are brief, with the majority of runners usually staying away from home from 3 days (50%) to 1 week. Forty percent return home on their own, with parents being the most successful of all others in finding those who do not return during this initial period (Kurtz et al., 1991). Some of these youngsters never return home. The incidence of runaway behavior has increased in recent years, particularly the multiple episode type of runaway. Multiple runaways may be associated with the pattern of prolonging adolescence as a developmental phase in this society (Morgan, 1982).

When they run, a large percentage of youth remain within their general community or region (Brennan, Huizinga, & Eliot, 1978). Most stay with a neighbor, peer, or relative. Only 5% of the running population are served by runaway houses in the receiving communities (most of whom are multiple episode, habitual, and noncrisis runaways) (Morgan, 1982). Staff at many shelters attempt to help the youngsters resolve their past and current problems while also encouraging them to return home. As surrogate parent figures, they try to protect the youth from any dangerous situations they may have become involved in since leaving home (Thompson, 1990).

Many other youth are homeless and simply live on the streets or in abandoned buildings. Because of the strong influence of peers at this stage and the desire for acceptance, they often go to localities where other runaways congregate. Rothman (1989) indicated that Los Angeles has been considered a gathering place for runaway and homeless teenagers for many years. Some go to places that help them live out their fantasies about growing up to become famous as actors or rock stars, for example. Others end up in cities and towns where they believe they can be anonymous.

The average age of youth who run away is 15 years. More females than males are runaways, at a ratio of approximately 2:1. The majority of all runaway teens are white (70%) (Kurtz et al., 1991; Nye & Edelbrock, 1980; U.S. Department of Health and Human Services [DHHS], 1983).

According to a report on the U.S. Congress' first effort to count runaways (Thompson, 1990), approximately 500,000 runaway youth are roaming this country's streets. That number is assumed to be undercounted; even so, the report is the most comprehensive study on runaway youth since 1976. Thompson (1990) noted that another 500,000 adolescents are in foster homes, detention homes, or mental health facilities and that many of those are runaways at some point. Other researchers place the number of homeless and runaway youth much higher; for instance, the Federal Office of Juvenile Justice and Delinquency Prevention estimated there are between 1.3 and 1.5 million in any given year (Subcommittee on Children, Family, Drugs, and Alcoholism, 1985). Other estimates of this population are as high as 4 million (Children's Defense Fund, 1988). It is important to note that these numbers of runaway or throwaway youth are separate from the population of homeless families with children and adolescents, which may range from 400,000 to 500,000 per year (Kozol, 1988, p. 3; "400,000 Children," 1987; Shane, 1989).

Reasons for Running Away

The reasons for running away are linked also with the development issues that confront all adolescents: separation from parents and the family of origin, friendship and loyalty concerns, love relationships with the opposite sex (or the same sex, for some teenagers), career planning, and identity (Freeman & McRoy, 1986). Running away is assumed to be an effort to solve intractable problems that develop out of interactions between developmental and environmental factors. It can be an effort to (a) prevent something from occurring (having to live with a new stepparent), (b) cause something to happen (causing the parents to love, trust, or allow the youth more autonomy), (c) remove a youngster from a danger or threat to survival (removing him or her from emotional, physical, or sexual abuse), or (d) exit a hopeless situation (escaping from school failure or from a parent's substance abuse problem) (Morgan, 1982; Moroz & Segal, 1990; Rothman, 1989).

Running away to achieve more autonomy and control, for instance, can be viewed within the context of separation from parents and attempts to establish an individual identity apart from the family and others. Similarly, running away from the threat or fact of sexual abuse is related to developing trust and love relationships with the opposite sex. Leaving forces the necessary physical separation from parents, but unfortunately it also blocks the resolution of emotional conflict and identity confusion, thus making the development of new and trusting attachments more difficult. In summary, running away is an aspect of some adolescents' development that is influenced by familial and environmental variables, along with characteristics of the runner.

Rothman (1989, p. 14) and other authors have summarized some of these variables and characteristics that can be found in the literature:

1. The intended length of stay away from home
2. Personal and social characteristics, including behavioral and attitudinal characteristics of runaways and/or their families, school success, and peer networks
3. Whether running away is self-initiated or youth are push-outs or throwaways
4. Whether there is an escalation of problem behaviors to criminal offenses
5. The degree to which the young person considers street life to be a desirable style of living (Boisvert & Wells, 1980; Brennan, 1978; Dunford & Brennan, 1976; English, 1973; Levine, Metzendorf, & VanBoskirk, 1986; United States DHHS, 1983).

Identification of these variables helps clarify the reasons for runaway behavior. It provides a framework for research on the phenomenon by identifying many of the relevant variables for study, thus suggesting that attention to the interplay between them is more important than a focus on any single variable (Kurtz et al., 1991). And in terms of designing interventions for addressing the runaway problem, the typology encourages a focus on the need to affect the individual, peers, family, and certain social institutions in the environment, such as the public schools. For both research and intervention purposes, the emphasis is on internal as well as external variables—for example, on attitudinal aspects *and* on the behaviors of the persons and systems involved.

What is missing from the typology is a focus on the role that race (ethnic group status), gender, and socioeconomic class may play in runaway behavior. It may be assumed, however, that youngsters who are coping with racial stress/racial identity issues, gender biases, and deprivation of food and shelter may be coping with additional factors that can precipitate turning away or homelessness. Another area missing from this typology reflects factors in the receiving community that can help escalate criminal offenses or enhance the desirability of street life for the runaway (the fourth and fifth variables listed above). These factors may provide additional reasons for *not* returning home and may reinforce the original reason for leaving. This dilemma suggests that a sixth variable should be added to reflect the potential for persons exploiting runaways within the communities to which they flee.

EXPLOITATION OF RUNAWAY AND HOMELESS YOUTH

Although not all teenage runaways are involved in drugs or other self-destructive behaviors, the nature of those experiences is serious enough to warrant special attention by society. Estimates are that the amount of alcohol and drug use among these youth ranges from 8% to 30%, similar to the range among the general population of adolescents (Conroy, 1988; Johnston, O'Malley, & Bachman, 1986; Schwartz, 1988; Smith, 1984). What is not clear is the percentage of homeless and runaway youth who also are involved in stealing, drug dealing, prostitution, assaults, and other crimes. Also unknown are the number involved in prostitution and other exploitative sexual activity, although some place the number at approximately 3% of runaway and homeless youth (Kurtz et al., 1991;

Morgan, 1982), or up to 150,000 youth per year. The conflicts and rupture of family relationships that can help precipitate the runaway behavior as well as the developmental need for acceptance make the adolescent particularly vulnerable to influences in the receiving community.

If adolescents are using alcohol and other drugs prior to running away, they may have been distracted from engaging in the vital developmental tasks that were discussed in the previous section and, as a consequence, may be arrested developmentally (Freeman, 1990). Their reasoning and decision-making abilities may not be adequate enough to prevent them from making poor judgments about the people they meet or about the consequences of their behavior. If they are not using drugs prior to leaving home, they may be enticed into drug use as a way of initiating and keeping them involved in drug dealing, robberies, assaults, burglaries, and/or prostitution.

Initial Contacts

James (1976) mentioned that other teenagers sometimes are used by adults to make the first contact with runaways, frequently in bus stations or video parlors, when these youngsters first enter a community (although some peers may develop informal networks with new runaways without ulterior motives). Often the adult provides the runaways with free drugs initially to get them addicted. The enticer is viewed as providing security in meeting the youngsters' needs; shelter and food may be provided in addition to drugs. If the youngsters have been involved in begging and stealing to obtain food, they may be even more grateful for this seemingly "no strings attached" offer of food and shelter. The youngsters quickly come to believe that this person in the only individual who has ever cared for them (James, 1976; Satterfield, 1981). The dependent relationship helps blur value differences about drug use and sales, as well as other criminal activities that may have been the focus of previous family conflicts. The need for acceptance in the dependent relationship and the use of physical abuse if the enticer feels it is necessary are two of the weapons used to force the youngsters into other criminal offenses, including prostitution (Schaffer & DeBlassie, 1984). Often youth may become involved in several of these illegal activities. Prostitution is discussed in more detail in the following section because it is frequently the "entry level" activity that leads to other crimes by some youth, such as stealing and drug dealing (Subcommittee on Children, Family, Drugs, and Alcoholism, 1985).

The Patterns of Teenage Prostitution

According to Satterfield (1981), most juvenile prostitutes are relegated to the streets under the supervision of a pimp. As many as 95% of prostitutes under the age of 20 have worked on the streets at one time. The hierarchy ranges from the streets, hotel bars, massage parlors, and bordellos to escort and call girl services. A priority is placed on recruiting young teenagers, with those as young as 14 being sought out in some areas of the country (Satterfield, 1981). Once the youngster has been enticed into prostitution, the pimp makes the contacts and manages the money, unless the runaway has entered prostitution without a pimp.

The control exercised by the pimp can be understood in light of the needs of young prostitutes. Many of the juvenile prostitutes who have been studied suffer from self-esteem problems, exhibit passivity, are vulnerable in their relationships, and lack sex education (Kurtz et al., 1991; Schaffer & DeBlassie, 1984). Their attachment to peers and others who entice them into prostitution is influenced by their perceptions of a lack of concern by family members and by the excitement they perceive in the life-style of their new environment. Although male and female runaways who become prostitutes have some of these needs in common, they are also different in the nature of their activities.

First, most of the males engage in homosexual rather than heterosexual contacts. They report that their primary motivation is money, and many identify themselves as heterosexual (Schaffer & DeBlassie, 1984). It is not known how many of them continue to engage in homosexual contacts on into adulthood, but it is acknowledged that some have full-blown identity crises in late adolescence, due possibly to these sexual experiences (Schaffer & DeBlassie, 1984). Second, fewer informal supports seem to be available among the male runaways. Satterfield (1981) noted that females are more likely to form some type of social network among themselves, whereas males generally do not.

The Addiction Process: Life-Style Issues

The previously discussed experiences involving prostitution, drug use and drug dealing, stealing, and other forms of nightlife represent an exciting, glamorous life-style that some misguided youth associate with growing up and becoming prosperous. In fact, Schaffer and DeBlassie (1984) indicated that money and a sense of self-importance are the prime motives for adolescents entering and continuing this life-style. Drugs such as alcohol, heroin, PCP, and cocaine (smoked in the form of crack or inhaled) cause youngsters to become drug dependent—one type of addiction.

A second type of addiction for some adolescents may be to the life-style itself (the risks and dangers of stealing and engaging in prostitution, for example). Often youngsters develop a sense of urgency for being continuously immersed in the life-style. The sense of urgency is accompanied by an adrenalin "high" akin to the physical and psychological reactions they experience from the drugs they are abusing. They may exhibit anxiety (a withdrawal symptom) when they are away from the life-style—for instance, when they are in jail, in drug treatment, or when they return home to their families.

Figure 3.1 illustrates this interlocking addiction process that develops in some runaways. The individual and environmental factors that maintain the addictions require interventions that are sufficiently powerful to help youth initiate recovery, resolve individual and family developmental issues, and disrupt dependency relationships with pimps or other negative role models.

SERVICES FOR CRISIS MANAGEMENT

Interventions for homeless and runaway youth can disrupt negative relationships by shifting their dependencies to more positive relationships and activities. The prognosis for change is probably less for some youth who are involved in drug dealing and other more serious crimes in addition to their drug use. Crisis work by helping professionals and community leaders can occur in a number of sites. The beginning work may need to take place on the streets of the receiving community and then, when possible, be shifted to specialized shelters for teenagers.

Street Services

Helping professionals employed by a number of organizations can be placed strategically in the communities to which runaways flee. These organizations include community centers, family service agencies, social organizations, protective and foster care services, shelters, the juvenile court system, school districts, public health agencies, hospital emergency rooms, churches, health maintenance organizations (HMOs), drug and alcohol treatment programs for youth, and mental health centers. Staff at many of these organizations have intermittent

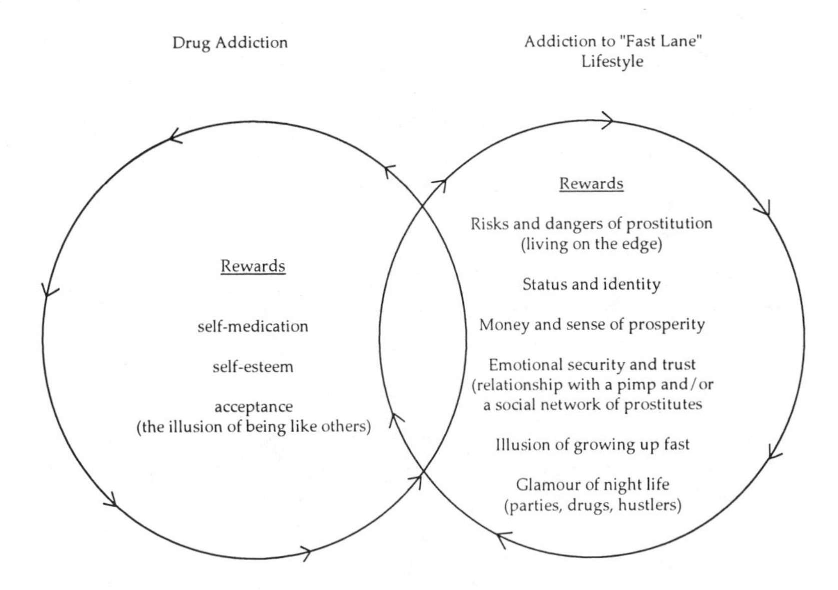

Figure 3.1. Dual Exploitation and Dual Addictions of Runaway and Homeless Youth

contact with runaway youth and a concern about their needs. For instance, hospital emergency rooms are used frequently for health care during crises involving drug overdoses, but staff in those settings have little opportunity for follow-up, given the structure of their present services.

Morgan (1982) noted that some other organizations have exacerbated the problem of runaways, and, consequently, they need to modify their crisis services. For example, Morgan recommended that juvenile courts eliminate their jurisdiction over status offenses such as running away. He indicated that this recommendation is "in line with the clear legislative intent of the Juvenile Justice and Delinquency Prevention Act (1974) and of Title III contained therein, The Runaway Youth Act" (p. 123). If this recommendation were followed, juvenile court staff then could be involved more therapeutically in meeting the needs of runaway youth. Their crisis management interventions, along with those of other organizations identified above, could be improved through a stronger network for coordinating services within each community.

In addition, the precrisis activities of social workers and other helping professionals from those organizations can involve the following:

- Informally identifying runaways in the community
- Determining the places where runaways congregate and/or live
- Identifying leaders of street gangs that steal; listing pimps and drug dealers who involve youth in their activities and reporting them to the police
- Studying the informal networks among runaway youth and learning about similarities between male and female runaways
- Becoming a participant-observer in terms of the teens' daily activities

A period of trust building is necessary during which youth can interact gradually with practitioners so that the latter can make use of crises situations for providing on-the-spot assistance. Crises often involve new and experienced runaways who need shelter and money for food, and those experiencing drug overdoses, drug withdrawal, physical and sexual assaults, suicide attempts, health problems such as AIDS or other sexually transmitted diseases, pregnancy, and depression (Bassuk & Rubin, 1987; Moroz & Segal, 1990; DHHS, 1983).

Crisis services include the following:

- Discussing alternatives for resolving the crises
- Identifying and using formal and informal resources
- Advocating for services when runaway youth are discriminated against or when organizational policies involve requirements that they cannot meet
- Providing emotional support
- Helping to negotiate a return to the family or to work out alternative living arrangements (e.g., with a relative or in foster care)

These services can help some teens shift their dependency on negative role models as their only resource to more positive relationships with individual practitioners on the street. The crisis work can provide opportunities for work on other, more long term issues, including addiction, trust, identity, separation conflicts, or employment. Relationships with pimps and drug dealers, as well as the stress of living on the streets, may become the focus for later problem solving. Clarifying the rewards of that life-style can be equally important in the process of change (see Figure 3.1, in which those rewards are noted). Some youth may strongly resist giving up the relationship with other street people, such as pimps, or working on recovery. Post-traumatic stress disorder, similar to the syndrome experienced by Vietnam veterans and other victims of repeated violence, may be a factor in their hopelessness about the possibility of change (Eth & Pynoos, 1985). (See Chapter 7 for a full discussion of PTSD and drug addiction). For other youth, drug addictions may cause them to deny the seriousness of their loss of control, while addiction to the risks involved in prostitution and other activities can compound that denial.

But the crisis management is also an important service in itself; it may become a bridge for working on these other long-term issues for some youth, but for others it may not. The Juvenile Justice Standards Project (1977) advocated for youth the development of crisis-oriented and longer term services that are locally based, accessible, and voluntary. Those services may help decrease multiple runaways and increase the number who make use of shelters specially designed for teenagers.

Shelter Services

To serve youth more effectively, shelter staff may need to enhance their present outreach and crisis management services because only about 5% of runaways currently use those services (Morgan, 1982; Thompson, 1990). Developing additional shelters and employing peer street workers to provide runaways with emotional security and information about shelters can be effective in lessening the dependency on pimps (Thompson, 1990). Peers who have been drug addicted and who have engaged in prostitution in the past may be particularly effective in sharing the pros and cons of their experiences. They can work in teams with social workers and other helping professionals on the street or in shelters. An alternative staffing pattern is to use teams of peer counselors on the street as a transition to helping professionals who work with runaways once they enter a shelter. The on-site use of professionals who are skilled in addiction counseling and work with adolescents is essential. The importance of these specialized skills and a knowledge of adolescent development for facilitating recovery has been documented (Deckman & Downs, 1982; Freeman, Logan, & McRoy, 1987).

The same types of crises management services that were discussed as part of interventions outside the shelters are relevant to work within the shelters. Some examples of shelter models are Covenant House in New York and other cities (Kandel, 1990) and Wyandotte House in Kansas City, Kansas (Thompson, 1990). Coordination of those services within the formal service network, informal tracking of the youth being served, and work on past family conflicts are important short-term goals as well.

SERVICES FOR STRENGTHENING FAMILIES

For youth who return to their homes, services are needed to help resolve previous family conflicts and to strengthen family functioning so that future runaways are prevented. A generic family systems approach (that combines components from several approaches) is useful for providing families with help in handling their relational issues (Hartman & Laird, 1983). This approach can be accomplished through problem-solving techniques that provide alternatives for alleviating stress and for communicating more effectively. Families are currently under much economic and psychological stress that often is compounded by the stress of parenting an adolescent. Less energy may be available for meeting the needs of the unit and the individual youth when those needs conflict. Parents may use substances to handle their stress and also subtly encourage that type of dysfunctional stress management in their children.

Alcoholics Anonymous (AA) and Narcotics Anonymous (NA) groups for teenagers are an important part of recovery because many of these youngsters and some helping professionals believe adult self-help groups are ineffective for this purpose (Freeman et al., 1987). The work of these self-help groups should be integrated with the services of specialized drug and alcohol treatment programs that serve teenagers. As part of the treatment program, or in addition to it, family groups and peer groups for teenagers can be used to discuss and experience alternative ways of managing stress. The participants can be actively involved in practicing relaxation exercises, family sculpting, communication exercises, and refusal skills related to substance abuse or sexual activity including prostitution.

Problem solving around real-life situations that previously precipitated runaway behavior can be addressed through the group process to aid in the discussion and resolution. Group members might be far more effective in confronting a youngster's denial of addiction or the possibility of relapse (Schwartz, 1988). Instances of youth ignoring intense feelings or expressing them inappropriately could be pointed out in a supportive manner by members with the help of the group facilitator. Members can be encouraged to use each other as a resource for crises outside the group through supportive contracts developed during group sessions. For instance, before running away again, a member would agree to contact the person he or she contracted with and use that person as a crisis manager. Parents could be expected to contract with and call on each other for help with their crises situations as well.

Peer counselors and helping professionals who provide services on the street and in shelters can lead discussions on how to strengthen family resources in problem solving. They can teach negotiation skills for handling differences about values, decision making related to peers, rules about curfews, or the use of substances. Even youth who have not been able to make the transition back home may be useful in warning group members about the hazards of running away, based on their experiences.

HOMELESS YOUTH: DEVELOPING ALTERNATIVE FAMILIES

The Needs of Homeless Youth

Youth who do not return home for various reasons may need a type of service different from those described in the previous section. Current forms of foster care and even small group homes may not be adequate for the needs of homeless and runaway youth. A study by Kurtz et al. (1991) found that only 30% of their sample of homeless youth returned to live with parents after leaving shelters for runaways ($N = 349$). Most lacked a stable, supportive family to which they could return. Thus family reunification or adoptive homes do not seem feasible for this segment of the population (Sims, 1988). As indicated by Dempsey (1983), "The majority of these youth simply age out of care with few personal or social resources for independent living" (p. 1).

If homeless youth have experienced addiction problems, drug dealing, stealing, and involvement in prostitution, the lack of independent living skills may make it more likely that they will continue that life-style. Such a life-style, coupled with earlier family dysfunctions and relational difficulties, can heighten their identity crises. And although physical separation from parents will have occurred, continued problems with emotional separation and individuation can be expected (Timberlake et al., 1987). Predictably a lack of clearly delineated boundaries between themselves and significant others will make adult, independent functioning difficult (see Figure 3.1, related to this developmental barrier).

The following case examples demonstrate the difficulties that some youth have in achieving adult, independent functioning without supportive family relationships.

Case Example 1

Leslie is a 16-year-old white male teenager. He ran away from home when he was 15 because his parents were alcoholic. They often locked him out at night if he was not there when they went to bed because they "forgot about" him. He felt unloved, he was failing in school, and he had problems from trusting peers too quickly and thoroughly until "they disappointed" him. He was from a rural area; when he ran away, he ended up in a large metropolitan area. He got involved in prostitution after a new friend talked him into using cocaine and then suggested he try prostitution as a way of "getting over." His earlier drug use soon led to addiction; he went into a shelter after two teens whom he had befriended assaulted and robbed him to get money for drugs. The shelter staff tried to get him to return home. When his parents refused to allow him to return home, Leslie was placed in a new foster care program designed to teach youth independent living skills. The placement was successful in providing him with job readiness skills and a sense of belonging.

Case Example 2

Maria is a 17-year-old Hispanic girl who ran away from home to escape sexual abuse by her stepfather. She had worked part-time to supplement the family's income and had attendance problems in school. Her parents said she should go to school, but if she did not, they accepted it. Maria used marijuana and alcohol before she ran away from home; she quickly increased her use after running away. She met another runaway who introduced her to a group of teenagers who were into shoplifting, stealing cars, and other crimes as a way to survive on the streets. Maria eventually was caught stealing by the police and was placed in a traditional group home when she refused to return to live with her parents. At the time, she had neglected to get medical care for a sexually transmitted disease, so placement helped her obtain the needed medical care. But Maria continued to believe that everyone was trying to use her. She declared that as long as she could "boost" things, she would never again have to work at a job. She eventually "aged out" of the group home without many of the independent living skills necessary for her to take care of herself and without recovering from her alcohol abuse.

These and other examples indicate a need for innovative, nontraditional programs to meet the needs of runaway and homeless youth.

A New Approach to Programming

A *strengths approach* to homeless youth can achieve two goals: (a) develop an alternative family support structure and (b) develop the skills of independent living. Resources may include creative and new ways of using foster care monies, private foundations, and federally funded demonstration grants. Small group homes could be used to implement the approach, although they need to be significantly different from traditional group homes. They could house only five or six youth, an older peer counselor and helping professionals would serve as coaches rather than experts, and addiction counseling would be a mandated on-site service.

In addition to the services of coaches and addiction counselors (including on-site AA and NA groups), other components of the approach would include the following (some components currently are included in existing programs, but not at this comprehensive level, nor has their effectiveness been evaluated to date):

- Educational and/or vocational services
- Workshops focused on independent living
- Self-assessment and self-monitoring of independent living skills
- Task groups
- Family meetings
- Mentoring by positive community role models (Deckman & Downs, 1982; Freeman & McRoy, 1986; Moroz & Segal, 1990; Timberlake et al., 1987)

The approach has family systems and cognitive, affective, relational, and behavioral aspects integrated throughout in terms of the above components. It consists of a combined cognitive-behavioral and task-centered family systems theoretical framework that allows an emphasis on building and enhancing strengths at various system levels. Services to males and females may be different or similar, depending on the circumstances. For instance, programs serving females with children would need to include child care and parenting skills. Sex education focused on knowledge and values is essential for services to both sexes. It can be provided as a separate component and/or integrated with the other components that have been identified.

Services may need to be more culturally specific for minority group teenagers and the young women in such programs. Each program component described below should be implemented with attention to these special needs. For example, the teaching of stress management and relaxation techniques should include discussions on sources of racial stress in the environment and alternative ways to cope other than substance abuse. Task groups should focus on the realities of racial and gender biases in employment and on strategies for affecting those systems on behalf of individual clients and at a policy level by program administrators. Family meetings can provide a rich emotional and educational process focusing on multicultural dynamics within the family group, as well as in life outside the independent living facility.

Tutoring, GED classes, and creative arrangements for apprenticeships with private industry and governmental organizations are examples of educational and vocational services. Periodic workshops that provide information in short, intensive segments can be used to address vocational skills, housing options, and independent living skills. The focus is not only on skills but also on knowledge and attitudes related to these areas. The approach in the workshops should be on learning and processing information by doing and on sharing reactions to the information with peers.

Self-assessment of independent living skills and psychosocial functioning, including responses to role changes, could help adolescents identify strengths and areas needing improvement. The process could include the construction of each youngster's life chronology (Anderson & Brown, 1980), highlighting and reviewing important events in the family and experiences since the running away. Drawings could be done to replace photographs and other mementos left with the family. This process can help probe barriers to leading a "straight" life away from the previous "fast" life-style and any unfinished family business that an adolescent is dealing with.

Self-assessment could be done early in a youngster's tenure in the group home and then periodically so that self-monitoring could be used to provide ongoing feedback. The feedback could be used to determine what interventions and activities need to be implemented by the coaches, as well as by the adolescents. Some instruments are available for assessing emancipation skills and psychosocial functioning (Sheagren, 1985; Timberlake, 1979), although they do not adequately monitor small and more subtle changes in these areas (Timberlake et al., 1987).

Task groups focused on identifying, discussing, and practicing skills for independent living for older adolescents living at home or in out-of-home placements have been found to be highly effective (Freeman & McRoy, 1986; Timberlake et al., 1987). These groups can address goal identification and planning, career development, job search, job maintenance, social network building, and life management tasks such as budgeting and consumerism. The groups also can help members sort out residual effects from their experiences of addiction and prostitution by encouraging them to compare what they learned in those experiences with current learning. Also taught and practiced in these groups are stress management techniques for handling stress that arises from these discussions and the role transitions they are involved in (see Figure 3.1, related to other sources of stress during recovery). The task groups, as well as other components of this strengths approach, can simulate family relationships, cohesiveness, and support.

Family meetings can help adolescents develop alternative family structures for resolving unfinished business about relationships and separation. Young people can negotiate new relationships in family groups involving their peers in the small group home, and they can work on current issues related to new or pending role changes. The coaches may need to assume a parental role and become a member of the family unit, similar to the use of family meetings in nuclear families (Hawkins, Catalano, Brown, & Vadasy, 1988). The purpose is to resolve problems that arise in living together as a family and to provide the emotional climate where feelings can be expressed and trusting relationships can be developed during recovery.

Finally mentors from the community can be used as positive role models who can help reduce the influence of street people, including pimps, in the community. These volunteers need to be trained in understanding the goals of the approach, but it is their natural helping skills and mentoring activities that are essential to the program. Natural leaders in social organizations, business leaders, professional athletes, ministers, and other community people are good candidates for the mentor role. Their work can be integrated with the work of coaches and other professionals. Mentoring may consist of giving emotional support, providing information, teaching social and vocational activities, finding alternative and positive leisure time activities, active listening, and networking for community or other resources.

IMPLICATIONS FOR PRACTITIONERS

A number of important implications are apparent from this discussion on services to runaway and homeless youth. First, emancipation should not occur when youth reach a particular "magical" age or as a result of someone else's arbitrary decision. Instead social workers and other clinicians may need to become comfortable with such decisions arising out of a youngster's self-assessment activities, along with input from peers, family, or an alternative family structure. Adolescents can learn by doing and experience mutuality in such decision-making experiences. This empowerment process may conflict initially with some clinicians' personal values.

In a similar manner, a worker's values may affect his or her ability to work with young people who are involved in drug or alcohol abuse, begging, stealing, and prostitution. The second implication is the need for the clinician to stay focused on encouraging youth to explore all consequences of their behavior in a neutral way, while realistically pointing out consequences that they may have ignored previously. This strategy can defuse conflicts between the practitioner and youth about the related values. It also provides an opportunity to help adolescents clarify their values—what they believe and desire—in comparison to their behavior and the potential outcomes.

The third implication involves the potential risks that can be associated with professional practice on the street or in the community. Violence may occur from youth under the influence of substances or from street people who object to police reports on their activities (Thompson, 1990). Drive-by murders and other forms of violence have been used by drug dealers against those who interfere with their activities. Burnout is another significant risk in this high-stress form of clinical practice.

These risks are implicit in many of the different roles that have been discussed in this chapter for helping professionals. Some of the roles are traditional ones for clinicians, such as strengthening the formal service network; others, such as crisis management on the street, are more typical of community workers' roles. These diverse roles can be integrated to improve the range of services provided.

CONCLUSION

The use of advocacy and brokering strategies and the need to affect social policies at state and national levels are a fourth implication related to the practitioner roles described above. Those macrostrategies have been discussed in this chapter as follows:

1. The development of social and public policies that strengthen families and their social support and education functions for children and youth (e.g.,

family leave provisions, national child care services, preventive parent education, preventive health care, job retraining and placements for families experiencing job loss from industry closures and technology changes, and preventive family alcohol and drug education)
2. The creation of nontraditional group homes that require structural changes in the child welfare system
3. The elimination of juvenile courts' jurisdiction over status offenses, such as running away, through clarifying the intent of existing legislation
4. The development of closer linkages with police departments, including the reporting of adults involved in enticing young people into drug use, drug dealing, prostitution, and other crimes
5. The reduction of youth unemployment and the enhancement of youth development through innovative job training and job maintenance programs aligned with public and private industry
6. The changing of discriminatory policies of social agencies and health organizations that are barriers to the growth and recovery of runaway and homeless adolescents
7. The restructuring of traditional drug treatment programs for teenagers so that their services help address developmental issues and addiction problems related to a fast life-style (such as the life-style involved in prostitution and drug abuse)
8. The strengthening of existing natural helpers in the communities of teenage runaways by involving those helpers in mentoring programs and providing ongoing supports for their activities

Provision of the crisis services, interventions for strengthening families, and services for independent living for homeless youth will not, in itself, totally resolve the problems addressed in this chapter. More structural, large-scale changes such as those described above are needed in combination with these other microlevel services. Many of the macrolevel changes will require a shift in societal values and resources in terms of how services are organized and provided in particular systems: the child welfare system, health care services, age-specific drug and alcohol treatment programs, and the juvenile justice system. Social workers, family therapists, addiction counselors, psychologists, and other helpers are involved in these and other relevant systems through their daily administrative and direct practice activities. They have a unique part to play, based on these roles and a commitment to serve vulnerable, high-risk population groups. Some of the current roles assumed by multidisciplinary helping professionals must be expanded to include advocacy strategies with legislators, new types of collaborative relationships with police and staff in homeless shelters, and skillful social network interventions.

REFERENCES

Anderson, J. E., & Brown, R. A. (1980). Life history grid for adolescents. *Social Work, 25,* 321-323.

Bassuk, E., & Rubin, L. (1987). Homeless children: A neglected population. *American Journal of Orthopsychiatry, 57,* 279-287.

Boisvert, M. J., & Wells, R. (1980). Toward a rational policy on status offenders. *Social Work, 25,* 230-234.

Brennan, T., Huizinga, D., & Elliot, D. S. (1978). *The social psychology of runaways.* Lexington, MA: Lexington.

Children's Defense Fund. (1988). *A children's defense budget FY 1989.* Washington, DC: Author.

Clayton, R. R., & Ritter, C. (1985). The epidemiology of alcohol and drug abuse among adolescents. *Advances in Alcohol and Substance Abuse, 4,* 69-97.

Conroy, R. W. (1988). The many facets of adolescent drinking. *Bulletin of the Menninger Clinic, 52,* 229-245.

D'Angelo, R. (1987). Runaways. *Encyclopedia of Social Work, 1,* 513-530.

Deckman, J., & Downs, B. (1982). A group treatment approach for adolescent children of alcoholic parents. *Social Work with Groups, 5,* 73-77.

Dempsey, S. C. (1983, October 9). Youths aging out of foster care posing a challenge. *New York Times,* pp. 1, 20.

Dio, J. (1987). "All the fools sailed away." *Dream evil album.* Burbank, CA: Warner Brothers.

Dunford, F. W., & Brennan, T. (1976). A taxonomy of runaway youth. *Social Service Review, 50,* 457-470.

English, C. J. (1973). Leaving home: A typology of runaways. *Trans-Action, 10,* 22-24.

Eth, S., & Pynoos, R. S. (1985). *Post-traumatic stress disorder in children.* Washington, DC: American Psychiatric Press.

400,000 children may be homeless. (1987, March 17). *Chicago Tribune,* p. 15.

Freeman, E. M. (1990). Social competence as a framework for addressing ethnicity and teenage alcohol problems. In A. R. Stiffman & L. E. Davis (Eds.), *Ethnic issues in adolescent mental health* (pp. 247-266). Newbury Park, CA: Sage.

Freeman, E. M., Logan, S., & McRoy, R. (1987). Treatment of teenage alcohol problems: Survey of mental health agencies. *Arete, 12,* 21-32.

Freeman, E. M., & McRoy, R. (1986). Group counseling program for unemployed black teenagers. *Social Work with Groups, 9,* 73-90.

Gullotta, T. P. (1978). Runaway: Reality or myth. *Adolescence, 13,* 543-549.

Harris, L. H. (1983). Role of trauma in the lives of high school students. *Social Work in Education, 5,* 77-88.

Hartman, A., & Laird, J. (1983). *Family-centered social work practice.* New York: Free Press.

Hawkins, J. O., Catalano, R. F., Brown, E. O., & Vadasy, P. F. (1988). *Preparing for the drug free years: A family activity book.* Seattle: Developmental Research and Programs.

James, J. (1976). Motivations for entrance into prostitution. In L. Crites (Ed.), *The female offender* (pp. 197-208). Lexington, MA: D. C. Heath.

Johnston, L. D., O'Malley, P. M., & Bachman, J. G. (1986). *Drug use among American high school students, college students and other young adults: National trends through 1985.* Rockville, MD: National Institute on Drug Abuse.

Juvenile Justice and Delinquency Prevention Act. (1974). 88 Stat. 1109-43 (codified in sections of 18.42 U.S.C.A. Supplement 1975). [The Runaway Youth Act is Title III of the full act.]

Juvenile Justice Standards Project. (1977). (Standards related to noncriminal misbehavior). Cambridge, MA: Ballinger.

Kandel, B. (1990, February 7). How Covenant House grew. *USA Today,* p. 2A.

Kozol, J. (1988). *Rachel and her children: Homeless families in America.* New York: Crown.

Kurtz, P. D., Jarvis, S. V., & Kurtz, G. L. (1991). Problems of homeless youths: Empirical findings and human service issues. *Social Work, 36,* 309-314.

Levine, R. S., Metzendorf, D., & VanBoskirk, K. A. (1986). Runaway and throwaway youth: A case for early intervention with truants. *Social Work in Education, 8,* 93-106.

Morgan, O. J. (1982). Runaways: Jurisdiction, dynamics, and treatment. *Journal of Marital and Family Therapy, 44,* 1231-1237.

Moroz, K. J., & Segal, E. A. (1990). Homeless children: Intervention strategies for school social workers. *Social Work in Education, 12,* 134-143.

Nye, I. F., & Edelbrock, C. (1980). Introduction: Some social characteristics of runaways. *Journal of Family Issues, 1,* 147-150.

Nystrom, J. (1989). Empowerment model for delivery of social work services in public schools. *Social Work in Education, 11,* 160-170.

Palenski, J. E., & Launer, H. M. (1987). The process of running away: A redefinition. *Adolescence, 22,* 347-362.

Rothman, J. (1989). Intervention research: Application to runaway and homeless youths. *Social Work Research and Abstracts, 25,* 13-18.

Satterfield, S. B. (1981). Clinical aspects of juvenile prostitution. *Medical Aspects of Human Sexuality, 15,* 126-132.

Schaffer, B., & DeBlassie, R. R. (1984). Adolescent prostitution. *Adolescence, 19,* 689-696.

Schwartz, S. (1988). School-based strategies for primary prevention of drug abuse. *Social Work in Education, 11,* 53-63.

Segal, E. A. (1991). The juvenilization of poverty in the 1980s. *Social Work, 36,* 454-457.

Shane, P. G. (1989). Changing patterns among homeless and runaway youth. *American Journal of Orthopsychiatry, 59,* 208-214.

Sheagren, J. (1985). Emancipation Social Functioning Scale. In Baltimore County Department of Social Services, National Catholic School Social Services, Institute for Social Services to Families, *Final report: Project for stepping out of foster care into a more self-sufficient independent living network* (Grant 90-CO-0223101). Washington, DC: U.S. Department of Health and Human Services, Children's Bureau.

Sims, A. R. (1988). Independent living services for youths in foster care. *Social Work, 33,* 539-542.

Smith, T. E. (1984). Reviewing adolescent marijuana abuse. *Social Work, 29,* 17-21.

Subcommittee on Children, Family, Drugs, and Alcoholism. (1985). *Exploitation of runaways* (Senate Hearing 99-323). Washington, DC: Government Printing Office.

Thompson, J. (1990, February 8). KCK leader asks senators to help runaways. *Kansas City Times,* p. C-7.

Timberlake, E. (1979). Child social functioning: A data base for planning. *School Social Work Quarterly, 1,* 229-240.

Timberlake, E. M., Pasztor, E., Sheagren, J., Clarren, J., & Lammert, M. (1987). Adolescent emancipation from foster care. *Child and Adolescent Social Work, 4,* 265-277.

To whom do they belong: Runaway, homeless and other youth in high risk situations in the 1990s. (1991). Washington, DC: National Network of Runaway and Youth Services.

U.S. Department of Health and Human Services (DHHS). (1983). *Runaway and homeless youth: National program inspection.* Washington, DC: Author.

Chapter 4

A CULTURALLY SPECIFIC APPROACH TO ETHNIC MINORITY YOUNG ADULTS

JACOB U. GORDON

Alcohol and other drug abuse, violence, and crime are a tragic plague on American communities. This epidemic does not discriminate. It is not bound by income, race, or gender; it does not favor urban or rural dwellers; it does not spare school children or the newly born; and it will not cure itself with time.

During the past several years, alcohol and other drug abuse has emerged as a critical problem affecting young people in America today. Authoritative estimates, provided by the United States government and other sources, consistently indicate that during the past decade, problems associated with alcohol and drug abuse have escalated to the point that now it is generally acknowledged that these problems represent one of the major threats to our nation. They affect all aspects of life in the United States and all strata of society (Clark & Midanik, 1982; Gary, 1980; Herrington, Jacobson, & Benzer, 1987; Okpaku, 1985).

An estimated 9-12 million Americans are directly affected by the abuse of alcohol and other drugs. One out of every three people participating in a recent survey reported that alcohol or other drugs had caused problems in his or her family (Office of Substance Abuse Prevention [OSAP], 1991). According to Herrington et al. (1987), accidents were responsible for 49,000 deaths and 150,000 cases of permanent disability in 1986, and 50% of those accidents were directly attributable to alcohol or other drugs. For the same period, 50% of all murders in the United States involved alcohol and/or other drugs, and

80% of people who attempted suicide had been drinking at the time. The suicide rate among alcoholics is approximately 600% greater than among the general population, and alcoholics have a life expectancy approximately 12 years shorter than that of nonalcoholics. The death rate from accidental falls is 500% higher for alcoholics than for nonalcoholics, and death in fires is 1,000% greater for alcoholics than for the general population as a whole (Herrington et al., 1987).

The economic consequences of substance abuse are enormous. The costs of medical care for alcohol- and other drug-related illnesses and injuries now exceed $7 billion per year, and another $7 billion is added to the bill for traffic accidents, fires, crimes, and related costs (National Institute on Drug Abuse [NIDA], 1991). Absenteeism and lost productivity are calculated to cost the country another $37 billion annually (Blackmon, 1985). In fact, data suggest that the total costs associated with alcohol and other drug abuse represent 25% of this country's current national debt. Official government estimates are that 10% of the drinking population consume 50% of the alcoholic beverages sold in the United States and that government agencies collect $17 million per day in taxes on alcohol (NIDA, 1991; OSAP, 1991).

Much of the current general literature addresses many of the above consequences of addiction for adults. The newly emerging risk-focused literature identifies risk and protective factors for children and adolescents, along with the special consequences of use and abuse for that population. Less attention has been directed toward the vulnerability of young adults to substance abuse problems and the related consequences. This 20 to 25-year-old age group often experience a range of developmental stresses as they gradually assume adult family, social, and career responsibilities. This chapter summarizes factors that influence alcohol and other drug abuse among young adults in general. It includes a discussion of use patterns and factors that influence those patterns in subgroups of ethnic minority young adults. Then the impact of cultural differences on treatment with such groups is described, along with examples of culture-specific treatment techniques for African-American young adults. Case examples are included of young adults who could benefit from the services.

CONTRIBUTORS TO YOUNG ADULT ALCOHOL AND OTHER DRUG USE AND ABUSE

Although the causes of addiction cannot be determined precisely, it is important that effective prevention and treatment strategies begin with an understanding of the many reasons why young adults start to use alcohol and other drugs. Historically, searches for explanations focused on the individual; researchers studied the personality traits, communication skills, and family use patterns, as well as the attitudes and beliefs of individuals, as factors related to alcohol and other drug use (Bailey, Habermann, & Sheinberg, 1965; Cahalan, Cisin, & Crossley, 1969). Later investigators observed that immediate environments are not all alike and that certain external conditions might make a person more or less likely to use alcohol and other drugs. Researchers studied the family and the social and community experiences that shape an individual's environment (Moos, Finney, & Gamble, 1985; Zucker, 1979). In the 1980s, investigators took a hard look at what are termed "distal," or more global, environmental influences relating to the legal, economic, and cultural circumstances that affect lives in general, as well as alcohol and other drug-using behavior specifically (Clarke & Midanik, 1982; Okpaku, 1985; Rogan, 1986). Without an understanding of the reasons why young adults use alcohol and other drugs, treatment programs become a "hit or miss" or "hit and run" activity. Understanding the underlying reasons, including cultural factors, leads to a more targeted treatment approach.

Although it is not news that individuals are influenced by the world in which they live, many treatment programs continue to concentrate solely on changing the individual, while ignoring environmental and cultural factors that may contribute to alcohol and other drug use. Other researchers indicated that this limited approach seldom results in long-term behavior change. Consequently treatment programs in general, especially programs for ethnic minorities, must begin to target elements of the environment and culture known to be associated with alcohol and other drug use (OSAP, 1989). Few treatment initiatives can target every factor to alcohol and other drug use simultaneously. Adopting a systems approach, however, such as a culturally specific family systems approach, does encourage the development of long-term, comprehensive treatment strategies that build over time. Figure 4.1 illustrates this multidimensional systems approach to the cultural, social, biological, family, and other environmental factors that influence whether young adults develop substance abuse problems.

INFLUENCES ON THE USE PATTERNS OF ETHNIC MINORITY GROUPS

Epidemiologic data from research funded by the National Institute on Drug Abuse (NIDA, 1987) indicate that the following use patterns

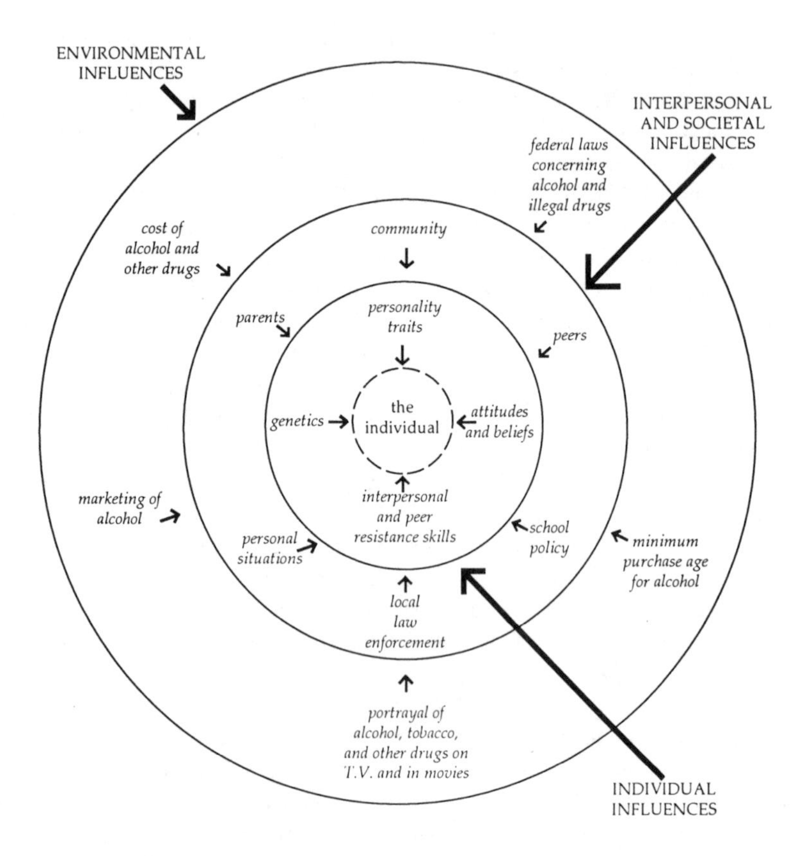

Figure 4.1. Factors That Influence Alcohol and Other Drug Use
SOURCE: From *Prevention Plus II* (p. 19) by Office of Substance Abuse Prevention, 1989, Washington, DC: Government Printing Office.

among blacks, Hispanics, and Native Americans have particular implications for young adults in those groups:

- Nearly 7.6 million blacks and 3.7 million Hispanics have used an illicit drug at least once in their lifetimes.
- Hispanic teenagers aged 12-17 years are more likely than white or black youth to have used cocaine at least once during their lifetimes, during the past year, or during the past month. Blacks aged 35 and above are more likely than whites or Hispanics of the same age to have used cocaine at

least once during their lifetimes, during the past year, or during the past month.

- Drug abuse is an important factor associated with the high rate of school dropouts among blacks, Hispanics, and Native Americans.
- Hispanics accounted for 22% of emergency room episodes due to inhalants—a significant overrepresentation of that ethnic group, compared with their numbers in the total population.
- Black and Hispanic clients in treatment for drug abuse are more likely than whites to report speedballing, the intravenous combination of heroin and cocaine.
- Between 1984 and 1987, cocaine-related deaths among blacks and other minorities tripled, compared with a doubling among whites.
- Among 12 to 17-year-olds, blacks and Hispanics are more likely than whites to see no risk associated with the occasional use of marijuana. Among the 18 to 25-year-olds, blacks are more likely than Hispanics and whites to see no risk associated with occasional use of marijuana.
- A higher rate of perceived risk-free cocaine experimentation was found among black and Hispanic males than white males in the 12-17 age category. Perceptions of the harmful effects of marijuana and cocaine are related to past-year drug use for each of these drugs.
- Although minority youth perceive less risk associated with drug abuse than do white youth, they are more likely to be responsive to drug education programs. Drug education courses or lectures in school appear to have a greater preventive impact on black than white students.
- Vulnerability and risk factors associated with the onset of drug use and the progression from use to abuse and dependency are complex and include interpersonal, intrapersonal, and environmental factors.

During the last 15 years, research to determine the precursors of drug abuse has progressed largely as a result of longitudinal studies of various cohorts of preadolescents and adolescents. These pathways may be interpersonal, intrapersonal, or environmental. Of particular importance is the early identification of high-risk children. Research suggests that initial markers of later problem behaviors can be identified as early as elementary school. The early emergence of conduct disorders and achievement problems in school have been shown to be predictive of later antisocial and delinquent behavior, including substance abuse, in adolescence (Schwartz, 1988).

Other social and behavioral markers of later drug abuse include (a) poor and inconsistent parental practices, (b) physical and/or sexual abuse, (c) low degree of social bonding, (d) positive beliefs and attitudes toward drug use, (e) high levels of sensation seeking, rebelliousness, shy, and aggressive behavior, (f) association with deviant-prone peers, (g) age of first use, and (h) an affinity for unconventional behaviors. A combination of these factors appears to place an individual at high risk for subsequent drug abuse (Hawkins, Catalano, & Miller, 1992; Vasquez, 1988). More recently, research has focused on biological and genetic factors that predispose individuals to the abuse of alcohol and other drugs. Special attention also has been directed toward the problems and special needs of children of alcoholics and addicted parents (Pilat & Jones, 1985). These findings are important for understanding how they and other cultural factors can influence the treatment process with members of ethnic minority groups.

CULTURAL INFLUENCES ON TREATMENT

Members of most cultural groups tend to use mental health and substance abuse treatment agencies as a last resort, only after they have exhausted resources in their natural support systems and the problems have become so chronic and severe that the outlook for treatment and alleviation of symptoms is poor. Therefore they are more likely to be at higher risk when they are seen. Rogan (1986) documented barriers to the substance abuse treatment of blacks and Native Americans, for example. This underuse of mainstream mental health agencies and substance abuse treatment programs stems from (a) language problems (verbal and nonverbal); (b) low awareness of community mental health programs; (c) limited access to mental health services; (d) stigma attached to needing such services; (e) negative past experiences with agencies that have created distrust, suspicion, fear of agencies, and unfavorable attitudes toward mental health care; and (f) mental health services' lack of interest in and sensitivity to the needs of culturally diverse clients so that clients have been "treated" without proper awareness or concern for cultural differences (Brisbane, 1992; NIDA, 1987). An understanding of the following list of cross-cultural differences is important for effective treatment of culturally diverse clients (Brisbane, 1992):

1. *Differences in attitudes toward receiving psychiatric or mental health care.* In some cultures, loss of status, fear of being seen as a failure, and shame accompany psychiatric help-seeking behaviors.

2. *Differences in verbal expressiveness in talking about one's family problems with a stranger.* Some cultures are very expressive, while others are much more closed.
3. *Differences in culture-specific intervention strategies.* Some cultures employ particular rituals and techniques to resolve an individual's problems.
4. *Differences in definitions of abnormal behavior.* What is perceived as psychopathology in one culture might be sanctioned, even encouraged, in others.
5. *Differences in explanations of the causes of abnormal behavior.* The underlying cause of abnormal behavior may be seen as physiological or psychological in nature, or the behavior may be viewed as the result of the actions of others (living or dead) or supernatural or spiritual forces.
6. *Differences in style of intervention preferred.* In general, cultures relying on internal controls promote insight-oriented therapy, while cultures relying on external controls are more amenable to directed therapies. For those oriented toward the "guidance-nurturant" approach, clients expect the counselor to take an active and directive role and to give them explicit directions on how to solve problems and bring immediate relief from their distress. To these people, the nondirective approach is seen as uncaring and indifferent. To reduce uncertainty, the counselor first must clarify what is planned in therapy and why. Counseling methods that rely on introspection, reflection, and extensive client verbalization do not meet the needs of these cultural groups.
7. *Differences in views of long-term versus immediate goals.* Some cultures are more present oriented, while others are more future oriented. Those with a present orientation will be frustrated by therapies focused on long-term, future-oriented change.
8. *Differences in individual versus group approaches to problem solving.* African Americans and Hispanics tend to stress cooperation among family and the community groups to help individuals in distress, whereas mainstream European Americans generally place greater value on individual solutions to problems.
9. *Differences in therapeutic agents or people whose help is sought for psychosocial disorders.*

In addition to the cross-cultural differences above, value differences are important influences in how cultural groups perceive and respond to substance abuse treatment. Table 4.1 helps illustrate important value differences between European Americans or Anglo Americans and other ethnocultural groups that may influence their treatment experiences. Because of these differences in attitudes toward counseling, it may be most effective to work through community-based health care agencies in ethnic minority communities in order to reach young adults.

Table 4.1
Comparison of Common Values

European or Anglo American	*Other Ethnocultural Groups*
Mastery over nature	Harmony with nature
Personal control over the environment	Fate
Doing-activity	Being
Time dominates	Personal interaction dominates
Human equality	Hierarchy/rank/status
Individualism/privacy	Group welfare/"collectivism"
Youth	Elders
Self-help	Birthright inheritance
Competition	Cooperation
Future orientation	Past or present orientation
Informality	Formality
Directness/openness/honesty	Indirectness/ritual/"face"
Practicality/efficiency	Idealism
Materialism	Spiritualism/detachment
Nuclear family structure	Extended family structure
Dominant culture status	Subculture or minority status
Use of mental health services	Reliance on traditional support system

Often such agencies have established effective mechanisms for trust building and getting acquainted with community members over time. They may have developed a reputation among residents for providing culturally relevant services at important early developmental transitions. That type of history can encourage the involvement of young adults in family-focused alcohol and other drug treatment services. These services should be characterized by the "seven *A*'s" (Gordon, 1983):

Availability
Affordability
Accessibility
Acceptability
Adaptability
Achievability
Accountability

In the history of human thinking, the most fruitful developments frequently occurred at those points where different lines of thought met. Those lines may have their roots in different cultures, in different times, and in different religious traditions. If these lines are allowed to meet, a new and interesting way of being will emerge.

The United States is a nation made up of many ethnic, racial, religious, and cultural groups. The concept of *the melting pot,* now outmoded, has been replaced by the recognition that this diversity lends strength and uniqueness to the fabric of this society. With this broad range of experiences that various parts of the population bring to everyday life in America comes the need for increased efforts at understanding and valuing the differences as well as the similarities. Because the culture in which each person is raised greatly influences his or her attitudes, beliefs, values, and behaviors, it is important to gain an awareness and knowledge of cultural determinants of these factors (Hale-Benson, 1988). Thus, when counseling a young adult from a cultural or ethnic group such as an African American, Asian American, Native American, or Hispanic/Latino, it will be important to assess the degree to which the client has become acculturated to mainstream America or has retained his or her ethnic/traditional ways. These variables are important in determining the appropriate techniques and methods of treatment. Understanding clients from the perspective of their own situation, however different that may be from the practitioner's culture, is necessary in helping them handle problems within their own culture and environment. These assumptions about culture-specific substance abuse treatment have been applied in the following sections to services for Native-American and African-American young adults.

Culturally Specific Treatment With Native Americans

In a cross-cultural relationship, Native Americans traditionally prefer noninterference, in that outside intervention is an encroachment on their personal lives and is regarded as disrespectful. *Self-reliance* is preferred, and outside help from a social service or substance abuse agency is the last resort. Reflecting this orientation, Native Americans have developed a natural helping system. Figure 4.2 presents sources of assistance in the order in which they are approached by Native Americans seeking aid (Lewis, 1975). As can be seen from this figure, the broader community health care system is the least significant source

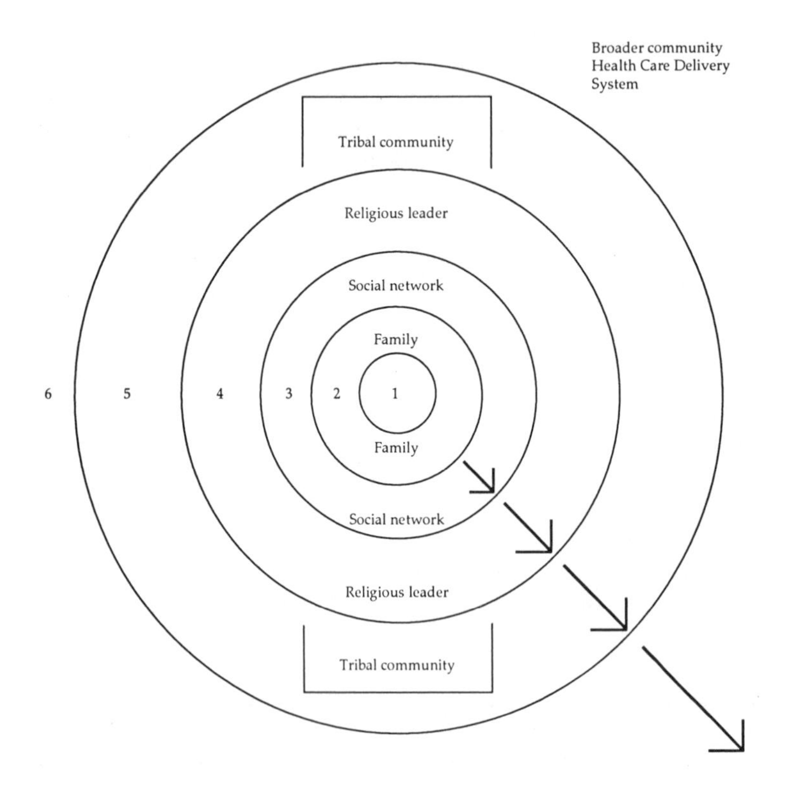

Figure 4.2. Schema: Individual Seeking Aid. Numbered in Order of Significance for Native American and Path Followed for Seeking Help

of help, with the most immediate culturally relevant sources of help for Native Americans being used as primary sources. Young adults from this ethnic group may be especially vulnerable to ethnic stress and to substance abuse in their attempts to handle conflicting values from larger society and their ethnic group related to help seeking, life-styles, and other important issues. Effective substance abuse services must, therefore, build on this system of natural helpers to meet the needs of young adults in this ethnic group. For example, using family, peer, religious, or tribal leaders to facilitate prevention services or to serve as consultants in treatment sessions is an important way to use this natural helping and culturally specific path to services.

Johnson et al. (1978), from the University of South Dakota, spelled out the following important factors in developing interpersonal relationships with Native Americans:

- Individual needs include handling one's own fears.
- Avoid good-bad judgments about Indian culture and life-styles.
- Have respect for the elderly.
- Give consideration to minimal eye contact.
- Give consideration to family influence.
- Respect the individuality of Indian people.
- Do not force a relationship.
- Spend considerable time in small talk.
- Allow plenty of time.
- Allow Indian persons to know who you are as a person.
- Find some small concrete service to provide.
- Learn how to work appropriately with Medicine Men and natural helpers.

Communication can be stressful and anxiety provoking if attitudes of superiority-inferiority are manifested in the treatment relationship. *Stress* is a daily experience for which the different ethnic groups have developed personalized coping mechanisms. Service providers should find Table 4.2 useful in their efforts to deliver services to Native Americans (Satala, 1981). The table is useful as well for understanding sources for coping with stress among African-American, Hispanic, and European-American young adults.

Afrocentric Family Systems Treatment

> Afrocentricity is a liberating ideology. A person who chooses to live an Afrocentric life will always transcend the mundane attitudes. It is a way of looking at yourself differently from the way other people may see you. It helps you to better understand and appreciate who you are and how you can improve yourself as an African American. To be Afrocentric is to be in touch with one's ultimate reality in every way. (Asante, 1980, p. 3)

An effective strategy for working with African-American young adults must include a service delivery model based on Afrocentricity and the importance of the family. Afrocentricity defines Africans and people of African descent in terms of their:

Table 4.2
Sources for Coping With Stress by Different Ethnic Groups

African American
Ministers
Root workers
Voodoo priests
Spiritualists
Family
Asian American
Herbalists
Family/friends/diviner
Latino/Hispanic
Curanderos/espiritistas/santerios
Native American
Medicine Man
Singers
European American
Counselors
Psychiatrists
Psychologists
Social Workers
Ministers

History
Spirituality
African personality
Social organizations
Economic/political organizations
Community well-being
Life-styles and health
Creative production (art, music, communications, literature, dance)
Values and practices

Overview of Afrocentric Values and Principles

Afrocentricity is rooted both in cultural values and in the practices of Africans and the African Diaspora (people of African descent who reside in the United States and the Caribbean). It includes the following African traditional principles of virtue:

Truth
Justice
Propriety
Harmony
Reciprocity
Balance
Order

These principles are embodied in the black value system (Nguzo Saba) created by Maulan Karenga. According to Karenga (Maulan, 1989), a *value system* is a set of principles that guides a person in his or her day-to-day life experiences. It helps determine what one should do and should not do. A person who has a positive value system is more likely to do positive things. The Afrocentric value system is based on the Nguzo Saba because it helps people of African-American descent work together, respect each other, and promote and celebrate their collective history, identity, and struggle against oppressive forces in American society.

Nguzo and *Saba* are Swahili words that mean "principles" and "seven," respectively. The following are the seven principles:

1. *Umoja* (unity)—To strive for and maintain unity in the family, community, nation, and race.
2. *Kujichaguilia* (self-determination)—To define ourselves, name ourselves, create for ourselves, and speak for ourselves instead of being defined, named, created for, and spoken for by others.
3. *Ujima* (collective work and responsibility)—To build and maintain our community together and to make our sisters' and brothers' problems our problems and to solve them together.
4. *Ujamma* (cooperative economics)—To build and maintain our own stores, shops, and other businesses and to profit from them together.
5. *Nia* (purpose)—To make our collective vocation the building and developing of our community in order to restore our people to their traditional greatness.
6. *Kuumba* (creativity)—To always do as much as we can, in the way we can, in order to leave our community more beautiful and beneficial than when we inherited it.
7. *Imani* (faith)—To believe with all our heart in our people, our parents, our teachers, our leaders, and the righteousness and victory of our struggle.

These Afrocentric values and principles provide a solid foundation for a culture-specific treatment program for African-American young adults. An effective treatment program must integrate these principles and values into the recruitment strategies and other aspects of the treatment program in order to reach the target population and use a culturally specific family systems approach.

Identifying and Reaching the Target Group. Young adults in the African-American community must be recruited through peers and the other key sources that they use for coping with stress, as identified in Table 4.2. Peers are likely to know others who need substance abuse treatment, and the key individuals are respected leaders within the ethnic group by virtue of their status and experience. In addition, other natural leaders can help identify potential or actual substance abusers among African-American young adults, including barbers and beauticians, indigenous community workers, members of local cultural and political organizations, and activists in anticrime organizations. Outreach can best be facilitated through a focus on many of the issues and concerns that young adult African Americans struggle with in addition to substance abuse. Thus the focus of outreach and systems-oriented treatment should address employment, education, family, cultural, and political/community involvement needs within an Afrocentric approach. The key individuals above can be used not only to identify young adults with existing and potential substance abuse problems but also to help with culturally relevant interventions that encourage the young adults to enter treatment.

The Afrocentric paradigm as a family systems approach is applicable to young adults from various socioeconomic, educational, and family backgrounds and levels of acculturation who are high risk or are involved in substance abuse behaviors. Gordon (1983) clearly identified five cultural subgroups within the African-American ethnic group that are distinguished by the following differences:

Educational levels
Socioeconomic levels
National origin (blacks from Third World countries)
Age
Religion
Rural versus urban residence
Skin color or degree of pigmentation
Degree to which they have become acculturated to the Eurocentric mainstream

Table 4.3 presents differences between the five subgroups in terms of acculturation and other important variables. In reaching out and designing treatment services for young adult African Americans, it is important to be aware of which subgroupings are represented in the target group. Also, among these subgroups, young adults from the inner cities are the most underserved. They generally are high risk for substance abuse, live in poverty, lack education, often have low self-esteem, exhibit unhealthful life-styles, and have little knowledge of African history. Their involvement in the Afrocentric family systems approach should provide a sense of identity leading to self-actualization, empowerment, and more nurturing ties with their families of origin and the families they are developing currently as young adults.

The following are case profiles of young adult clients who could benefit from the Afrocentric family systems treatment model.

Case Example 1

April is a young 19-year-old African-American female from a low-income family. Her parents were divorced when she was 5 years old. She became pregnant as a young adolescent (at age 15) and thereafter married a 20-year-old African-American male, David. David is from a family with a history of alcohol and drug abuse. He began drinking at the age of 12 and is now an alcoholic. They both experienced racial discrimination at an early age. April managed to complete high school, but David is a high school dropout. They had three children within 4 years of their marriage. David is unable to maintain a regular job because of his alcohol addiction. April has to stay home to take care of the children. Domestic violence is becoming a serious problem in the household.

Case Example 2

Johnson is a 22-year-old inner-city African-American male who was raised with traditional African-American values. At age 18 he received a scholarship to attend college. While in college, he fell in love with a white girl named Joyce. Joyce was raised in Louisiana. Her parents were angry about her love affair with Johnson, especially when she became pregnant. Two years after the baby, a boy, was born, Joyce and Johnson decided to get married, against the wishes of Joyce's parents. Following the marriage, Johnson left for Africa as a Peace Corp volunteer. On his return, he found Joyce pregnant, apparently by a man named Victor. Victor was a white male alcoholic who was married to an African-American female. Johnson became angry about the problems in his marriage, racial conflicts,

text continued on page 88

Table 4.3
Characteristics and Needs of African-American Young Adults in Five Cultural Subgroups

Groups[*]	*Traits*	*Values*	*Human and Spiritual Needs (love, religion, self-identity, etc.)*	*Survival Needs (politics, economics, education, standards, etc.)*
Acculturated Blacks	1. Reject the general attitudes, behaviors, customs, rituals, and stereotypic behaviors associated with being black. 2. Use rationalizations as defense mechanism. 3. Often well-educated. 4. Usually middle class.	1. Linguistic patterns, music, art, entertainment, food, and dress are indistinguishable from those of middle-class whites. 2. Assimilate into the mainstream white culture.	1. Middle-class white environment. 2. Interracial dating and marriages. 3. White church, usually Episcopal or Catholic.	1. White context
Bicultural Blacks	1. Pride in racial identity. 2. Comfortable operating in the white world. 3. Seek out diversity and integrated living environments. 4. Experience emotional pain from cultural or racial schizophrenia. 5. Usually middle class.	1. Linguistic patterns, music, art, entertainment, food, and dress are usually bicultural.	1. Either black or white. 2. Both black and white simultaneously. 3. Comfortable with interracial dating and marriages. 4. White church, usually Episcopal or Catholic.	1. Black and/or white.
Subcultural Blacks	1. Generally referred to by nonblacks as "militant." 2. Often angry and distrustful of whites. 3. Articulate issues of black oppression and racism.	1. Linguistic patterns, music, art, entertainment, food, and dress are identifiable as from the black subculture. 2. Reject white values and culture.	1. Needs are met in an exclusively black frame of reference. 2. Black church, but frequently Muslim.	1. Situationally met in a black or white context. 2. An all-black context is preferred.

Third World Blacks	1. Recent African and Caribbean immigrants. 2. Pride in racial identity and national origin. 3. Comfortable operating in the white world. 4. Seek out racial diversity and integrated living environments. 5. Often accepted by white middle class. 6. Experience emotional pain from black American rejection/disregard/ignorance of African/Caribbean culture. 7. Usually middle class and assertive.	1. Linguistic patterns, music, food, art, entertainment, and dress are identifiable as African, Caribbean, European, and American. 2. Advocate the preservation of African culture and values. 3. Appreciative of other cultures and values.	1. Euro-African context. 2. Black and white context. 3. Extended family. 4. Comfortable with interracial dating and marriages. 5. Euro-African religions.	1. Extended family context. 2. Black/white context. 3. International context.
Traditional Blacks	1. Neither reflect nor accept black identity. 2. Limited contact outside black community. 3. Carriers of the essence of black American culture. 4. Usually older, roots in the South, rural and/or poverty background. 5. Strong commitment to extended family.	1. Linguistic patterns, music, food, art, entertainment, and so on are tied to the black community and the church. 2. Values, morals, artifacts, language, customs, and history of blacks are vested in the traditional black person.	1. Exclusively black context. 2. The black church, usually AME or Baptist. 3. Quasi extended family.	1. Most often met in the white context. 2. Quasi extended family.

NOTE: *These cultural groupings are fluid rather than static.

and his inability to finish college. He sought to solve his problems by joining a street gang; he eventually became a drug dealer and drug addict. His family could benefit from an Afrocentric substance abuse treatment approach.

Case Example 3

Abubaka is a 25-year-old African American from a middle-class family. He is married to Angela, a graduate from a predominantly white institution of higher learning. Abubaka is studying to become a physician. They have two children, a boy and a girl. Angela's three best friends are single parents who are heavily engaged in alcohol and drug abuse. Angela has become an alcoholic. Abubaka is seeking a divorce and custody of the children. Angela's parents also wish to have custody of the children. The children currently are neglected, and their futures seem bleak because of the custody struggle and the mother's alcoholism.

Format and Content of the Afrocentric Approach. The format of treatment provided in the Afrocentric family systems approach covers a wide range of areas. The important elements of Afrocentricity have been stated clearly in the previous sections. The use of the Afrocentric model depends on the needs of the target group (see Table 4.3). For example, communication styles of inner-city young adults are different from those of rural dwellers. The same is true of their values, educational achievement, life-styles, and socioeconomic status. The best approach is to use an individualized assessment with special attention to family and cultural needs related to substance abuse recovery. The assessment will help in determining the number of sessions, the type of Afrocentric exercises, and the content of the treatment for clients such as April and David, Angela, and Johnson and Joyce.

Afrocentric treatment should be combined with conventional family systems approaches based on the outcomes of the family/cultural assessment (e.g., combined with intergenerational, strategic, or structural family systems treatment). In the case of Abubaka and Angela, on the one hand, an intergenerational approach could be useful for addressing the child custody, divorce, and substance abuse issues. On the other hand, the problem-solving family systems treatment approach could be combined with Afrocentric treatment in sessions with Johnson and Joyce, who are confronted with substance abuse, family conflicts, and Johnson's involvement in a street gang (the latter may represent his effort to solve his problems).

The content of treatment sessions should include alcohol and drug education, along with a focus on family and cultural strengths and problems that may affect recovery. In addition, treatment should focus on many of the Afrocentric elements identified previously. The following summary of the major elements of Afrocentricity has been drawn from the works of many scholars (Brisbane, 1992; Kunjufu, 1987; Myers, 1988; Nobles, 1985).

Important Elements of Afrocentricity

Afrocentric Patterns	*Treatment Applications*
Nonverbal Communication Styles	
Use eye contact and body language effectively.	Pay attention to other forms of nonverbal behaviors.
Expect elderly to be treated with respect.	Address elderly more formally than younger clients.
Verbal Communication Styles	
Oral delivery as an opportunity to engage in a textual as well as a contextual search for harmony.	Conduct session in black English or standard English when appropriate.
Hesitant to disclose personal or family information to a stranger.	An initial period of friendly, informal conversation or chatting before discussing problems often helps avoid appearing unfriendly or discourteous.
Females emotionally expressive, but males do little expression of feelings.	

Views Toward Counseling

Low use of mental health services:	
Believe that the system is culturally insensitive.	Provide culturally appropriate care.
Believe services are organized and operated to serve middle-class European-Americans.	Convey acceptance of clients through verbal and nonverbal means.
Live in urban areas and lack transportation to get to clinics.	Aid in lining up transportation services or take services to them in neighborhood clinics.
There is often an absence of African-American therapists.	Have a qualified Africanist available.

Rely on folk healers and African traditional values for many emotional problems because these healers are perceived as more effective than mainstream health workers.	Incorporate these healers and African traditional values into treatment when appropriate.
Mental illness implies stigma and loss of respect. For males it is viewed as weakness.	Reassure clients regarding problems they are experiencing. Reassure the males of their masculinity.
Prefer direct, tangible, and action-oriented approaches over introspective "talk and listen" methods.	Help clients define specific actions they can take to cope with their problems.
Males may be uncomfortable with female counselors because of traditional sex role expectations. However, homosexual or bisexual males may have difficulty discussing sexual problems with another male.	Team same-sex counselor with client if possible except when counseling males regarding homosexuality or bisexuality.
Feeling of being outside mainstream American society may be basis for many problems.	Work toward helping clients resolve conflicts by clarifying and understanding their options within their cultural context.

Family

Family Structure

The strongest and most valued institution is the family, which includes the extended network of blood relatives, close friends adopted as godparents, and in-laws. This respect for the traditional family is called *community.* Functions and responsibilities of the family include financial and emotional support, care for the elderly and ill, care and protection of the children, and a sense of belonging.	Involve significant members from the extended family and the community in the counseling or treatment plan. Female members of family play an especially important role in health matters and should be included.

Family Dynamics

Traditionally prescribed sex roles: Male—head of household; dominant authority figure; key decision maker in matters outside the home; gives strength, honor, and protection to female; disciplinarian but few other responsibilities for child rearing.	Be aware of roles each plays when counseling couples. Any suggestions to break with traditional roles should be considered according to level of acculturation. Consider impact of chronic illness on male client with these cultural expectations.
Female—nurturer; household responsibilities, child rearing, and education; mediator between authoritarian father and the children.	
Elderly—well respected; care for children and help in their rearing.	Address with respect and include them when possible in the treatment plan.
Children—considered to be a priority; parents make personal sacrifices for them; longer period of dependence on parents; older children expected to follow in parents' footsteps; consult parents for advice on important issues.	Respect young adult's admiration of parents but encourage developmentally appropriate independent actions. Incorporate parents when possible in counseling.

Health and Illness

Illness traditionally has its roots in physical imbalances or supernatural forces that include God's will, magical powers, evil spirits, powerful human forces, or emotional upsets.	Encourage clients to talk about why they feel they are "ill," "depressed," etc.
There is no differentiation between physical and emotional illnesses.	Client may present with physical complaints when, in fact, there is an emotional problem. Probe for cause of physical complaints.
	Involve the spiritual healers and ministers in crisis intervention and therapy.
Fatalistic world view.	Explore ways clients can participate in determining their own fate.

Spirituality

A direct search for harmony is at the base of African-American spirituality. Faith in God or Allah. Strong identification with ancestor worship and Rasfar.	Explore ways clients can express their spirituality and practice their faith.

Aesthetics

Art, music, literature, dance, poetry, drama, oratory, folklore, sculpture

Black expressiveness that reveals and analyzes the artistic and creative experiences of black life. Emotionalism, spontaneity, and rhythm is a thread that runs through the fabric of black culture.	Engage client in appropriate aesthetic activities, for example, art and music therapy. Productive activities are very effective.

History

The cradle of civilization is Africa, the ancient kingdoms, modern Africa, the transplantation of the African way of life, and the New World experience.	Relate to the rich African roots and American heritage of African-American clients. References to history must be positive and factual. Selected African proverbs that reflect African people can be helpful.

Dietary Patterns

Soul foods (greens, black-eyed peas, corn bread, fried chicken, candied yams, sweet potato pie, etc.). African foods and mainstream American foods are generally acceptable, depending on socioeconomic status. Soul food is usually heavily seasoned.	Be familiar with client's eating habits and food content when addressing life-style, health, acculturation, values, and intercultural issues.

Afrocentric Exercises. As noted in the discussion under "Aesthetics" and other sections under "Treatment Applications," the active involvement of young adult African-American clients in treatment at an experiential level is extremely important. A number of Afrocentric exercises can be used to accomplish this goal during substance abuse treatment and in aftercare services. As in treatment and aftercare services in general, it is important to involve family members (from the family of origin or current family as indicated) and members of the young adult's support network (community) in these Afrocentric exercises (Perkins, 1989). This strategy reinforces the family systems aspects of the treatment approach. The examples of exercises address issues of ethnic identity, self- and cultural esteem, the family history, and service to the community that can affect substance abuse recovery. Moreover, the issues addressed by these exercises are developmentally appropriate for young adults who often are leaving the family of origin at this stage, as well as establishing their own families and identities.

AFROCENTRIC EXERCISES

Ethnic Identity

This exercise may be used in individual or group treatment sessions. It is useful to have each client write out his or her answers to the questions before discussing them. A brief introduction to the exercise should emphasize the significance of identity.

> The identity of a person is very important. It helps to know who you are and who you are not. It also helps acknowledge your heritage and culture. Persons of African descent have been given many identities, including:

1. African
2. Afro-American
3. African American
4. Black
5. Negro
6. Slave
7. Colored
8. Minority

1. Which one of the above best describes who you are?
2. Why did you make this choice?

3. Name three people in your life who have had the greatest influence on you.
4. Name three African Americans whom you admire, and explain why.
5. What do you like most about being a person of African descent?
6. What would you like to be when you become an adult? Why?
7. What do you know about the civil rights movement? Explain.
8. What do you know about the black power movement? Explain.
9. Name three things you like to do most.
10. What are your three favorite subjects?
11. Name five African countries.
12. Name three of your favorite books.
13. Name three of your favorite television shows.
14. Name three things that make you feel good.
15. Name three things that make you feel bad.

This second exercise, focused on identity, relates African principles to daily life situations that can, as a result of enhanced identity, become less threatening to recovery. The discussion on these principles may be used to contract with young adult clients concerning use of family members and other supports for finding additional ways to apply the principles to their lives.

Describe below how you might include each principle of the Nguzo Saba in your daily experiences.

1. Umoja
2. Kujichaguilia
3. Ujima
4. Ujamma
5. Nia
6. Kuumba
7. Imani

Self- and Cultural Esteem

This exercise on self- and cultural esteem is useful in family treatment sessions. It can help members understand how their self- and cultural esteem may reflect differences in the members' levels of acculturation (see Table 4.3). *Self-esteem* helps tell how individuals feel about themselves. People who have high self-esteem generally feel good about themselves.

A self-esteem that is guided by Afrocentric principles will help you:

Be proud of who you are and your heritage
Feel positive about yourself
Never feel inferior to anyone else
Do well in school and become motivated
Achieve in all your endeavors
Have respect for yourself and others

To help you judge your Afrocentric self-esteem, answer the following questions.

Yes____ No____ 1. People of African descent are a minority in the world.
Yes____ No____ 2. People of African descent built the world's first great civilizations.
Yes____ No____ 3. I believe I'm a very special person.
Yes____ No____ 4. I'm as good as people of other races.
Yes____ No____ 5. I can be a good student if I want to be.
Yes____ No____ 6. I like my skin color the way it is.
Yes____ No____ 7. I have pride in my race.
Yes____ No____ 8. I believe I can accept difficult challenges.
Yes____ No____ 9. I have pride in myself.
Yes____ No____ 10. I can feel good about myself without using tobacco, alcohol, and other drugs.

Family Tree

Since the publication of Alex Haley's (1976) best-selling book *Roots,* there has been an increased interest among African Americans to trace their family heritage. In his book, Haley traced his family heritage over seven generations to a small village named Juffure in Gambia, West Africa. Although few people can achieve what Haley accomplished, it is possible for many African-American young adult clients to trace their family trees over two or three generations. In traditional African societies, the family tree was also known as the *extended family* because it included all persons who had some direct blood relationship in the family. Constructing a family tree from an Afrocentric perspective can be educational, fun, and therapeutic. This exercise may be done as an in-session or out-of-session task. Family members may assign themselves specific tasks and/or collaborate on others. If the individual client is working on the family tree alone, homework assignments can provide a reason for him or her to connect or reconnect with family members from whom he or she is estranged. In either case, family and cultural strengths, as well as instances of chemical addictions over the generations, are likely to be clarified. Tracing a family tree may begin in several ways, some of which are listed below:

1. If any of your grandparents are living, ask them to tell you about their parents.
2. If your grandparents are not living, ask your parents to tell you about them.
3. Ask your aunt, uncle, or other elders in your community to tell you about your parents.
4. Contact the elders in your church, siblings, and/or cousins to tell you about your parents.
5. Consult the National Archives. It contains a wealth of information about individuals whose names appear in federal records.
6. Check the following documents:
   Family Bible
   Old letters and diaries
   Birth and death certificates
   Deeds and wills
   Marriage and divorce records
   News clippings about family members
   Church and cemetery records

Afrocentric Community Service

One of the most important features of Afrocentricity is that it is *collective* in purpose, thought, and actions. This feature means that young adult African Americans must help others in their communities as they help themselves. Community service helps them fulfill this principle and expresses the value of Kuumba. The following are suggested community service projects:

- Do errands for the elderly.
- Help clean up your neighborhood.

- Volunteer to help the sick and/or poor.
- Tutor youngsters.
- Protect your environment.
- Volunteer to help your church, school, or social agency.

CONCLUSION

A culture-specific approach to substance abuse treatment offers the most effective method for reaching young ethnic minority adults and for enhancing their self- and cultural esteem. Two examples of such family-focused and culture-specific approaches have been described in this chapter for Native Americans and African Americans. The Afrocentric counseling/treatment model relies on the strength of the African and African-American cultures. The African-American culture has a rich legacy, heritage, and tradition. Its roots can be traced to the oldest organized cultures in human history. It is a culture that has contributed outstanding art, literature, poetry, agriculture, music, architecture, science and mathematics, dance, religion, and philosophy to the world. It is a culture that shines with creativity, celebrates, entertains, and educates so that its people can always be proud. It also expresses not only the joys but also the pains that people of African descent have experienced. Some of those pains, and those of other minority groups, are related to oppression and have been coped with through substance abuse. The cultures of such groups can be a source for healing during treatment. The poem "Lift Every Voice and Sing," written by James Johnson (1900), has been put to music and is now the black national anthem. It expresses the essence of the black experience.

> Lift every voice and sing
> Till earth and heaven ring
> Ring with the harmonies of Liberty;
> Let our rejoicing rise
> High as the listening skies,
> Let it resound loud as the rolling sea.
> Sing a song full of the faith that the dark past has taught us,
> Sing a song full of the hope that the present has brought us,
> Facing the rising sun of our new day begun
> Let us march on till victory is won.

REFERENCES

Asante, M. (1980). *Afrocentricity: The theory of social change.* Buffalo, NY: Amulefi.

Asante, M. (1985). *African culture: The rhythms of unity.* Westport, CT: Greenwood.

Asante, M. (1987). *The Afrocentric idea.* Philadelphia: Temple University Press.

Asante, M. (1990). *Afrocentricity and knowledge.* Trenton, NJ: African World Press.

Asante, M. (1991). Multiculturalism: An exchange. *American Scholar, 60,* 267-276.

Bailey, M., Haberman, P. W., & Sheinberg, J. (1965). *Distinctive characteristics of the alcoholic family.* New York: National Council on Alcoholism.

Berg, W. E. (1992). Evaluation of community-based drug treatment programs: A review of the research literature. In E. M. Freeman (Ed.), *The addiction process: Effective social work approaches.* White Plains, NY: Longman.

Blackmon, B. (1985) Networking community services for elderly clients with alcohol problems. In E. M. Freeman (Ed.), *Social work practice with clients who have alcohol problems* (pp. 189-201). Springfield, IL: Charles C Thomas.

Brisbane, F. (1992). *Working with African Americans: The professional's handbook.* Chicago: HRDI International.

Cahalan, D., Cisin, I., & Crossley, H. (1969). *American drinking practices.* New Brunswick, NJ: Rutgers Center for Alcohol Studies.

Clark, W. B., & Midanik, L. (1982). Alcohol use and alcohol problems among U.S. adults: Results of the 1979 national survey. In *Alcohol consumption and related problems* (pp. 40-50). (Alcohol and Health Monograph 1, DHHS Publication No. ADM 82-1190). Washington, DC: Government Printing Office.

Gary, L. E. (1980). Role of alcohol and drug abuse in homicide. *Public Health Reports, 95,* 553-554.

Gordon, J. U. (1983, April). Black cultural groupings: A theoretical model. Paper presented at the Annual Conference of the Popular Culture Association, Wichita, KS.

Haley, A. (1976). *Roots.* Garden City, NY: Doubleday.

Hawkins, J. D., Catalano, R. F., & Miller, J. W. (1992). Risk and protective factors for alcohol and other drug problems in adolescence and early adulthood: Implications for substance abuse prevention. In State of Washington Division of Substance Abuse, *Planning the future of prevention II in Washington State* (pp. A1-11). Olympia, WA: Developmental Research and Programs.

Herrington, J., Jacobson, E., & Benzer, M. (1987). *Alcohol and drug abuse handbook.* St. Louis: Warren H. Green.

Johnson, J. (1975). Lift every voice and sing. In R. R. Davis, *Lexicon of Afro-American history* (p. 108). New York: Simon & Schuster.

Kunjufu, J. (1987). *Lessons from history: A celebration in blackness.* Chicago: African-American Images.

Lewis, D. K. (1975). The black family: Socialization and sex roles. *Phylon, 36,* 221-237.

Maulan, K. (1989). *Introduction to black studies.* Los Angeles: University of Sankore Press.

Moos, R. H., Finney, J. W., & Gamble, W. (1985). The process of recovery from alcoholism II: Comparing spouses of alcoholic patients and matched community controls. In E. M. Freeman (Ed.), *Social work practice with clients who have alcohol problems* (pp. 292-314). Springfield, IL: Charles C. Thomas.

Myers, L. (1988). *Understanding an Afrocentric worldview: Introduction to an optimal psychology.* Dubuque, IA: Kendall/Hunt.

National Institute on Drug Abuse (NIDA). (1987). *Drug abuse among ethnic minorities* (DHHS Publication No. ADM 87-1474). Washington, DC: Government Printing Office.

National Institute on Drug Abuse (NIDA). (1991). *Drug abuse and drug abuse research: The third triennial report to Congress from the Secretary, Department of Health and Human Services* (DHHS Publication No. ADM 91-1704). Washington, DC: Government Printing Office.

Nobles, W. (1985). *Africanity and the black family: Development of a theoretical model.* Oakland, CA: Black Family Institute.

Office of Substance Abuse Prevention (OSAP). (1989). *Prevention plus II* (DHHS Publication No. ADM 89-1649). Washington, DC: Government Printing Office.

Office of Substance Abuse Prevention (OSAP). (1991). *Prevention plus III* (DHHS Publication No. ADM 91-1817). Washington, DC: Government Printing Office.

Okpaku, S. O. (1985). State of the art on the multiply addicted: Treatment models for blacks. *Alcoholism Treatment Quarterly, 2,* 141-154.

Perkins, U. E. (1989). *Afrocentric self-inventory and discovery workbook for African-American youth.* Chicago: Third World Press.

Pilat, J. M., & Jones, J. W. (1985). A comprehensive treatment program for children of alcoholics. In E. M. Freeman (Ed.), *Social work practice with clients who have alcohol problems* (pp. 141-159). Springfield, IL: Charles C Thomas.

Rogan, A. (1986). Recovery from alcoholism: Issues for black and Native-American alcoholics. *Alcohol Health and Research World, 2,* 42-44.

Primm, B. J., & Wesley, J. E. (1985). Treating the multiple addicted black alcoholic. *Alcoholism Treatment Quarterly,* 2(3/4), 155-178.

Satala, T. J. (1981). Multicultural skill development in the aging network: An Indian perspective. In J. U. Gordon (Ed.), *Cross-cultural perspective in gerontology* (pp. 00-00). Topeka: Kansas Department on Aging.

Schwartz, S. (1988). Primary prevention of drug abuse. *Social Work in Education, 11,* 53-63.

Vasquez, J. A. (1988). Contexts of learning for minority students. *Educational Forum, 52,* 243-253.

Zucker, R. A. (1979). Developmental aspects of drinking through the adult years. In H. T. Blane & M. E. Chafetz (Eds.), *Youth, alcohol, and social policy* (pp. 00-00). New York: Plenum.

Chapter 5

ALCOHOL ADDICTION AND CODEPENDENCY

CLAYTON T. SHORKEY
WILLA ROSEN

The concept of *codependency* has its roots in the theory of alcoholism as a family disease. Wegscheider (1976), using systems theory as an organizing framework, described the progressive influence of untreated alcoholism on members of the alcoholic family. Under the stress of the alcoholic's dysfunctions, family members shift roles and behaviors in an attempt to bring balance, stability, and survival to the family system. Wegscheider (1976, 1981) described five survival roles that develop in various forms and combinations in the spouse and children of the chemically dependent family member. As the addiction of the chemically dependent person progresses, so does the involvement of other family members. The survival roles include the chief enabler, family hero, lost child, mascot, and scapegoat. Significant changes occur in the thinking, emotions, and behavior of the family members who adopt these roles. Wegscheider (1976) coined the phrase "family trap" to describe the situation when family members become enmeshed in painful and ineffective patterns of interactions that may result in dysfunctional behaviors or a primary addiction.

These serious consequences affect not only family members in the current generation but also how the children in these families continue the same dysfunctional patterns in their families of procreation (Smalley, 1982). Breaking the cycle of cross-generational dysfunction can be accomplished by treatment of codependent and addictive behavior patterns within families. This chapter begins with traditional and alternative definitions of *codependent* or *co-alcoholic* relationships that lay a foundation for family and individual treatment. We present a rationale for caution in extending the definition of this label beyond the area of chemical dependency until additional empirical investigation is completed. A family systems problem-solving approach for assessment and treatment of codependent behavior is presented along with case examples throughout the chapter to highlight the process of family treatment. In this chapter the definitions of *family* and, consequently, descriptions of family treatment are not restricted to traditional definitions due to cultural/ethnic, sexual preference, and socioeconomic factors.

VARIED PERSPECTIVES ON CODEPENDENCY

Alcohol-Related Perspectives

Greenleaf (1981) used the term *co-alcoholic* to describe an adult who "assists in maintaining the social and economic equilibrium of the alcoholic person" (p. 3). The co-alcoholic may be the spouse, lover, friend, or parent of the alcoholic person. A dynamic of this type of relationship is the co-alcoholic stepping in and assuming roles and responsibilities abandoned by the alcoholic in order to keep the system functional. Efforts to maintain the integrity of the family system result in perpetuation of the addiction.

Greenleaf (1981) also contributed the term *para-alcoholic* to describe the role of children in the alcoholic family. These children learn ways of thinking, feeling, and behaving from the alcoholic and the co-alcoholic and thus tend to resemble both. Using the concept of *volition and mobility,* Greenleaf presented a compelling rationale for differentiating between adults involved with an alcoholic and children in the alcoholic family. Greenleaf (1981) wrote: "Children have neither the choice nor the mobility to enter into or exit from the parent-child relationship. The adult may feel trapped; the child is trapped" (p. 6). The special problems of children in chemically dependent families have been explored in detail by other authors and clinicians such as Claudia Black (1981), Charles Deutsch (1982), Janet Woititz (1983), and Robert Ackerman (1983). Although Wegscheider (1981) viewed chemical dependency from a disease model and Greenleaf (1981) described it from a behavioral perspective with no connotation of mental illness, both authors agree on the significant effects of chemical dependency on family members. A mediating framework using aspects of both the disease and behavioral models of alcoholism was presented by Whitfield (1984) in his definition of *co-alcoholism* as "ill health or maladaptive, problematic, or dysfunctional behavior that is associated with living, working with, or otherwise being close to a person with alcoholism" (p. 16). This view of co-alcoholic behavior is described further in the following case vignette.

Case Example 1

Barbara is a 30-year-old white female seeking services from a medical social worker in an urban community hospital. She was referred to meet with the social worker by the staff internist who was treating her husband for internal injuries resulting from a one-car accident. On admission to the emergency room, Bob, a 36-year-old white male, had registered a blood alcohol level of .23, more than twice the legal limit for alcohol intoxication. In addition to the injuries sustained during the accident, routine blood tests indicated the preliminary stages of liver disease.

During the initial meeting, the social worker finds Barbara to be an attractive woman, neatly dressed, and appearing significantly younger than her age. Barbara reports to the social worker that she is experiencing bouts of anxiety and is finding it difficult to concentrate on her work as a teacher's aide in a special education program and to attend to the needs of her husband and her two sons, aged 10 and 12.

On inquiry from the worker, Barbara states that Bob has been experiencing difficulties in finding employment as a construction subcontractor and that she has been financially responsible for the household for the past 18 months. She describes their relationship as being very close, with Bob needing lots of her support and understanding to get through the rough time. In addition to working, Barbara tends to most household and parenting responsibilities, including dealing with behavioral problems of the eldest son in school.

When the worker asks about Bob's drinking patterns, Barbara replies hesitantly, "I haven't really thought about it. Sure, he drinks a lot sometimes, but he's not an alcoholic." When asked to describe in detail how much and how often Bob uses alcohol, Barbara becomes withdrawn and blankly replies that Bob has had so much trouble getting work recently that he probably has been drinking a little more than normal. Also, she says, "Since I've been so tired and edgy, I've been nagging Bob too much about finding work and not giving him enough encouragement." Barbara then tries to change the topic by saying with noted hostility, "I don't understand why we're talking about this. His drinking isn't the problem. I'm here to help him get better and go back to work."

Exploring resources for Bob and Barbara, the worker learns that Bob has not had contact with his family for many years and that Barbara's parents, who live nearby, dislike Bob because of an argument several years back. Barbara and Bob live in a remote area outside of town, and Barbara expresses concern about commuting to get Bob to appointments. Barbara states that the children ride the bus to school and are old enough to take care of themselves until she gets home from work.

As seen in this example, Barbara has absorbed many roles and responsibilities of both marriage partners. The progression of Bob's alcoholism is compromising his ability to contribute to the family system and is adding increased emotional and financial strain. The wife denies that his drinking is the primary cause of their difficulties and continues to view his drinking as a result of vocational problems and her inability to be sufficiently supportive. Yet Barbara resents the social worker challenging her perception of the source of the problems that exist in her family and clings to her viewpoint despite evidence to the contrary.

Barbara's unwillingness to change her perception of her husband's addiction and the nature of her relationship to him will, no doubt, result in future enabling behavior. This behavior will allow Bob to continue his drinking and to increase his dependence on Barbara. Increased dependence can breed resentment, and Bob may begin to blame Barbara for his circumstances. Barbara's unsuccessful attempts to support and control Bob will result in stress, irritability, and feelings of hopelessness for her. This typical pattern of dysfunctional behavior and isolation will cause Barbara, Bob, and their children to be caught increasingly in this family trap.

As discussed by Cermak (1986), the term *co-alcoholic* was transformed to *co-dependency* in the early 1980s as a more inclusive term for individuals involved in a relationship with a chemically dependent person. Cermak (1986) suggested that what begins as adaptive behaviors and attitudes in the co-dependent individual to maintain family stability can become dysfunctional, rigid habits of coping with life issues. Over time the co-dependent person may lose his or her sense of identity and may focus habitually on protecting and meeting the needs of other people. Even the ability to conceptualize personal goals may be lost as feelings of anxiety and guilt result when the fulfillment of personal needs is considered. For many co-dependent persons, the family trap of chemical dependency provides a certain sense of security because it is familiar and predictable. Concerns about being entrapped are often replaced by feelings of loss when the relationship terminates or the partner begins to recover and improve his or her functioning. Co-dependent persons, unprepared for these major changes in their social and emotional environment, may experience devastating fear, anxiety, resentment, and depression as the familiar is replaced by the unknown.

Case Example 2

Maria is a 38-year-old Mexican-American female who was referred by her manager to a social worker with the Employee Assistance Program (EAP) at a large electronics company because of excessive use of sick leave. She is a production supervisor and has been a much-lauded employee until the past year or so. During the initial session, Maria tells the social worker that she is having difficulty focusing due to repeated crying spells on the job, and her performance has dropped in the past 6 months. Maria states that she and her lover of 12 years, Jerri, have not been getting along well and that she is afraid she is about to lose this relationship. Jerri is a 42-year-old Anglo woman who has been clean and sober from polysubstance abuse of alcohol, marijuana, and methamphetamines for the past 18 months; she is actively involved in a same-sex-oriented group of Alcoholics Anonymous.

During the next session, the worker discovers that Maria began experiencing difficulties when Jerri became more active in her work as editor for a local newspaper and expanded her interests to include new friends, jogging, and volunteering in a local political campaign. Jerri is not at home much anymore and does not include Maria in her new activities. At the same time, Maria stays home, watches television by herself, and rarely goes out of the house. Maria has been isolated from her family for many years and feels shunned by her parents after she told them she was a lesbian. Over the years, Maria has lost track of her old friends as she invested heavily in her relationship with Jerri.

In this example, Jerri's recovery from polysubstance abuse has allowed her the opportunity to become involved in a variety of new activities. She is developing new friendships and is pursuing interests to improve her physical health and to increase her social involvement within the community that seems threatening to the family's survival from Maria's perspective. Jerri is an outgoing and talented person, and, because of her work with the newspaper, she is regularly invited to participate in local events. Jerri also expends much energy in working on her recovery process and is helpful to other women struggling with chemical dependency. Jerri remains very grateful to Maria for her financial and emotional support and companionship in the past, but she has placed high priority on achieving stability, sobriety, and making necessary life changes.

Maria consequently feels neglected, abandoned, and rejected. She has been experiencing increased anxiety because she fears that Jerri no longer wishes to maintain their relationship and the family unit. Maria realizes that she must begin to develop some of her own interests as well as be open to new friendships. Maria now has the opportunity to test a renewed relationship with her family of origin but fears experiencing another form of rejection.

The common thread among the concepts of co-alcoholism, codependency, para-alcoholism, and adult children of alcoholics is the progressive impact that chemical addiction in one family member can produce in the functioning of other family members. This conception places codependent individuals into the context of a traditional or alternative family system and clearly associates the development of dysfunctional behavior with the chemical dependency.

Family-of-Origin Perspectives

One broad perspective about codependency involves the need for people to be connected to significant others. Smalley (1984), citing Alfred Adler, believes that codependency emerges from the human pursuit of belonging: "It is a dependence on people and things outside of the self along with neglect of the self to the point of having little self identity" (p. 3). Another perspective states that rigid codes of conduct within the family-of-origin system can cause codependent behavior. Subby and Friel (1984) defined *codependency* as "a dysfunctional pattern of living and problem solving which is nurtured by a set of rules within the family system . . . these rules make healthy growth and change very difficult" (p. 3). Friel, Subby, and Friel (1984) suggested that codependency is the product of dysfunctional families in which children cannot develop a clear identity. Yet another perspective focuses on real or perceived abuse and neglect as the cause of codependency. Mellody (1989) described codependency as a primary disease resulting from dysfunctional parental behavior that she termed "child abuse," which can include parent-child boundary violations, whether physical, verbal, emotional, or spiritual. The term *child abuse* is not used in the traditional sense, but it is equated with any behavior, attitude, or action deemed as "less than nurturing" to the child. These alternative conceptions of codependency can be described as the "family-of-origin" framework in which individuals reared in dysfunctional families fail to develop a clear and coherent sense of personal identity.

It is interesting to note that although codependency is viewed by some popular authors as a result of dependency, poor self-identity, child abuse, and rigid family rules, only characteristics associated with more socially acceptable emotional disorders are emphasized as products of these situations.

Research Gaps Related to Codependency

Codependency has been expanded without empirical documentation by several authors to include enabling relationships with disturbed individuals who are not necessarily alcoholics or drug addicts. Ackerman and Pickering (1989) suggested that the term applies to women in relationships with battering partners. Beattie (1987) believes that the concept of *codependency* is also applicable to any person intimately involved with an individual who has a serious illness or who displays destructive, compulsive behaviors. However, we agree with the conclusions drawn by Cermak (1986) and Gierymski and Williams (1986): that the usefulness of the concept of *codependency* for describing relationships with chemically dependent people should be investigated empirically before being applied to relationships with individuals who have any type of serious dysfunctional behavior patterns.

Only one study concerning the appropriate use of the term *codependency* was identified in the literature on addictions, and no studies were found in literature for other areas. Asher and Brissett (1988) conducted intensive interviews with 52 women married to alcoholics to determine their level of psychosocial functioning and their understanding of the term *codependency*. These authors found a broad range of responses by these women to their husbands' alcoholism. Although some of these women reported what are widely acknowledged to be codependent patterns, others appeared to reject this label and its connotations. For many individuals in a relationship with a chemically dependent person, the label is neither useful nor appropriate. As Asher and Brissett (1988) pointed out, the utility and appropriateness of the concept of *codepend-*

ency in work with individual clients is determined by the clients' acceptance of the label and by the types of characteristics they believe are appropriate to their situation. Additional research is needed in this area to provide clarity about appropriate treatment approaches for effective work with chemically addicted and codependent family members. This faddish conception of mental health appears to focus primarily on individuals, such as adult children of alcoholics or others with neurotic symptoms, who would be expected to be good clients and to shy away from those who would be more difficult clients. Very little attention is focused on individuals from dysfunctional homes who exhibit narcissistic, schizoid, and/or antisocial characteristics.

Harper and Capdevila (1990) noted that billions of dollars in health insurance coverage is spent on private alcoholism treatment and that many members of the chemical dependency field would like to fit codependency into a diagnostic and reimbursable category. Gomberg (1989) wrote, "The term 'codependency' has been expanded without any consideration of its meaningfulness or its contribution to theory and practice, so that it encompasses virtually the entire population of the United States" (p. 120). It should be noted that more than a few organizations and individuals have profited successfully from codependency literature, workshops, and treatment based on these alternative definitions of codependency.

A FAMILY SYSTEMS PROBLEM-SOLVING APPROACH

We propose a way to view codependency through a family systems problems-solving approach. This type of systems approach involves a set of procedural steps in an orderly sequence to resolve family conflicts or to reach goals. From a problem-solving perspective, an individual in a family with a chemically dependent member attempts to eliminate the blocks and obstacles to the systems goals that are adversely affected by the behavior of the addicted person. Ineffective problem solving, or "doing all the wrong things for all the right reasons," is characterized by an increased assumption of the chemically dependent member's role responsibilities by others in order to maintain the family system (O'Neill & O'Neill, 1989, p. 26). These ineffective methods of problem solving enable the continued substance abuse patterns of the addicted person and interfere with the autonomous self-development of the codependent members. A family systems problem-solving framework is useful not only for conceptualizing how codependency develops but also as a guide to assessment and treatment with families having a chemically addicted member (D'Zurilla & Goldfried, 1971; Nezu & D'Zurilla, 1981). This approach includes a variety of methods for developing a knowledge base about addictions and codependency. The emphasis is on assessing the individual and system goals of the members of the family unit and on identifying the source of blocks to goal attainment. These obstacles should be related to the dynamics of addiction, cultural differences, and environmental conditions such as poverty. This approach builds in ways to develop effective strategies for both the individual and the family system to attain their goals.

Individual and Family System Goals

In an ideal family or two-person relationship, each member chooses individual life goals and participates in the process of choosing and prioritizing goals for the system. Effective functioning requires each member to value and support the attainment of personal life goals of its members, to negotiate compromises between or among conflicting goals, and to work cooperatively toward individual and group goal attainment. Interdependence between members of the system increases the likelihood that each member will satisfactorily attain his or her life goals (Shorkey & Crocker, 1981).

In families with an addicted member, persons may become dysfunctional to the degree that group goals as well as life goals of nonaddicted members lose priority. Goals related to controlling, compensating for, or dealing with the negative consequences of addiction gradually assume the highest priority in such families (Wegscheider, 1976). Displacement of both group goals and goals of individual family members increases as the dysfunctioning of the addicted individual progresses. As the capacity for positive functioning diminishes, the goals of the family also will become more and more basic in terms of Maslow's hierarchy of needs (1970), listed in Table 5.1.

Because many families may not have satisfied their basic needs for self- and other-esteem, love, and belongingness, the increased dysfunctional behavior of the chemically dependent person causes family members to pursue other needs. Maintenance of basic physical needs, such as nutrition, shelter, medical care, and rest, may become the main focus of goal attainment by family members as a result. Although each family

Table 5.1
Maslow's Hierarchy of Needs

Need	*Satisfied by*
Self-Esteem	achievement, competence, confidence, independence
Other-Esteem	dignity, importance, recognition, appreciation
Love	exchanging love, affection, sexuality
Belonging	satisfying relationships, a secure place within a family or group
Safety	stability; predictability; dependence; freedom from fear, anxiety, chaos, death
Physical	food, shelter, rest, medical care

system may have a different level of initial functioning, the progression of chemical dependency will contribute almost always to some loss of functioning (Wegscheider, 1981).

Family members may experience many frustrations or blocks and obstacles to the attainment of personal or group goals. These blocks typically result from the actions, attitudes, or behaviors of the addicted person and from responses to the situation by other family members. As continued problem-solving efforts fail, the codependent individual may suffer increasing emotional disturbances as a result of repeated frustrations. This process often will continue until one or more family members develop an emotional disorder that requires treatment, the family system breaks up, someone dies, or the chemically dependent family member begins to take steps toward recovery (Woititz, 1983).

The Dynamics of Chemical Dependence and the Effects on Problem Solving

An important question remains: Why do so many people choose similar yet ineffective problem-solving strategies to attain personal or family goals? The primary cause may be a lack of knowledge about the dynamics of an addicted family system. Most codependent individuals do not understand that addiction to alcohol or other drugs is a bio-psychological disorder that, left untreated, will progressively destroy the individual's life functioning capabilities and ultimately cause his or her death.

Codependent persons often share in the denial of the addicted person; they believe that the problem will magically cease, that life circumstances will mitigate against the problem, or that the addicted person suddenly will recognize the problem and change his or her behavior (Whitfield, 1984). Many codependent persons use problem-solving strategies that proved effective in prior situations in which a member of the family system was temporarily unable to carry out his or her roles due to illness, accident, or pursuit of alternative goals that were given temporary priority. Without knowledge or awareness of the chronic nature of chemical dependency, codependent persons become fixated in use of solutions that become progressively maladaptive as the system's functional level decreases.

Cultural Factors: Special Considerations in Problem Solving

The societal belief that alcoholism is a moral weakness ties in with the vow of the spouse to love and cherish the other: for better or for worse; in sickness and in health; "till death do us part." The marriage vow is maintained as the cornerstone of the reality for many couples and families. The cultural beliefs of families are important also as determinants of enabling behaviors in family systems, often reflecting dominant Christian religious principles and an ethnic group's value system. It is important to note that a person's culture defines which problem-solving strategies and goals are likely to be chosen and valued. Krestan and Bepko (1990) noted that many theories about the functional or "ideal" family structure are based on white, patriarchal, middle-class systems. These theories assume that all families, regardless of cultural or ethnic differences, should fit the same model. With little resemblance to the broad range of contemporary family structures, compositions, and value systems, these narrow and limited family frameworks lack the cultural sensitivity needed in our increasingly pluralistic society. In Mexican-American family systems, the value placed on maintaining the family as a unit supersedes the importance placed on the individual welfare of its members (McRoy, Shorkey, & Garcia, 1985). Emphasis on maintenance of the family system directs the efforts of the codependent partner toward protecting and caring for chemically dependent members and assuming their responsibilities within the system. Such cultural patterns can be observed in the following example.

Case Example 3

Anna is one of several daughters from a large Mexican-American family. She was seen by the social worker at a psychiatric facility for an adjustment disorder with depressive features following the death of her husband, Jorge, who had died at age 52 from liver failure as a result of years of alcohol abuse. Since Jorge's death, her eldest daughter, son-in-law, and their children have moved from Anna's home, leaving only 17-year-old Frank, the youngest son. During the past 10 years, Anna and Jorge had survived on his social security disability check, which they received because Jorge was unable to work due to his alcoholism. Currently Frank is the only person receiving government benefits, which are due to terminate on his 18th birthday. Anna had taken care of her daughter's young children while her daughter was at work and had looked after Jorge. Various members of Anna's family, including her parents and sisters, helped out with transportation, did home repairs, and provided a great deal of social and emotional support.

During the past several months, Anna, who has never held any form of paid employment, was forced to find her first job in food service. She has found this work to be both stressful and tiring but does not have the education, training, or experience to obtain a better job. Her life and that of her children had revolved around her husband. Although she admits that Jorge had been physically abusive at times, she had a purpose to her life and had family around her. At age 48, she does not believe that she has either the energy or the interest to create a new life-style. She reports feeling lost and afraid.

In Mexican-American families, many members of a large extended-family system may assume such responsibilities as providing temporary housing, baby-sitting, and nursing care. Through the *compadrazgo* system, individuals who are not related to the family through blood ties but who are co-parents or close friends may also contribute toward meeting the basic needs of members of the chemically dependent family (McRoy et al., 1985). Mexican-American families generally have a strong commitment to providing both material and emotional support for their members, and many show an unwillingness to draw on outside supports for resources or solutions to family problems (Dillard, 1987).

Mexican-American families are generally stable, two-parent households. Over 75% are headed by married couples, and the divorce rate is lower than that of any other ethnic group (Becerra, 1988). Because of the shared nature of codependent roles in these Mexican-American families, the immediate negative impact on the chief codependent adult is reduced. Sharing the burden throughout the system helps the immediate and extended family members, but often the chemically dependent person is further enabled to continue to use alcohol or drugs. However, other needs of the chief codependent person, such as esteem and intimacy, may not be met adequately. Although the overall survival of the family unit is assured, the chemically dependent member often will experience the consequences of chronic addiction with increased health problems, incarceration, or death. The tragedy in families such as Anna's is that the shared responsibilities of maintaining the family stability serve to reduce the impact on her as the chief enabler, but the alcoholic husband's disease progressed as a consequence until he died. In many cases, serious illness or significant criminal justice problems that also threaten the integrity of the family are the only other factors that may induce change in such systems.

Like Mexican-American families, black families place a strong emphasis on maintaining the family unit. As identified by Boyd-Franklin (1989), characteristics of strong black families include achievement orientation, adaptability of family roles, strong kinship bonds, and a high degree of religious orientation. A high priority is placed on the care of children, and family aspirations often center around the children's future accomplishments. Family strength is not contingent on traditional white family structure (McRoy, 1990; McRoy & Shorkey, 1985). Some black family units differ from other ethnic groups in that they may have a multigenerational component sometimes combined with a single-parent head of household. It is interesting to note that 47% of all black households are headed by females, an increase of 130% in the last decade. Unemployment, pressures from discrimination, urban living, and poverty have caused black fathers to either never marry or leave the household (Staples, 1988). Other families may include various relatives, boarders, or members of another household (Dillard, 1987). Therefore enablers of chemically dependent family members sometimes may include siblings, grandparents, or even individuals who do not live in the same residence. An example:

Case Example 4

Gene is a 23-year-old black man seeking services in a publicly funded chemical dependency treatment program. He is looking for help in getting his sister Tammy into treatment. Tammy is a 23-year-old black, single mother of three who is severely addicted to crack cocaine. Gene has been living with Tammy for the past 2 years, since their mother died. Numerous relatives on their mother's side of the family live in the same town.

During the last 8 months, Tammy has changed from an energetic, creative woman who worked as a salesperson in a retail clothing store to a destitute crack addict. Gene worries about Tammy because he knows she sometimes steals and has prostituted herself to obtain money for drugs. Gene reports that he has held down two jobs since they no longer have an income from Tammy and is doing his best to care for Tammy's children. Aunt Colleen comes over regularly to help with the cooking and cleaning, and her daughter helps with baby-sitting from time to time. Gene and his family are very concerned about the welfare of Tammy's children and the effect that her addiction will have on them.

The social worker notes that Gene gradually has given up his personal life, has lost contact with his friends, and has not had any form of personal relationships during this time. He reports that between work and family, he does not have time or energy to do anything else. Gene says that he is afraid that Tammy probably will be arrested or die if her drug abuse continues.

Although Gene, Aunt Colleen, and others have taken over the role responsibilities of mother, homemaker, and wage earner previously filled by Tammy, they recognize that they must take action to intervene in her self-destructive behavior to protect the family system from further deterioration. The family members have tried to convince Tammy to stop using crack and encouraged her to change her life-style before something drastic happens. They are concerned about her health and her safety on the streets, in addition to the deleterious effect on her children. Unaccustomed to seeking help outside the family, Gene contacts a local drug treatment program because he has no other alternative. However, Gene has little concern for himself and is focused primarily on the needs of Tammy and her children. His ineffective but earnest problem-solving efforts must be clarified during initial and ongoing contacts as Gene and the social worker become engaged in the treatment process.

The Family Systems Problem-Solving Process

The Initial Phase. Many clients receiving services from helping professionals such as psychologists, addiction counselors, and social workers are in relationships with significant others who are at various stages of chemical dependency. These clients frequently are seen in inpatient and outpatient medical programs, probation and parole programs, mental health facilities, child and family service agencies, alcohol and drug treatment programs, and public welfare programs. Clients may have family members who are currently chemically addicted, such as Barbara and Gene in a previous section. Even when separated from the chemically dependent members, clients may experience a continuation or change in problems associated with their past codependent relationships, such as the experience of the recent widow, Anna. Other clients may have family members who are in the process of recovering from substance abuse, as in the example of Maria. Many codependent clients initially seek services for someone other than themselves, as in the case of Barbara asking for health care assistance or Gene wanting help in finding treatment for his sister Tammy. Some clients come to the worker for services for themselves, as in the case of Maria, who wanted help in coping with emotional distress at work and at home, or Anna who wanted help in dealing with anxiety and adjustment after her spouse's death.

After the presenting problem has been identified, the worker assists the client in procuring needed resources, referrals, and services, while fostering the supportive relationship to encourage the client to explore other aspects of his or her individual, family, and environmental situation. Barbara's worker may find affordable health care in her area for Bob. Gene's worker will try to help him get Tammy admitted to a women's treatment center, and if possible, one that serves minority women with children. Maria's EAP social worker may choose to refer her to a psychiatrist for a physical and psychiatric examination to rule out biological factors in her anxiety or to a Hispanic-oriented 12-step program. Or in Anna's case, the worker may look into obtaining some form of public assistance to supplement her income. By meeting clients' identified needs for themselves or others, the helper facilitates continued exploration of broader aspects of the presenting problem.

It is important to note that after meeting initially identified needs, clients may choose to terminate their contact with the worker even after the problems related to addiction and codependency have surfaced. When this is the case, information about relevant referrals for services and programs can be provided and clients can be invited to contact the agency or worker if other concerns arise or if they decide to accept treatment at a later date. What occurs can be viewed in a linear fashion; that is, a client may decline services, and there is little that the worker can do to promote change. This prospect can be seen in Barbara's case, in that she denies the existence of any problem with the exception of Bob's need for medical care. The process also may be viewed as circular in terms of systems theory: If the client does opt for further help, the problem-solving process can continue to the next phase, building on the initial work that has taken place.

The Second Phase. Codependency issues can begin to be addressed during the second phase of the treatment process because the client has been assisted with services to cope with the presenting problem. The client has an opportunity to ventilate and express thoughts, feelings, and problematic issues. The worker and client also can examine the current goals for the client system as a whole and can explore problems related to achieving these goals. The goals of the client system may include the desire to obtain treatment for the chemically dependent family member or to obtain services for other members who are affected, such as children or adolescents within the family.

The worker should take steps to educate the client on the impact of alcoholism and drug dependence on partners or other members of the family system. This educational process can occur within a variety of contexts. The worker may choose to explain the dynamics of a chemically dependent system directly to the client, recommend reading an appropriate self-help book, or refer the client to a workshop or lecture that focuses on these issues. In the case of Barbara, whose husband was hospitalized after a car accident, the worker may suggest that she read *Codependent No More* (Beattie, 1987) and then discuss during future sessions her relevant personal experiences as they pertain to the book. The worker may recommend that Maria attend a workshop on communication and then examine differences in Maria and Jerri's communication patterns since Jerri has been sober. This ongoing educational process serves to give the client the knowledge base needed to gain insight into his or her unique personal and family issues.

Information and support may be provided to the client to obtain the services of alcohol and drug abuse professionals who specialize in working with families. Such interventions are designed to motivate the chemically dependent person to accept help through guided confrontation by family members and concerned others (Miller & Rollnick, 1991). Self-help books such as *Chemical Dependency and Recovery: A Family Affair* (1987) and videotapes such as *The Enablers* (1984) and *The Intervention* (1979), available from the Johnson Institute, may be useful to the client who is attempting to persuade the chemically dependent person to accept treatment. For Barbara, her worker may suggest that she have her children assessed for emotional disturbances caused by the family situation. For Gene, his worker may discuss the progressive nature of addiction. The worker also may confront the possibility of Tammy's actions having severe consequences and emphasizing Gene's lack of control of her choices and consequences.

As the treatment progresses, the worker and client may agree to a detailed assessment of the client's codependent behavior and the impact on the whole family system. Recently professionals in the chemical dependency field have devised a number of procedures and tools to facilitate this assessment of people who may be confronted with codependency issues. Procedures include use of genograms for gathering information on the extended family system. As detailed in McGoldrick and Gerson (1986), genograms can be useful in revealing transgenerational patterns of behavior and the presence or impact of chemically dependent and other compulsive persons within the family system. As Smith (1988) described, the impact of alcoholism can skip a generation, and grandchildren of alcoholics often suffer from severe codependency issues. Genograms are useful in identifying cultural factors relating to social roles, perception of chemical use and abuse, individual and family goals, and religious beliefs within the system.

Another way codependency can be assessed is through self-report inventories. The range of treatment and program marketing materials can provide somewhat objective measures of behaviors and attitudes associated with codependency. The Co-dependent Relationship Questionnaire (Kritsberg, 1989) consists of 25 yes/no questions that describe numerous behaviors associated with codependency. This tool may be used in conjunction with other interactive techniques, especially structured interviews, to give the worker some idea of the degree to which codependent behavior patterns have affected the client's life.

Once the client has identified the need for specific services related to codependency issues, the worker then should link the client to appropriate self-help support groups. The most prevalent type of support group is 12-step programs based on the recovery approach of Alcoholics Anonymous. Within the past two decades, there has been a proliferation of 12-step groups that address the needs of individuals from alcoholic families. These groups include Al-Anon, Alateen, Families Anonymous (FA), Codependents Anonymous (CoDA), Narc-Anon, Coc-Anon, Sex and Love Addicts Anonymous (SLAA), and Emotions Anonymous (EA). In AA groups it is acknowledged that the alcoholic is powerless over alcohol, but in these other 12-step support groups the codependent person's powerlessness over another person and his or her own destructive behavior pattern is acknowledged. Maria may best be served by a referral to a gay/lesbian-sensitive or women-only meeting. Anna may feel more comfortable at a Spanish-speaking meeting. Gene may benefit more from a group with African-American members or from a men's group.

It is our belief that any helping professional, regardless of the field or specialization, should be familiar with the operations of 12-step programs. We highly recommend that helpers read *Alcoholics Anonymous* (1976) and other 12-step literature and attend AA and Al-Anon meetings in their area; most of these groups are open to the public and welcome observers. By taking this initiative, practitioners can more easily facilitate making appropriate referrals for their clients.

When referring a client to a 12-step program, it is important for the social worker, psychologist, or other practitioner to take time to explain the basic concepts of these support groups, as they may be confusing to the client. Many codependent persons are not accustomed to discussing their personal ideas, beliefs, and feelings with anyone, much less a large group of strangers. This situation is terrifying for all newcomers to these groups, so precautions should be taken to facilitate a client's involvement with the support groups. It is usually advisable to make available a list of meetings, including dates, times, and places. Also, because different meetings have different foci, such as women's, black, Hispanic, gay/lesbian, or atheist issues, it is advisable to refer clients to a meeting that can meet their specific needs.

The Third Phase. After the client has begun to participate in a self-help support group and has broken through his or her denial system, there may be a need for a third phase of treatment. The helper may continue to work with the client's problem-solving system by using cognitive, behavioral, or expressive-emotive techniques within a family systems framework to address issues not dealt with elsewhere. One of the most effective vehicles for treatment with codependent clients is the use of social group work. These groups can be designed as multiple family groups or as peer groups for codependent individuals that focus on family and individual issues. Groups provide an environment in which clients and family members are encouraged to listen and contribute to discussions about codependency and the experience of being involved with a chemically dependent person. This involvement can be extremely beneficial to family members, especially to the codependent individual, in that they tend to operate under the three rules of dysfunctional families—don't talk, don't trust, don't feel (Black, 1981). Being in a group environment helps break through these dysfunctional rules and forges a more adaptive pattern of relating to others.

The worker may integrate techniques from a variety of treatment approaches with the family systems framework to accomplish these goals in family treatment, individual sessions, or group work. Gestalt therapy techniques can be used to develop a new self-awareness and to help create adaptive behavior patterns in the individual or whole family. Members can be encouraged to talk with absent family members, dialogue with parts of themselves, work on boundary issues, and deal with unfinished business (Blugerman, 1986). A second benefit of treatment in the group context is the potential for clients to observe functional behavior and more effective problem-solving strategies that are modeled by the facilitator and other group members. Gene's worker may aid him in recognizing which of his needs are not being met due to his difficulty in setting limits with Tammy and her children. The group's service as a medium for developing and testing new knowledge and skills for identifying personal goals is a third benefit of this modality. This benefit is especially important in situations in which treatment of the codependent member leads to a disruption of the family because the addicted member refuses treatment. In those situations the self-actualized formerly codependent member can use the group as a transition before building a new social support system outside the group.

Behavioral methods also can develop more effective problem-solving, communication, listening, and assertiveness skills. Behavioral techniques such as modeling, behavior rehearsal, positive reinforcement, and corrective feedback can be used to develop and strengthen new behavior patterns among family and group members. Initially the worker can model basic social skills such as approaching someone, making eye contact, and introducing oneself; the worker then may use behavior rehearsal to help the client practice these skills. Homework assignments can be used to generalize new behaviors to many life situations and problematic family relationships. The worker can use a behavioral contract to delineate the parameters of the assignment and family relationships/boundaries, such as what behavior each client will complete, where it will happen, how long it will last, and how many times the behavior will be performed (Lerner, 1988). After practice on basic social skills with the worker, Anna may be given an assignment to attend, unescorted, an annual festival at her church and to stay for at least half an hour, during which she will have to introduce herself to at least three people. Anna will monitor her behavior in this situation and, on completion of the activity, will likely get positive reinforcement from the people she encounters and, it is hoped, will experience some self-reinforcement. This support is important because it is uncomfortable for a widow in a traditional Mexican-American community to meet new people as an unattached person. The skills she develops from this work can help Anna overcome her shyness and become more assertive.

Cognitive-behavioral techniques based on rational emotive therapy are especially effective in confronting belief systems that encourage shame and guilt and in teaching new belief systems about autonomy and new strategies for coping with stress (Ellis, 1975; Ellis, McInerney, DiGiuseppe, & Yeager, 1988). Maria's worker may challenge her notions about taking responsibility for herself and may emphasize the need for taking risks as a step toward achieving personal goals. The worker may help Maria examine her perceptions of her family's reaction to her because of her same-sex life-style. Maria reports that she "feels shunned" by her family and as a result isolates from them. The worker can show Maria that she may be projecting her own lack of self-acceptance onto her family members. The worker initially would use cognitive-behavioral methods to increase her acceptance of herself with her sexual preference. When she feels more comfortable with herself, she can begin to develop a more interactive relationship with members of her family of origin and with Jerri as her current family.

The Final Phase. After the client has become involved in either a self-help or a family treatment group, the social worker and client system may choose to continue their working relationship to examine their current life situations and to explore more advanced personal goals beyond codependency issues. A person may become more self-actualized and may make changes as a result of increased self-esteem, better problem-solving skills, and more focused individual and system goal attainment. Clients may be encouraged to participate in continuing their growth and development through classes and other educational activities to promote the development of social skills and assertiveness abilities and to further clarify their values and belief systems. Gene, for example, may go back to school to work toward his goal of becoming a teacher. Most communities offer a broad range of opportunities that clients can learn to use. Maria could develop a personal interest and take classes in folk dancing and become involved with a local dance group. Through continued use of available resources within the community, clients can strengthen their ability to function more effectively and autonomously in pursuit of personal goals and family/interpersonal relationships. Maria may meet her goals by becoming involved in the singles group at her church. These changes should lead to more autonomy rather than dependence or need for control in interpersonal relationships.

CONCLUSION

Work with codependent groups and families presents many challenges for effective clinical practice. This chapter has summarized traditional, family-of-origin, and problem-solving perspectives about the codependency process. The first two perspectives may encourage the labeling and generalizing of assumptions about individual clients, and they ignore the unique dynamics in each client's person-situation. These perspectives challenge helping professionals' abilities to remain objective and nonjudgmental about clients' values, whereas the proposed family systems problem-solving perspective is more consistent with a culturally specific view of the codependency process that encourages a focus on the unique ways in which clients solve problems in interaction with significant others.

A major implication flows from the case examples and the discussion about diversity among families with an addicted member: diversity in race, sexual preference, family structure, and age. Social workers, family therapists, addiction counselors, psychologists, and others must be attuned to factors of diversity that interact with issues of codependency and thus should become more knowledgeable about those interactional effects and the need for individualized treatment planning. For instance, treatment should focus on the positive aspects of cultural supports and social networks in black and Hispanic families, while addressing the isolation associated with family biases against same-sex, codependent relationships. By virtue of professional training and their professions' value orientations, social workers and other practitioners are capable of meeting and responding to such challenges.

REFERENCES

Ackerman, R. J. (1983). *Children of alcoholics.* Holmes Beach, FL: Learning Publications.

Ackerman, R. J., & Pickering, S. E. (1989). *Abused no more: Recovery for women from abusive or co-dependent relationships.* Blue Ridge Summit, PA: Tab Books.

Alcoholics Anonymous. (1976). *Alcoholics Anonymous* (3rd ed.). New York: Alcoholics Anonymous World Services.

Asher, R., & Brissett, D. (1988). Codependency: A view from women married to alcoholics. *International Journal of the Addictions, 23,*(4), 331-350.

Beattie, M. (1987). *Codependent no more.* New York: Harper/Hazelden.

Becerra, R. M. (1988). The Mexican American family. In C. H. Mindel, R. W. Habenstein, & R. Wright, Jr. (Eds.), *Ethnic families in America: Patterns and variations* (pp. 141-159). New York: Elsevier.

Black, C. (1981). *It will never happen to me.* Denver: M.A.C.

Blugerman, M. (1986). Contributions of gestalt theory to social work treatment. In F. J. Turner (Ed.), *Social work treatment: Interlocking theoretical approaches* (3rd ed., pp. 69-90). New York: Free Press.

Boyd-Franklin, N. (1989). *Black families in therapy: A multisystems approach.* New York: Guilford.

Cermak, T. L. (1986). *Diagnosing and treating co-dependence.* Minneapolis: Johnson Institute Books.

Deutsch, C. (1982). *Broken bottles, broken dreams: Understanding and helping the children of alcoholics.* New York: Teachers College Press.

Dillard, J. M. (1987). *Multicultural counseling: Toward ethnic and cultural relevance in human encounters.* Chicago: Nelson-Hall.

D'Zurilla, T. J., & Goldfried, M. R. (1971). Problem-solving and behavior modification. *Journal of Abnormal Psychology, 78*(1), 197-216.

Ellis, A. (1975). *How to live with a neurotic.* New York: Crown.

Ellis, A., McInerney, J. F., DiGiuseppe, R., & Yeager, R. J. (1988). *Rational-emotive therapy with alcoholics and substance abusers.* New York: Pergamon.

Friel, J., Subby, R., & Friel, L. D. (1984). *Co-dependency and the search for identity.* Deerfield Beach, FL: Health Communications.

Gierymski, T., & Williams, T. (1986). Codependency. *Journal of Psychoactive Drugs, 18*(1), 7-13.

Gomberg, E. (1989). On the terms used and abused: The concept of "codependency." *Drugs and Society, 3*(3-4), 113-132.

Greenleaf, J. (1981). *Co-alcoholic, para-alcoholic: Who's who and what's the difference?* New Orleans: 361 Foundation.

Harper, J., & Capdevila, C. (1990). Codependency: A critique. *Journal of Psychoactive Drugs. 22*(3), 285-292.

Johnson Institute (Producer). (1979). *The Intervention* [Film]. Minneapolis: Johnson Institute.

Johnson Institute (Producer). (1984). *The Enablers* [Film]. Minneapolis: Johnson Institute.

Johnson Institute. (1987). *Chemical dependency and recovery: A family affair.* Minneapolis: Author.

Krestan, J., & Bepko, C. (1990). Codependency: The social reconstruction of female experience. *Smith College Studies in Social Work, 60*(3), 216-232.

Kritsberg, W. (1989). *Am I in a co-dependent relationship?* Deerfield Beach, FL: Health Communications.

Lerner, R. (1988). *Boundaries for co-dependents.* Center City, MN: Hazelden.

Maslow, A. H. (1970). *Motivation and personality.* New York: Harper & Row.

McGoldrick, M., & Gerson, R. (1986). *Genograms in family assessment.* New York: Norton.

McRoy, R. G. (1990). Cultural and racial identity in black families. In S. M. L. Logan, E. M. Freeman, & R. G. McRoy (Eds.), *Social work practice with black families: A culturally specific perspective* (pp. 97-111). New York: Longman.

McRoy, R. G., & Shorkey, C. T. (1985). Alcohol use and abuse among blacks. In E. Freeman (Ed.), *Social work practice with clients who have alcohol problems* (pp. 202-213). Springfield, IL: Charles C Thomas.

McRoy, R. G., Shorkey, C. T., & Garcia, E. (1985). Alcohol use and abuse among Mexican Americans. In E. M. Freeman (Ed.), *Social work practice with clients who have alcohol problems* (pp. 229-241). Springfield, IL: Charles C Thomas.

Mellody, P. (1989). *Facing co-dependence.* New York: Harper & Row.

Miller, W. R., & Rollnick, S. (1991). *Motivational interviewing: Preparing people to change addictive behavior.* New York: Guilford.

Nezu, A., & D'Zurilla, T. J. (1981). Effects of problem definition and formulation on decision making in the social problem-solving process. *Behavior Therapy, 1,* 100-106.

O'Neill, J., & O'Neill, P. (1989). *How to get help: When someone else's drinking or drugging is hurting you.* Austin, TX: Creative Assistance.

Shorkey, C. T., & Crocker, S. B. (1981). Frustration theory: A source of identifying concepts for generalist practice. *Social Work, 26*(5), 374-379.

Smalley, S. (1982). *Co-dependency: An introduction.* New Brighton, MN: SBS.

Smalley, S. (1984). *Co-dependency: An intimacy dilemma.* New Brighton, MN: SBS.

Smith, A. W. (1988). *Grandchildren of alcoholics: Another generation of co-dependency.* Deerfield Beach, FL: Health Communications.

Staples, R. (1988). The black American family. In C. H. Mindel, R. W. Habenstein, & R. Wright (Eds.), *Ethnic families in America: Patterns and variations* (pp. 303-324). New York: Elsevier.

Subby, R., & Friel, J. (1984). *Co-dependency and family rules: A paradoxical dependency.* Deerfield Beach, FL: Health Communications.

Wegscheider, S. (1976). *The family trap. . . . No one escapes from a chemically dependent family.* Minneapolis: Johnson Institute.

Wegscheider, S. (1981). *Another chance: Hope and health for the alcoholic family.* Palo Alto, CA: Science & Behavior Books.

Whitfield, C. L. (1984). Co-alcoholism: Recognizing a treatable illness. *Family and Community Health, 7*(2), 16-28.

Woititz, J. G. (1983). *Adult children of alcoholics.* Deerfield Beach, FL: Health Communications.

Chapter 6

TREATMENT FOR DUALLY DIAGNOSED CLIENTS

MARSHA R. READ
ELIZABETH C. PENICK
ELIZABETH J. NICKEL

The term *dual diagnosis* in the addictions field usually refers to the co-occurrence of one or more substance use disorders with one or more nonsubstance use mental disorders. The concept has begun to take on a life of its own (Attia, 1988; Daley, Moss, & Campbell, 1987). Dual diagnosis treatment units are springing up throughout the country. Dual diagnosis symposia are being held everywhere. Numerous technical and nontechnical publications address the subject of dual diagnosis. Clinicians now state that they are in the dual diagnosis field. Yet scientifically reliable knowledge about dually diagnosed individuals is still skimpy. This paucity is particularly true about the natural long-term course of these disorders and which kinds of treatments are most effective for which dually diagnosed conditions.

In a recent comment about dual diagnosis, Lehman, Myers, and Corty (1989) noted that the National Institute of Mental Health's Epidemiologic Catchment Area Study (ECA) indicated that 19%-30% of the general population are at lifetime risk for developing some type of identifiable mental disorder and that 15%-18% of the general population are at risk for developing a substance use disorder. Of those at risk for developing a substance use disorder, 12%-16% will suffer from alcohol abuse and

AUTHORS' NOTE: The preparation of this chapter was supported, in part, by NIAAA Grant IR21- AA07539-01

5%-6% will suffer from some other type of drug abuse problem. Helzer and Pryzbeck (1988) reported that when compared to community individuals who had never abused alcohol or any other drug, individuals from the community in the ECA study who satisfied diagnostic criteria for a lifetime alcohol problem were also significantly more likely to satisfy diagnostic criteria for one or more additional mental disorders. This same ECA study found that the majority of surveyed community residents with substance use disorders and other mental disorders had never received treatment for either problem (Shapiro et al., 1984). The problem is exacerbated when one considers the number of family members affected directly by dually diagnosable members who are represented in this untreated segment of the population.

A recent review of the research literature on dual diagnoses (Penick, Nickel, et al., 1990) pointed out that when structured criterion-referenced interviews were used for diagnostic purposes, 30%-70% of individuals in treatment for alcohol and drug-related problems also will satisfy definitional criteria for at least one additional mental disorder. In some studies, about half of the dually diagnosed clients were found to have two or more additional co-existing mental disorders besides the substance abuse problem, a fact that suggests the term *dual diagnosis* is less accurate than *multiple diagnosis*. The flip side to the finding that many clients seeking help for a substance abuse problem also will fulfill definitional standards for another mental disorder is that larger-than-expected numbers of individuals receiving treatment for other mental disorders also have been found to abuse one or more substances at some point in their lives. These other mental disorders with elevated rates of substance abuse include the schizophrenias, the mood disorders, the anxiety disorders (especially post-traumatic stress disorder; see Chapter 7), the eating disorders, antisocial personality disorder, and some of the other personality disorders.

Moreover, substance abuse is a frequent complicating factor to many of the most devastating social problems, such as persistent crime, domestic violence including spouse abuse and child abuse, job loss, family dissolution, suicide, and fatal accidents (Goodwin, 1981; Holden, 1987; National Institute on Alcohol Abuse and Alcoholism [NIAAA], 1983, 1987). Such recent findings suggest that dual diagnosis conditions are common both in the community-at-large and in specialized programs that serve those who abuse substances, those who suffer from other kinds of mental illness, and those who are socially dysfunctional. Most helping professionals will encounter the dual diagnosis problem again and again in the public and private sectors and in all clinical treatment settings.

There are several good reasons why social workers, mental health therapists, addiction counselors, psychologists, and psychiatrists should become familiar with the idea of dual diagnosis. First, it is a frequent cause of personal suffering, social impairment, and physical disability that can be easily overlooked when attention is focused too exclusively on certain disruptive behaviors or on other specific health and social problems. Second, these helping professionals often serve as gatekeepers to people in trouble. The ability to recognize dual diagnosis problems should increase clinicians' chances for obtaining the best treatment possible for their clients. Third, a thorough understanding of dual diagnosis would allow practitioners to evaluate more intelligently the quality of treatment being provided to their clients. Fourth, recognition of the appalling lack of resources for clients suffering from a dual diagnosis should stimulate practitioners to lobby for change in the agencies they represent and influence. Fifth, an increased sensitivity to dual diagnosis should facilitate the clinical effectiveness of helpers in their work with individual clients and families. Family approaches provide guidelines for how to involve and strengthen family and other social support networks in the community. Family approaches are also consistent with an ecological perspective that helps practitioners maintain a focus on the person-and-environment. Accurate information about what is known and is not known about dual diagnosis can only enhance the professionalism of social workers in their interactions with their clients and family/community resources. And last, incorporation of knowledge about dual diagnosis into the curriculum and training of future generations of helping professionals should increase their effectiveness as teachers, clinicians, administrators, and researchers.

In this chapter we summarize state-of-the-art developments in the description and assessment of dual diagnosis conditions, along with information about prevalence rates and the etiology of the conditions. Family systems prevention and treatment strategies are presented in relation to the professional roles required for effective work with individuals, peer networks, and families. Case examples illustrate how such strategies can be used effectively.

DESCRIPTION AND ASSESSMENT OF DUAL DIAGNOSIS CONDITIONS

Diagnostic Criteria or Standards

Most clinicians are familiar with the diagnostic standards published in the 1980 and 1987 editions of the *Diagnostic and Statistical Manual of Mental Disorders* (American Psychiatric Association [APA], 1980, 1987). Social worker Janet B. W. Williams was actively involved in the development, organization, and testing of those diagnostic standards and has written extensively about them (Williams & Spitzer, 1980, 1982). The *DSM-III* and its revision represent a dramatic shift in the way mental disorders are "officially" conceptualized and defined in the United States (Blashfield, 1984; Othmer, Penick, Powell, Read, & Othmer, 1989; Spitzer & Klein, 1978). Reflecting the descriptive, syndromatic approach to psychopathology, the *DSM-III* manuals present empirically derived "operational" clinical criteria to define the various mental disorders. The definitional criteria were designed especially to be neutral or "agnostic" with regard to the many widely circulating, but essentially unproven, theories of mental illness and psychopathology. The large-scale acceptance of the *DSM-III*s by mental health scientists and practitioners provided for the first time a set of explicit, uniform, and reliable diagnostic standards that all disciplines could use with ease.

When these contemporary diagnostic standards have been systematically applied to clinical and nonclinical research samples, the results have revealed what many clinicians previously suspected but were unable to document accurately—that individuals who abuse psychoactive substances also will often fulfill lifetime diagnostic criteria for another mental disorder (Fowler, Liskow, Tanna, & Van Valkenburg, 1977; Hesselbrock, Meyer, & Kenner, 1985; Powell, Penick, Othmer, Bingham, & Rice, 1983; Regier, Farmer, & Rae, 1990; Ross, Glaser, & Germanson, 1988; Rounsaville, Weissman, Kleber, & Wilbur, 1982). The concept of *dual diagnosis* resulted from the recognition that when "official" definitional standards were applied systematically without any particular bias, many individuals satisfied standards for both a substance use disorder and at least one other mental disorder. The growing interest in dual diagnosis also resulted from the recognition that many drug- and alcohol-dependent individuals and their families fail to benefit from conventional, individually focused substance abuse programs (Holden, 1987).

Acknowledgment of treatment failures in even the most sophisticated treatment programs led some clinicians to suggest that a portion of those failures might be due to the fact that the therapeutic effort did not deal vigorously enough with other co-occurring mental disorders and the effects on family and other social relationships. The hope that a better understanding of dual diagnosis conditions might result in more effective and broadly focused treatments is a major reason for the widespread interest in the area of dual diagnosis (Wallace, 1986).

Table 6.1

Illustration of *DSM-III-R* Diagnostic Criteria for Major Depression

A. At least five of the following symptoms have been present during the same two-week period and represent a change from previous functioning; at least one of the symptoms is either (1) depressed mood or (2) loss of interest or pleasure. (Do not include symptoms that are clearly due to a physical condition, mood-incongruent delusions or hallucinations, incoherence, or marked loosening of associations.)
   (1) depressed mood (or can be irritable mood in children and adolescents) most of the day, nearly every day, as indicated either by subjective account or observation by others
   (2) markedly diminished interest or pleasure in all, or almost all, activities most of the day, nearly every day (as indicated either by subjective account or observation by others of apathy most of the time)
   (3) significant weight loss or weight gain when not dieting (e.g., more than 5% of body weight in a month), or decrease or increase in appetite nearly every day (in children, consider failure to make expected weight gains)
   (4) insomnia or hypersomnia every day
   (5) psychomotor agitation or retardation nearly every day (observable by others, not merely subjective feelings of restlessness or being slowed down)
   (6) fatigue or loss of energy nearly every day
   (7) feelings of worthlessness or excessive or inappropriate guilt (which may be delusional) nearly every day (not merely self-reproach or guilt about being sick)
   (8) diminished ability to think or concentrate, or indecisiveness, nearly every day (either by subjective account or as observed by others)
   (9) recurrent thoughts of death (not just fear of dying), recurrent suicidal ideation without a specific plan, or a suicide attempt or a specific plan for committing suicide

B. (1) It cannot be established that an organic factor initiated and maintained the disturbance.
   (2) The disturbance is not a normal reaction to the death of a loved one (Uncomplicated Bereavement).

   Note: Morbid preoccupation with worthlessness, suicidal ideation, marked functional impairment or psychomotor retardation, or prolonged duration suggest bereavement complicated by Major Depression.

C. At no time during the disturbance have there been delusions or hallucinations for as long as two weeks in the absence of prominent mood symptoms (i.e., before the mood symptoms developed or after they have remitted).

D. Not superimposed on Schizophrenia, Schizophreniform Disorder, Delusional Disorder, or Psychotic Disorder NOS.

SOURCE: American Psychiatric Association: *Diagnostic and Statistical Manual of Mental Health Disorders, Third Edition, Revised.* Washington, DC, American Psychiatric Association, 1987. Reprinted by permission.

For illustrative purposes, Table 6.1 presents a summary of *DSM-III-R* diagnostic criteria for major depression. It can be noted that while the *DSM-III-R* definitional criteria are relatively straightforward, there is room for individual interpretation that might result in clinical disagreement or lowered reliability (Kendell, 1975; Spitzer, Endicott, & Robins, 1978; Spitzer, Skodol, Williams, Gibbon, & Kass, 1982; Othmer & Othmer, 1989; Othmer et al., 1989).

Structured Diagnostic Interviews

To reduce idiosyncratic clinical interpretations, diagnostic instruments have been constructed that reflect *DSM-III* definitional standards. The most widely accepted instruments of this kind are the structured diagnostic interviews that are designed to "rule in" or "rule out" certain of the more common and better researched mental disorders. Two of the most recent interview guides were designed for practitioners as well as clinical researchers. The first, which we co-wrote, is the Psychiatric Diagnostic Interview-Revised (PDI-R) (Othmer et al., 1989). The PDI-R systematically reviews 18 basic psychiatric syndromes and 4 derived syndromes from both a current and a lifetime perspective. Constructed to resemble a "guided conversation" with considerable give-and-take between the interviewer and client, the PDI-R consists of carefully tested questions that capture the essence of the broader, more abstract diagnostic criteria. For example, Table 6.2 presents the questions used by the PDI-R to review the syndrome of depression. It includes the explicit PDI-R rules that are provided to score the depression syndrome as positive or negative—that is, ever present or never present.

An independent recording booklet and guidelines for obtaining current and lifetime diagnoses are also components of the instrument. The PDI-R yields a diagnosis for almost 100% of those individuals receiving treatment in a substance abuse program and over 90% of those who seek help from a general mental health treatment setting.

A less structured but numerically more representative diagnostic interview developed for clinicians and researchers is the Structured Clinical Interview for *DSM-III-R* Disorders, or the SCID (Spitzer, Williams, Gibbon, & First, 1988). The SCID encompasses all of the *DSM-III-R* personality disorders and several other disorders not reviewed by the PDI-R. Because of its relative newness, the SCID has not been as extensively tested for reliability and validity as has the PDI-R. Unlike the PDI-R, the SCID assumes that the user has had experience

text continued on page 131

Table 6.2

Questions and Criteria Used to Identify Major Depression in the *Psychiatric Diagnostic Interview—Revised (PDI-R)*

Cardinal Questions:

1. Have there ever been times when you felt unusually depressed, empty, sad, or hopeless for several days or weeks at a time?

Syndrome should be reviewed regardless of any explanations.

2. Have there ever been times when you felt very irritable or tired most of the time for hardly any reason at all?
3. (If yes to either Item 1 or 2) How long do these feelings usually last? (If less than 2 weeks) What is the longest they have ever lasted? (If less than 2 weeks) Have these feelings ever stayed with you most of the time for as long as 2 weeks?

Mark Item 3 if the mood lasted 2 weeks or longer. This criterion is fulfilled if the patient was hospitalized for depression. Fluctuations in mood can occur.

If one or both Items 1 and 2 plus Item 3 are positive, the patient has met the criterion for this section. If positive, proceed to the Social Significance questions.

If the criterion for this section was not met, proceed to Item 1 of the next syndrome, Mania.

Social Significance Questions:

4. Did these depressed feelings ever cause you any problems or discomfort in your life?
5. Did these down moods ever interfere with your schoolwork, your job, or your chores around the house?

This item is marked if the patient was hospitalized for depression.

6. Did they ever cause you problems with your family or cause your family to worry about you?
7. Did they ever interfere with your social life or friendships?
8. Did you ever receive treatment or medication because of these feelings?
9. (If yes on Item 8) Were you ever hospitalized for this?
10. How old were you when these feeling caused you the most trouble in your life?

If any one or more of Items 4 through 9 are positive, the patient has met the scoring criterion for this section. If positive, proceed to the Auxiliary questions.

If the criterion for this section was not met, proceed to the next syndrome, Mania.

Auxiliary Questions:

When you have been most depressed or down, did you ever:

Group A

11. Lose your appetite?
12. Lose weight without trying to diet? (If yes) How much weight did you lose? How long did it take to lose this much? Was your weight loss caused by a medical illness?

Mark Item 12 if the patient lost 10 pounds or more in 1 year or 2 pounds a month and the weight loss was unrelated to physical illness.

continued

Table 6.2
Continued

13. Find that your appetite increased?
14. Gain weight? (If yes) How much weight did you gain? How long did it take you to gain this weight?

Mark Item 14 if patient gained 15 pounds or more in 1 year or 1 pound or more a month.

Group B

15. Have trouble falling asleep?
16. Tend to wake up a lot during the night?
17. Wake up early in the morning and find it hard to get back to sleep?
18. Feel like you wanted to sleep a lot more than usual?

Group C

19. Feel drained, as though you had hardly any energy at all?
20. Become tired easily and have to force yourself to do things?
21. Feel as though you could hardly move at times?

Group D

22. Talk or move more slowly than usual?
23. Get tense and restless and have a hard time relaxing?
24. Become more impatient, angry, or short-tempered?
25. Sometimes start to cry for practically no reason?
26. Feel slowed down and find it hard to get going?
27. Find it very hard to get things done?

Group E

28. Tend to lose interest in things you usually enjoy?
29. Tend to withdraw from other people?
30. Have less interest in sex than usual?
31. Feel so down that almost nothing could cheer you up?
32. Practically stop taking good care of yourself?

Group F

33. Feel hopeless about the future?
34. Feel that you were worthless and no good?
35. Almost completely lose confidence in yourself?
36. Feel that others might be better off without you?
37. Feel very guilty and ashamed about things that usually don't bother you that much? Assumes a clearly exaggerated sense of guilt.

Group G

38. Have trouble concentrating and keeping your mind on one thing?
39. Notice that your thoughts seemed slow or mixed up?

continued

Table 6.2
Continued

Group H

40. Think more about death or dying?
41. Wish you were dead?
42. Think seriously about killing yourself?
43. Try to kill yourself?

To meet the scoring criterion for this section, five or more of the eight Groups A through H must have at least one item marked. The Syndrome, Depression, is positive if all 3 Sections are positive.

If positive, proceed to the Time Profile questions.

If the criterion for this section was not met, proceed to the next syndrome, Mania.

Time Profile Questions:

44. How old were you when you were first bothered by these depressed feelings?
45. How old were you when you were last bothered by these feelings?
46. Have you been bothered by many of these same feelings in the last month?
47. Have you been bothered by many of these same feelings sometime in the last 2 years?

in applying *DSM-III-R* criteria in clinical settings. In contrast, the PDI-R was designed so that, with training and supervision, even paraprofessionals can reliably administer and score the interview. Of course, the more clinical experience a person has, the better any diagnostic tool will be in his or her hands.

Two other widely used, structured, diagnostic interviews are the Schedule for Affective Disorders and Schizophrenia (SADS) (Endicott & Spitzer, 1978, 1979) and the Diagnostic Interview Schedule (DIS) (Robins, Helzer, Croughan, & Radcliff, 1981). Both of these instruments are quite complex to administer. However, because their reliability and validity have been extensively investigated, they often are used for research. Most recently, Schuckit and colleagues have proposed a brief structured diagnostic interview for use with substance use samples—the Alcohol Research Center (ARC) Intake Interview (Schuckit, Irwin, Howard, & Smith, 1988). This interview, composed of items from other instruments, was developed to examine a limited number of possible co-occurring psychiatric disorders in clinical settings that largely provide treatment for alcoholic men.

It should be emphasized that the only purpose of such diagnostic interviews is to determine whether an individual is suffering currently or has ever suffered from one or more of the recognized mental disorders. Diagnostic interviews based on *DSM-III* and *DSM-III-R* were not designed to do anything else. They do not, nor do they claim to, evaluate the whole person or important environmental aspects such as family relationships and resources. This highly focused but narrow concentration on the mental disorders of an individual is one of the main strengths of the structured diagnostic interviews. Their concentrated focus also is considered to be a weakness by some who adopt a very different view of mental illness, and, as a consequence, they may be used in combination with other more broadly focused screening and assessment procedures by persons with such a view.

Models of Psychopathology

At present there are essentially two ways of looking at the behaviors, thoughts, and feelings that are commonly thought to reflect mental illness or psychopathology. These two models of mental disorder differ enormously in the assumptions they make about disordered behavior, in the methods they use to record and assess such behaviors, and in what they will or will not accept as fact and proof (Othmer et al., 1989). One such approach to psychopathology, the one on which the *DSM-III*s are based, is usually referred to as the *descriptive, or neo-Kraepelin, model of mental disorder* (Blashfield, 1984). The second model of psychopathology goes by different names. It often is referred to as the *interpretative model of mental disorder* because the practitioners of this persuasion typically do not simply describe the behaviors of their clients but go well beyond description to speculative theories of causality. The interpretative approach to psychopathology is reflected in the different schools of family therapy and psychotherapy (especially those following a psychodynamic perspective), as well as the nonpsychometric theories of personality. Despite its former dominance among the mental health professions in this country, the interpretive approach to psychopathology essentially was rejected by the *DSM-III*s. Table 6.3 briefly contrasts the descriptive and interpretive models of psychopathology.

The *descriptive approach* confines itself to the methods of science, with an emphasis on what can be observed reliably and consistently.

Table 6.3
Two Contrasting Approaches to Understanding Psychopathology

Descriptive
Qualitative focus
Categorical measurement
Objective, reproducible knowledge
Verification by methods and procedures of science
Avoids nonoperational concepts

Interpretive
Quantitative focus
Dimensional measurement
Intuitive knowledge
Verification by recurring themes arising in psychotherapeutic interactions
Relies on nonoperational concepts

Theories or speculations that cannot be formally tested and rejected by the scientific method generally play a relatively minor role in the descriptive model. Traditionally the descriptive approach to psychopathology has assumed the existence of different and separate mental disorders that usually are referred to as diagnostic entities. Consequently the descriptive model emphasizes a categorical and criterion-referenced approach to the measurement of psychopathological behaviors. The *categorical approach* to measurement relies on a minimum threshold to identify the presence of a syndrome or a mental disorder. This approach to definition focuses on what can be observed and reported without concern for possible underlying causes that are acknowledged as being currently unknown by the descriptive practitioner.

For example, as seen in Table 6.1, to satisfy minimal diagnostic criteria for major depression in *DSM-III-R,* the client must manifest dysphoric mood and/or loss of pleasure for at least 2 weeks and also must experience symptoms in at least five of the nine symptom groups that essentially define this condition. The use of a minimum threshold to define psychiatric syndromes or mental disorders does not mean that all people who satisfy definitional standards for a particular disorder will suffer equally or be equally impaired by it. Instead the *minimum threshold method* of producing a categorical diagnosis in mental health simply informs the clinician that the course and treatment response of a particular client who has satisfied criteria for a particular mental disorder is likely to resemble composite study groups that have been defined in the same way.

The relatively straightforward descriptive approach to psychopathology differs greatly from the interpretive approach because the interpretive models typically de-emphasize the reliable observation of overt behaviors. The interpretive models have been especially preoccupied with discovering the underlying causes of normal and abnormal behavior through intuitive knowledge generated mostly from interactive, interpersonal psychotherapies (Penick, Read, et al., 1991). The intuitive approach to understanding usually produces a series of elegant and intriguing ideas about human behavior that generally cannot be operationalized or subjected to the scrutiny of science (Goodwin, 1986, chap. 6, pp. 40-47; Popper, 1962).

As a rule the interpretive schools of psychopathology do not make sharp categorical distinctions between sick and well, normal and abnormal, mentally ill and not mentally ill. The interpretive practitioner thinks in terms of dimensions, not categories. When attempting to assess or clinically evaluate a client, the interpretive practitioner typically emphasizes quite complex hypothetical dimensions, such as ego strength or reality testing or unconscious conflicts or the strength of object relations. The development of dimensional measures of psychopathology was influenced by the previously dominant interpretive approach to psychopathology and was reinforced by the enormous success of psychometric instruments that were constructed to assess various intellectual and cognitive functions.

How does this digression about the two major models of diagnosis in the mental health field relate to dual diagnosis? Quite simply, for clinicians to best help their dual diagnosis clients, they first must be able to identify and assess the conditions accurately. A clinician may or may not intellectually accept the descriptive approach to psychopathology represented in the *DSM-III-R* (Mirowsky & Ross, 1989), but he or she should be aware that this is the way dual diagnoses currently are defined. Because the definition of *dual diagnosis* is based on categorical diagnostic concepts, not on dimensional diagnostic concepts, the clinician must be very careful not to confuse these two different approaches to assessment (Blashfield, 1984). Most of the self-administered paper-and-pencil tests, such as the Michigan Alcoholism Screening Test (MAST) (Selzer, 1971), the Minnesota Multiphasic Personality Inventory (MMPI) (Hathaway & McKinley, 1943-1982), the Symptom Checklist-90-R (SCL-90-R) (Derogatis, 1977), and the Beck Depression Inventory (BDI) (Beck, Ward, Mendelson, Mock, & Erbaugh, 1961), are based on a dimensional concept of psychopathology. Similarly most of the rating scales currently used in clinical practice also are based on a dimensional concept of psychopathology. These include the Brief Psychiatric Rating Scale (BPRS) (Overall & Gorham, 1962) and the Hamilton Rating Scale for Depression (HAM-D) (Hamilton, 1960).

Such frequently used and often very helpful instruments cannot be translated easily into a categorical *DSM-III-R* diagnosis. It is important to keep this fact in mind. To "translate" a dimensional measure of psychopathology into a categorical diagnosis, some sort of "cutoff point" or "cutting score" must be developed and clinically validated. The development of diagnostic cutting scores is surrounded by controversy because such scores ultimately are dependent on a categorical model of psychopathology. It is clear that the process of establishing a cutting score from dimensional measures to achieve a categorical diagnosis is excessively indirect and makes little sense when closely examined (Othmer et al., 1989). Projective and semiprojective tests, such as the Rorschach ink blots (Exner & Clark, 1978) or the human figure drawing tests (Hammer, 1978), are barely capable of producing a reliable, contemporary, categorical diagnosis because their clinical applications are derived from a model of psychopathology that differs from the model on which *DSM-III-R* was based.

Another disadvantage of the dimensional psychometric instruments in identifying dual diagnosis clients is the fact that many of these instruments are keyed to assess events that were experienced in the recent past, usually within the past week for mood-disturbance scales and within the past 6 months to 1 year for the substance abuse scales. Although a time frame of 6 months to 1 year is less problematic, a time frame of 1 week is very problematic when trying to establish a dual diagnosis for individuals who recently have entered into treatment for substance abuse. When most drug- or alcohol-dependent people enter into treatment, their affective distress, behavioral deviance, and cognitive dysfunction are likely to be at an all-time high as a direct result of the substance abuse. Therefore, when substance-abusing clients first enter into treatment, dimensional measures that focus on the immediate past are not especially good indicators of other lifetime mental disorders.

If the practitioner interested in dual diagnosis wants to employ a formal procedure when assessing his or her clients, one of the structured *DSM-III-R*-compatible diagnostic interviews is recommended, supplemented when it becomes available, by the person-in-environment (PIE) system that has been proposed by the National Association of Social Workers (NASW) (Karls & Wandrei, 1992). For social workers, psychologists, or other mental health professionals engaged in research or evaluation, use of a structured, diagnostic interview to identify dual diagnosis conditions is virtually mandatory because questions still remain about what the term *dual diagnosis* really means.

Validity of the Dual Diagnosis Concept

Although the definitional standards of the *DSM-III* have become widely accepted since its initial publication more than a decade ago, the concept of *dual diagnosis* is not nearly so well accepted. Why not, if the *DSM-III* standards for the substance use disorders and other major mental disorders are so well accepted? Is it not logical to assume that the combination of two or more *DSM-III-R* disorders into dual diagnosis categories would be equally well received? The logic is sound, but the conclusion is inaccurate. Many professionals in the substance abuse field who readily accept *DSM-III-R* diagnostic standards do not fully accept the idea of dual diagnosis. One reason for the nonacceptance of dual diagnosis is the same reason that many dimensional assessment instruments of psychopathology are not very helpful in determining a dual diagnosis at the time an individual enters into treatment. Those who question the validity of the dual diagnosis idea correctly point out that all of the psychoactive drugs of abuse, including alcohol and nicotine, can mimic or produce almost all of the symptoms of the other mental disorders, especially during the phases of acute intoxication and withdrawal (Schuckit & Monteiro, 1988).

Once the acute phase of intoxication and withdrawal ends, many of the symptoms suggestive of another mental disorder will disappear completely or become markedly reduced. It is this time-locked association between the phases of intoxication and withdrawal and the symptoms of other mental disorders that creates skepticism in the minds of many professionals about the validity of the *dual diagnosis* concept. Schuckit (1985, 1986, 1989) and Schuckit and Monteiro (1988), for example, urged caution in a too-willing acceptance of dual diagnosis by the substance abuse field. Schuckit, like others, proposed a primary-secondary distinction where the terms *primary* and *secondary* refer to the temporal relationships between two mental disorders. The disorder that begins first in the life of an individual is called the *primary mental disorder;* the disorder that begins after the first disorder is called the *secondary mental disorder.* Schuckit believes that the primary-secondary distinction is important in distinguishing "true" co-occurring mental disorders from "pseudo" mental disorders that he believes are only secondary effects of the substance abuse. That author would reserve the concept of *dual diagnosis* to those individuals who clearly developed another mental disorder independently of their substance abuse problems.

Allen and Frances (1986) described four possibilities that could account for the co-occurrence of substance use disorders with other mental disorders:

1. The additional mental disorder could be a direct result of the pharmacologic and behavioral consequences of the substance abuse, a position held by Schuckit (1985, 1986, 1989) for those mental disorders that begin during or after the onset of a substance use disorder.
2. The substance use disorder could be a direct result of another preexisting mental disorder, such as depression or panic disorder, an idea closely resembling a "self-medication hypothesis."
3. The presence of a substance use disorder with another mental disorder could be simply coincidental, an option that is increasingly difficult to accept because recent studies have shown that the risk of almost all of the mental disorders is elevated among people with any lifetime history of drug or alcohol abuse.
4. Both the substance use disorder and the co-occurring mental disorder could be the result of a third, currently unidentified, common etiological factor that might be biological, familial, or social in nature.

At this point, not one of these four highly complex hypotheses has been fully supported or fully disconfirmed by research, although the fourth possibility is more consistent with an ecological, systems perspective. Doubts about the validity of the *dual diagnosis* concept will continue until one of the four possibilities is confirmed by research.

In a recent review, we acknowledged that the concept of *dual diagnosis* is a good deal fuzzier and more vulnerable to disproof than many of its more avid supporters would like to believe (Penick, Nickel, et al., 1990). At the same time, there is by now considerable support for the clinical validity of many dual diagnosis conditions; that is, the presence or absence of another mental disorder in addition to a substance use disorder frequently seems to make a substantial difference in what has happened and in what will happen to those individuals who suffer from both. In instances where the substance abuse accompanies a chronic psychosis, the combination seems to make a very large difference indeed (Caragonne & Emery, 1987). Overall, the presence of one or more mental disorders in addition to a substance use disorder has been associated with the following characteristics:

Increased rates of mental disorder and psychopathology, including increased rates of substance abuse, among immediate family members and other close relatives

Earlier age-of-onset of the abuse of substances

Greater symptom severity and a more malignant clinical course

Greater psychosocial, legal, and interpersonal complications

Increased risk for accidents, acts of violence, and serious medical problems

Poorer compliance with and response to traditional treatment programs for substance abuse and mental illness

Higher likelihood of relapse for both the substance use disorder and the co-occurring mental disorder

Greater probability of the individual becoming homeless and/or totally and permanently disabled

It is important to note that there are exceptions to this list of associated characteristics, and certainly not all dual diagnosis combinations are equally devastating. But in general, the dually diagnosed client will experience more personal suffering, will create greater grief and concern to family members and others, and will respond less well to efforts of assistance than clients who satisfy definitional criteria for only a single substance use disorder.

PREVALENCE RATES AND ETIOLOGICAL ISSUES

It would be especially helpful for readers new to this field if a simple summary table could be presented to show the lifetime rates of the different mental disorders, among groups of people who abused different substances, by the usual sociodemographic breakdowns of age, gender, race, education, income, geographic residence, and the like. Unfortunately, at this time, it is not possible to create such a table with confidence. The concept of *dual diagnosis* is too new and the information is too fragmented and unstandardized to allow an accurate summary of that kind. Table 6.4 presents the combined results of two large studies of male veterans who had sought help for an alcohol problem from one of six VA medical centers (Penick, Nickel, et al., 1990).

Table 6.4
Co-Occurrence of Major Mental Disorders in 928 Alcohol-Dependent Male Veterans

Positive Psychiatric Syndrome	*Percentage*[*]
Depression	36.4
Antisocial Personality Disorder	24.0
Drug Abuse	17.1
Mania	16.1
Panic Disorder	9.5
Obsessive-Compulsive Disorder	8.6
Phobia	6.7
Schizophrenia	3.2
Organic Brain Syndrome	1.8
Somatization Disorder	0.1

NOTE: *Total greater than 100% because each individual could have more than one additional disorder.

The Psychiatric Diagnostic Interview (PDI) was used to assess the co-occurrence of additional mental disorders. Findings indicate that major depression and antisocial personality disorders were the most common disorders, followed by drug abuse and mania. Although the large sample size suggests that these findings are likely to be quite stable, clearly the data should not be generalized to nonwhite or non-male populations.

Prevalence of Major Mental Disorders

The following "facts" about prevalence rates appear more or less established at this point. As noted previously, the absolute rates for virtually all of the major mental disorders, including most of the personality disorders, appear to be significantly higher among those who abuse one or more substances when compared to those who have never abused any substance in their lifetimes (Helzer & Pryzbeck, 1988; Penick, Nickel, et al., 1990). Yet the relative rates of the different mental disorders among substance abuse groups appear to be very similar to the relative rates found in sociodemographically comparable non-substance-abuse groups; that is, the rank order of co-occurring disorders in substance abuse groups closely resembles the rank order of the same disorders in more general samples where substance abuse is not a problem or not the major problem. For example, the mood disorders are more common in substance abuse groups than are somatization disorder, anorexia nervosa, schizophrenia, or mental retardation, which are relatively rare. Similarly the mood disorders are more common in the general population and in mental health and other adult clinic setting than are somatization disorder, anorexia nervosa, schizophrenia, or mental retardation.

Gender-Associated Differences

Another more or less well-established fact is that gender-associated differences in the prevalence of the different co-occurring additional mental disorders is similar to gender-associated differences in the prevalence of the same disorders among male and female non-substance-abusers. For example, just as antisocial personality disorder (ASP) is more common among male non-substance-abusers than among female non-substance-abusers, ASP is also more common among male substance abusers than female abusers, even though the absolute rate of ASP is higher in both male and female substance abuse groups. Similarly major depression is more common among women nonabusers than men nonabusers, and it is also more common among all female than male substance abuse groups. In general, the "epidemiology" of co-occurring mental disorders in the different substance abuse groups seems toclosely resemble the "epidemiology" of the same mental disorders in non-substance-abuse groups except that the absolute rates of the different co-occurring mental disorders is greater in substance abuse groups than in non-substance-abuse groups. Although clearly in need of verification, if this proposal is correct, it could allow planners to anticipate the probable future treatment needs of the next generation of dually diagnosed clients.

A Secular Trend in Prevalence Rates

A third "fact" that has received empirical support is a special cause for concern. Often referred to as a "secular trend" in the epidemiology of mental disorders, this evidence suggests that the more recently born, younger individual may be at greater risk for developing multiple mental disorders than the older individual born at an earlier time (Klerman et al., 1985; Reich, Cloninger, Van Eerdewegh, Rice, & Mullaney, 1988). If this concept is accurate, the prevalence of dual diagnosis and the personal and familial suffering associated with these conditions is likely to increase substantially. If that trend continues, the need for dual diagnosis treatment facilities and trained personnel probably will become more urgent in the next several decades.

Important Knowledge Gaps

Some especially important gaps in knowledge about dual diagnosis must be pointed out. At present, there is insufficient good, comparative information about the long-term outcomes of most dual diagnosis types, especially the most extreme types. Thus it is not clear what the long-term outcomes are for subgroups of substance abusers with a chronic psychosis, severe manic-depressive illness, severe depression, severe anxiety disorder, or severe personality disorder. Moreover, little is known about the long-term outcomes of these extreme dual diagnosis subtypes when the co-occurring mental disorders have been treated adequately with conventional methods. Until very recently, the most systematically studied dual diagnosis subtypes have not included these more severe forms of co-occurring mental illness (Penick et al., 1984).

There is also a great lack of information about the long-term outcomes of dual diagnosis subtypes among females, minorities, the elderly, and those residing largely in rural areas. Typically, dual diagnosis research has focused on the white, urban, lower middle-class male high school graduate in his early 40s who has sought treatment from a public facility. In a related area, very little is known about how family members react to and cope with the immediate and long-term effects of a member with a dual diagnosis. It would be useful to know whether coping patterns and issues of concern vary across these different types of families and what family systems approaches and other modalities tend to be effective across these different family and mental disorder types. It is important also to close these knowledge gaps so that the field can more effectively set about studying the relative efficacy of "old" and "new" treatments for the different dual diagnosis subtypes in general, a research strategy commonly referred to in the substance abuse field as the "matching patients-treatment" approach (Miller & Hester, 1986).

The Causes of Dual Diagnosis Conditions

What about the etiology of dual diagnosis? What are the causes? It is a temptation to state simply and forcefully that the etiology of most mental disorders, including the substance use disorders, is presently unknown. This statement is absolutely true if one means by *etiology* the scientific proof for one or more causes of the condition or disorder under consideration (Goodwin & Guze, 1989). Although the cause or causes of the various mental disorders have not been proven scientifically, many theories of causation are available that the unsophisticated person can easily confuse with fact. Hunches and speculations derived from clinical practice and woven together, sometimes brilliantly, into theoretical systems remain just that—hunches and speculations that must be submitted to empirical scrutiny before they can be accepted as true (Penick, Read, et al., 1991). No such scientifically proven theory of causation exists either in the substance abuse or mental health fields.

The most widely accepted etiological theory of the substance use disorders is the bio-psychosocial model, possibly because its ecological perspective offers a little bit of something to clinicians of every theoretical persuasion (Zucker, 1987). The bio-psychosocial model reflects the thinking of many specialists—clinicians and researchers alike—who believe that the ultimate cause of the substance use disorders will be multifactoral in nature. Biological, psychological, and sociocultural influences are all now thought to contribute and interact in complex and yet unknown ways to produce the different substance use disorders.

Familial, twin, and adoption studies strongly suggest that genetic and/or biological factors affect the risk for developing a substance use disorder and other mental disorders as well. For example, adopted-away sons of alcoholics and adopted-away children of schizophrenic mothers are more likely to suffer from alcoholism or schizophrenia than are the adopted-away children of psychiatrically well biological parents, regardless of the kind of home in which the adopted-away children were reared (Goodwin, 1988; Gottesman & Shields, 1982). Moreover, many studies have shown that the biological children of alcoholics differ from the biological children of nonalcoholics along many genetically related dimensions well before those children approach the age of risk for alcoholism (Tarter, Alterman, & Edwards, 1985). The contribution of psychosocial influences also has been demonstrated in studies of families on the precursors of substance abuse. For example, disruptive and disorganized families most lacking in cohesiveness and personal warmth seem to produce children who are most likely to develop some type of mental illness and/or substance abuse later in life (Vaillant, 1983).

Finally the effect of sociocultural influences on the use and abuse of substances has been known for years. Such influences would include costs of the substances, government regulations, per capita income, cultural and religious beliefs, institutional racism and discrimination practices, occupational affiliations, and local as well as national norms (Goodwin, 1981, 1988). The bio-psychosocial model has been used to "explain" the substance use disorders and the other mental disorders separately. However, no theoretical system exists currently that was specifically designed to address the development of dual diagnosis subtypes. The concept of *assortative mating* from our research may account for the co-occurrence of other mental disorders with the substance use disorders (Read et al., 1990), but these studies need to be replicated carefully before that conclusion can be accepted. At the present stage of knowledge from research, it must be concluded that the cause or causes of dual diagnosis conditions are completely unknown.

FAMILY SYSTEMS PREVENTION AND TREATMENT APPROACHES

The Status of Prevention Efforts

When the proximate cause or causes of a particular condition are not known, efforts to prevent that condition are unlikely to succeed. Currently no primary prevention efforts have been designed to reduce the occurrence of dual diagnosis subtypes. The concept is too new to have been approached in this way. However, there have been many efforts in the last decade to prevent or reduce alcohol and drug abuse. It seems reasonable to assume that a significant reduction in the prevalence of substance abuse could lead to a reduction in the prevalence of dual diagnosis conditions, an assumption that could turn out to be wrong. At this point, however, it is not possible to evaluate this hypothesis because evidence for the effectiveness of primary substance abuse prevention programs is, at best, mixed and unconvincing (Hawkins & Catalano, 1988). In an attempt to increase the effectiveness of primary substance abuse prevention, some programs are beginning to target "high-risk" groups for specialized early attention (Silverman, 1989). These high-risk groups include children with a mentally ill or substance-abusing parent or children from disruptive families who are beginning to demonstrate some form of behavioral deviance. Such highly targeted groups of children may be especially at risk for developing a dual diagnosis. Until the results of those studies become available, the prevention of dual diagnosis disorders remains a hope, not a reality.

Current Treatment Approaches

What about treatment for dual diagnosis clients systems? Surprisingly little is known about how most effectively to treat individuals and their families with a dual diagnosis (Polcin, 1992). For many historical reasons, treatment systems for the substance abuser and treatment systems for the mentally ill each developed in parallel fashion, largely independent of each other and sometimes in competition (Penick, Nickel, et al., 1990; Ridgely, Goldman, & Willenbring, 1990; Wallace, 1986). As a result, individuals suffering from both kinds of disorder frequently "fell between the cracks" and were often unwelcome in both treatment systems. Many mental health personnel felt and still feel uncomfortable with treating the mentally ill client who also chronically abuses alcohol or other drugs. And many substance abuse personnel felt and still feel uncomfortable with caring for the chronic substance abuser who also suffers from a recognizable mental illness. This unfortunate and totally unnecessary situation has changed slowly in the last 5 years. Nevertheless the effects of the earlier neglect of the dually diagnosed client continues to be evident and probably will be for quite some time. The following example points to this continuing problem:

Case Example 1

Jerry is a 25-year-old biracial man who was diagnosed as having schizophrenia when he was 20. At that time he became very withdrawn, and his personal appearance and self-care abilities deteriorated dramatically. When he became suicidal, his parents had him admitted to a psychiatric hospital. Jerry had used alcohol and cocaine heavily, so the parents assumed that his changed behavior was a result of his alcohol and drug abuse. After detoxification, Jerry was placed on psychotropic medication and received individual psychotherapy. He was released in a month and returned to his college classes and his own apartment. Since that time, Jerry has been hospitalized twice for his mental disorder and has lived periodically with his parents.

He has not been able to work regularly except in a sheltered workshop or to continue his education. Jerry's main goal is to move out of the transitional housing where he lives presently, but he has problems coping with the stresses of daily living, including peer supports and relationships. When he feels pressured, Jerry stops taking his prescribed medication and writes bad checks to obtain money for alcohol and drugs. (He is currently on probation for that reason.) When he uses these substances, his psychiatric symptoms worsen (hallucinations, disorientation, abrasiveness). His family (parents and two older siblings) tries to be supportive, but Jerry interprets their interest as an effort to interfere in his life. Jerry's father is white; his mother is black. They wonder whether some of his problems could be due to internal conflicts about his racial background. It is interesting to note that Jerry has never been in a treatment program for his substance abuse, and when he has been hospitalized because of his psychiatric symptoms, he simply has been detoxed medically without additional interventions for the problem of substance abuse. Nor have family members been involved in treatment sessions, although they often transport Jerry to the hospital and have maintained regular contacts with the hospital staff, including Jerry's multidisciplinary team. The staff in the psychiatric hospital recognize that Jerry abuses substances and that he is frequently noncompliant in taking his psychotropic medication. They are not trained to treat substance abuse or to do family treatment, but they also have not referred him elsewhere for those specialized services.

The neglect of dual diagnosis has resulted in too few treatment facilities, too few trained personnel, and too little knowledge about what does and does not work for the different combinations of mental illness and substance abuse. A number of practitioners recently have shared their thoughts and experiences in treating individuals who have dual diagnoses (Borant, 1992; Evans & Sullivan, 1990; Fariello & Scheidt, 1989; Harrison, Martin, Tuason, & Hoffman, 1985; Hellerstein & Meehan, 1987; Kaufman, 1989; Kofoed, Kania, Walsh, & Atkinson, 1986; Minkoff, 1989). Anecdotal clinical reports such as these form a useful beginning but cannot replace systematic and controlled treatment efficacy trials.

At present there are very few controlled studies of treatment provided to dual diagnosis clients, and those studies often do not agree. For example, there is currently no proof that psychotropic medication is differentially helpful in the rehabilitation—not detoxification—phase of certain dual diagnosis subtypes (Liskow & Goodwin, 1987; Meyer, 1989; Miller, Frances, & Holmes, 1989), although many experienced clinicians recommend psychotropic medications during the rehabilitation phase for certain co-occurring conditions (Gallant, 1986, 1988; Linnoila, 1989; Osher & Kofoed, 1989). Similarly there is no convincing proof that individual counseling or family therapy or social support groups such as Alcoholics Anonymous (AA) are differentially effective in treating dual diagnosis disorders.

One research study suggests that, for certain groups of opiate abusers, brief individual psychotherapy is more effective than drug counseling and methadone maintenance alone. The researchers for that study reported that brief psychotherapy was significantly more useful for drug abuse clients showing moderate levels of psychiatric severity in the recent past than for drug abuse clients showing mild or severe psychiatric severity in the week before entering treatment (McLellan, 1986; Woody, Luborsky, McLellan, & O'Brien, 1986). A group of researchers at Yale University, however, found little benefit from individual psychotherapy for dual diagnosis, opiate abuse subtypes (Rounsaville & Kleber, 1985). Clearly a great deal more work needs to be done in the area of treatment evaluation, particularly evaluations of family-focused services (see Chapters 10 and 11 in this volume).

When the very limited treatment outcome research is examined closely, only one conclusion can be drawn: No one is certain about what kinds of treatment work best for the different kinds of dual diagnosis subtypes. Until more empirical data become available, how should the concerned practitioner proceed to help his or her client? Frances and Allen (1986) wrote:

> Patients who present with substance abuse and psychopathology have a poorer prognosis than those who have a single substance disorder without accompanying psychiatric disorders; however, they respond to treatment better when the multiple problems are addressed in a treatment tailored to their needs. *It is better to cut the shoes to fit the feet rather than the other way around.* (p. 436)

Until proven otherwise, common sense and clinical experience indicate that efforts to help the dual diagnosis client should focus first on the substance abuse itself. Beyond that point, however, there is little agreement about how the practitioner should best proceed. Are psychotropic medications appropriate for the co-occurring mental disorder? If so, how soon after the detoxification phase is completed should they be prescribed? Should the practitioner initiate psychosocial and/or psychoeducational therapies directed toward the co-occurring disorder—such as cognitive therapy for depression or behavior therapy for an anxiety disorder? Is it best to address through family therapy the current and cumulative intergenerational effects of familial distress and dysfunction? Is a focus on the childhood antecedents of the maladaptive adult behaviors useful? Should the therapeutic effort be narrowed to one or two issues that seem to be of critical importance to a particular client, such as uncontrolled aggression, cultural or value conflicts, fears of intimacy, low self-esteem, gender or sexual preference issues, inadequate social skills, or vocational deficits? Is it better to emphasize the networking of group experiences with significant others such as family members and peers rather than one-to-one treatment experiences with a single professional? All of these therapeutic options have been considered and tried. But no one knows for certain which of these treatment options is likely to provide the greatest benefit for particular dual diagnosis clients. No general consensus about treating dually diagnosed clients has emerged from clinicians who routinely try to assist them.

A Comprehensive Family-Focused Approach

We and others usually begin treatment by concentrating efforts on the substance abuse, using all of the conventionally accepted methods for detoxification, crisis management, psychoeducation, family treatment and involvement, and relapse prevention (Osher & Kofoed, 1989; Schuckit, 1989). This comprehensive, ecological approach is based on a theory base that includes a task-centered family systems model, crisis intervention, and cognitive-behavioral strategies. The task-centered strategies involved in this family systems approach can be particularly useful as concrete steps to be taken by various family members whose typical interactions with dually diagnosed individuals involve either "blame-shame" messages or overly protective behaviors. Because most currently active dual diagnosis clients are so medically, psychiatrically, cognitively, and socially dysfunctional when they seek treatment, it has been easier to address all of the complications associated with their disorders in residential or inpatient treatment settings. The typical dual diagnosis client will need more services, more intensively, for longer periods of time than most individuals who suffer from a substance abuse problem alone.

In the case described previously, Jerry would have been appropriate for many of these long-term intensive services. For instance, crisis management could be used to teach him and family members how to cope with his reactions to the stresses of daily living as well as particularly stressful periods. The family systems approach would be useful in identifying boundary conflicts about which of these aspects should be Jerry's responsibility and which ones family members could assist with. Psychoeducation could improve his medication compliance by helping him and family members understand the effects of discontinuing the medication at the points where it could be most useful to him. The dangers of mixing the medication with alcohol and other drugs could be highlighted. This work could be done after or simultaneously with addictions counseling focused on helping him become abstinent and find alternative methods for coping. The work also could help Jerry develop a peer support network by means of a self-help group to replace the supports previously provided by family members, once family sessions are used to help them clarify more appropriate adult-to-adult family relationships with Jerry.

Residential and/or inpatient settings also provide the best opportunity to confirm or reject the presence of an additional mental disorder by allowing the staff opportunities to observe the client closely and to obtain a careful history from family members and others who know the client well (Schuckit, 1989). Because dual diagnosis clients usually have many different problems, a multidisciplinary approach is almost always required. Often the clinical social worker has a key role on such teams in keeping the focus on the multiple factors that may be interacting in each situation. This holistic and ecological perspective also encourages a focus on helping the team identify client and familial strengths. Such a step is critical in the social worker's and team's treatment with the client and his or her family because it is easy to become focused on the mostly dysfunctional aspects of these clients' situations.

It is the rare dually diagnosed client who does not need a variety of services from a variety of professional helpers. Once the acute intoxication-withdrawal phase is completed and the client is physically stable, it has been helpful to devise a highly individual long-term treatment plan that usually will include the following components:

- A strong continuation of the initial psychoeducational thrust focused on the substance abuse problem and the other co-occurring mental disorder(s)
- Systematic involvement of family members and/or other significant people in family treatment sessions and in the psychoeducational process in order to provide them with support, to reduce their tendency to blame, and to facilitate the development of more constructive and useful patterns of social support
- If possible, psychopharmacologic interventions that are designed to directly reduce the risk of substance abuse relapse, such as Antabuse for alcohol abuse or methadone maintenance and naltrexone for opiate abuse
- When appropriate, carefully planned and monitored trials of psychoactive medications to reduce symptomatic distress associated with the co-occurring mental disorders such as chronic psychosis, significant mood disturbance, or a debilitating anxiety disorder that persists well beyond the detoxification phase

- Maximization of all possible social support systems, which can range from day-hospital facilities at one extreme to financial support for the pursuit of an advanced degree on the other
- The availability of supportive contacts over extended periods of time with a knowledgeable and flexible professional who assumes responsibility for coordinating and implementing the treatment plan and modifying it when necessary in order to provide the dually diagnosed client with an important consistency in his or her life that usually has been missing for a long time

The implementation of these components related to the family systems, task-centered approach is illustrated in the following case situation.

Case Example 2

Sylvia is a 38-year-old white female who works as a social worker in an abused women's shelter. She was referred to one of us because she was suffering from feelings of depression and anxiety.

On the PDI-R, Sylvia fulfilled criteria for alcohol abuse, major depression, and generalized anxiety. She stated that she had been drinking about 6-8 or more glasses of wine per day. She had blackouts; she admitted that it was difficult not to drink and that drinking was an important part of her day; she had not missed work because of her drinking and did not consider herself to have a drinking problem; however, she would let things go at home, and friends occasionally suggested that she was drinking excessively. On a few occasions recently, she would start drinking early in the day on Saturday and continue drinking throughout the weekend. She acknowledged that sometimes she felt that she could not get through the day without drinking. She has had no work-related drinking problems, nor has she ever gotten into trouble with the law. Sylvia reported that her drinking increased to the present level about 3 years ago.

Sylvia complained of symptoms of depression occurring over the past year, in which she had a depressed mood with irritability, decreased sleep including intermittent and terminal insomnia, decreased appetite with a weight loss of approximately 8-10 lbs, decreased energy, difficulty getting things done, loss of pleasure, feelings of hopelessness, loss of self-esteem, decreased concentration, thoughts about death and wishes that she were dead, but no suicidal thoughts, plans, or attempts. Sylvia had a severe episode of depression 15 years ago during a period when she was not drinking heavily. At that time she was admitted to a hospital and was treated with electroconvulsive therapy (ECT). She thought that the ECT was effective but wanted a less invasive method of treatment this time.

> Generalized anxiety symptoms are continually present, with feelings of anxiety, tenseness, inability to relax, feeling jittery and jumpy, being easily startled, becoming easily tired, feeling achy from the tension, tightness in her face, increased perspiration, becoming suddenly pale, having an upset stomach, racing heart, trouble breathing, excessive worry, feeling that something terrible is about to happen, difficulty sleeping, feeling on edge, being irritable, and having trouble concentrating. A psychosocial family history indicated that her father was an alcohol abuser and her mother suffered from depression. Her brother abuses alcohol and other drugs.
>
> Sylvia's current family of 10 years involves a lesbian relationship and her partner's two adolescent children, who have created some difficulty in the home recently. She believes that this problem in her family relationships, coupled with a very demanding job in a shelter for abused women, has placed a great deal of stress on her and is responsible for her current depression and anxiety.

Sylvia was referred to a psychiatrist in the clinic. It was agreed that even though she was currently drinking, her past history of depression indicated that she should be given a trial on antidepressant medication. The psychiatrist prescribed Prozac, 20 mg per day. Sylvia's initial response was not very good, in all likelihood because she continued to drink. In a series of psychoeducational therapy sessions, the interaction of alcohol with depression and anxiety was explained to her. As she became more convinced that her drinking was impeding her chances of getting better, she agreed to go to AA. A gay and lesbian AA group was available. She attended and found that she knew two of the members, who lent further support for her decision to stop drinking. After she stopped drinking (with less trouble than she had expected), she continued to have symptoms of depression. It was decided to increase the Prozac to 40 mg per day, and within a few weeks she began to feel considerably better.

Sylvia was seen in individual sessions for diagnosis-specific psychotherapy in which education about the disorder and issues around her problems with her partner were the therapeutic focus (Penick, Read, Lauchland, & Laybourne, 1991). As her depression diminished, many of the problems with her partner also were resolved. Her relationships with the children were not so stormy, and she was able to accept their adolescent behavior with more equanimity and the use of some cognitive behavioral relaxation strategies. Later conjoint family treatment sessions with her partner were set up to work on some of their relationship issues. Homework assignments and specific interrelated tasks were assigned to each to improve family relationships and roles between Sylvia, her partner, and the children. The children were not included in these family sessions because the problems seemed to be ironing themselves out. It was made clear, however, that if the need arose later, total family involvement was available. She also is considering attending an Adult Children Of Alcoholics (ACOA) group to work on some issues regarding her own family of origin that seemed to be affecting her current family relationships.

After she stopped drinking and began to respond to the Prozac, Sylvia's anxiety diminished. In her case, antidepressant medication adequately treated the anxiety. However, such treatment is not always effective. Despite the controversy in this area, we have used anxiolytics such as Librium, Xanax, Klonipin, and even Valium with success. Contrary to common wisdom, cross-tolerance or dependence was not found to be a problem in any but a few cases, which were easily taken care of by stopping the drug.

In Sylvia's case, her problem with alcohol abuse was of fairly short duration, and she was able to modify her drinking behavior with very little difficulty. In people who have much longer periods of abusive drinking or drug use, improvement may not be as quick or as great. Continued substance abuse may negate the efficacy of medication, at which time in-hospital detoxification and treatment may be necessary, as in Jerry's case, to effectively reach the client. What is important is (a) to examine the various facets of the client's functioning, including important family relationships or other social supports, and (b) to attempt to address all areas that are relevant. In Sylvia's case it was possible to use medical (psychiatric) treatment, individual and conjoint or family psychotherapeutic treatment, and community support groups, including AA and possibly ACOA.

CONCLUSION

Does the approach outlined above work? It seems to work for many dual diagnosis clients whom we have treated, but certainly not for all. Maintaining the dually diagnosed client and the active involvement of family members or peers in some kind of treatment program is frustrating and often unsuccessful. Helping professionals need to know much more about this group of people and what is most helpful for them. One thing does appear clear: The profession must keep trying. If conventional treatments do not work with dually diagnosed clients, new approaches that are effective must be sought out and implemented. The combination of substance abuse with a mental disorder results in too much suffering by individuals and their families to be ignored any longer.

REFERENCES

Allen, M. H., & Francis, R. J. (1986). Varieties of psychopathology found in patients with addictive disorders: A review. In R. E. Meyer (Ed.), *Psychopathology and addictive disorders* (pp. 17-38). New York: Guilford.

American Psychiatric Association (APA). (1980). *Diagnostic and statistical manual of mental disorders* (3rd ed.). Washington, DC: Author.

American Psychiatric Association (APA). (1987). *Diagnostic and statistical manual of mental disorders* (3rd ed. rev.). Washington, DC: Author.

Attia, P. R. (1988). Dual diagnosis: Definition and treatment. *Alcoholism Treatment Quarterly, 5,* 53-63.

Beck, A. T., Ward, C. H., Mendelson, M., Mock, J., & Erbaugh, J. (1961). An inventory for measuring depression. *Archives of General Psychiatry, 4,* 561- 571.

Blashfield, R. K. (1984). *The classification of psychopathology.* New York: Plenum.

Borant, D. (1992). Long-term outpatient support groups for dual diagnosis patients. *Substance Abuse, 13,* 21-27.

Caragonne, P., & Emery, B. (1987). *Mental illness and substance abuse: The dually diagnosed client.* National Council of Community Mental Health Centers, 12300 Twinbrook Parkway, Suite 320, Rockville, MD.

Daley, D. C., Moss, H., & Campbell, F. (1987). *Dual disorders: Counseling clients with chemical dependency and mental illness.* Center City, MN: Hazelden.

Derogatis, L. R. (1977). *SCL-90-Revised version.* Baltimore, MD: Johns Hopkins University School of Medicine.

Endicott, J., & Spitzer, R. L. (1978). A diagnostic interview: The Schedule for Affective Disorders and Schizophrenia. *Archives of General Psychiatry, 35,* 837-844.

Endicott, J., & Spitzer, R. L. (1979). Use of the research diagnostic criteria and the Schedule for Affective Disorders and Schizophrenia to study affective disorders. *American Journal of Psychiatry, 136,* 52-56.

Evans, K., & Sullivan, J. M. (1990). *Dual diagnosis: Counseling the mentally ill substance abuser.* New York: Guilford Press.

Exner, J. E., & Clark, B. (1978). The Rorschach. In B. B. Wolman (Ed.), *Clinical diagnosis of mental disorders: A handbook* (pp. 147-178). New York: Plenum.

Fariello, D., & Scheidt, S. (1989). Clinical case management of the dually diagnosed patient. *Hospital and Community Psychiatry, 40,* 1065-1067.

Fowler, R. C., Liskow, B. I., Tanna, V. L., & Van Valkenburg, C. (1977). Psychiatric illness and alcoholism. *Alcoholism: Clinical and Experimental Research, 1,* 125-128.

Frances, R. J., & Allen, M. H. (1986). The interaction of substance-use disorders with nonpsychotic psychiatric disorders. In R. Michels & J. O. Cavenar, Jr. (Eds.), *Psychiatry* (Vol. I, pp. 425-437). New York: Basic Books.

Gallant, D. M. (1986). The use of psychotropic medications in alcoholism. *Substance Abuse, 7,* 35-47.

Gallant, D. M. (1988). Diagnosis and treatment of the depressed alcoholic patient. *Substance Abuse, 9,* 147-156.

Goodwin, D. W. (1981). *Alcoholism: The facts.* New York: Oxford University Press.

Goodwin, D. W. (1986). *Anxiety.* New York: Oxford University Press.

Goodwin, D. W. (1988). *Is alcoholism hereditary?* (2nd ed.). New York: Ballantine.

Goodwin, D. W., & Guze, S. B. (1989). *Psychiatric diagnosis* (4th ed.). New York: Oxford University Press.

Gottesman, I. I., & Shields, J. (1982). *Schizophrenia: The epigenetic puzzle.* Cambridge, UK: Cambridge University Press.

Hamilton, M. (1960). A rating scale for depression. *Journal of Neurology, Neurosurgery and Psychiatry, 23,* 56-61.

Hammer, E. F. (1978). Projective drawings: Two areas of differential diagnostic challenge. In B. B. Wolman (Ed.), *Clinical diagnosis of mental disorders: A handbook* (pp. 281-310). New York: Plenum.

Harrison, P. A., Martin, J. A., Tuason, V. B., & Hoffman, N. G. (1985). Conjoint treatment of dual disorders. In A. I. Alterman (Ed.), *Substance abuse and psychopathology* (pp. 367-390). New York: Plenum.

Hathaway, S. R., & McKinley, J. C. (1943-1982). *Minnesota Multiphasic Personality Inventory.* Minneapolis: University of Minnesota Press.

Hawkins, J. D., & Catalano, R. F. (1988, October). *Risk and protective factors for alcohol and other drug problems in adolescence and early adulthood: Implications for substance abuse prevention.* Paper presented to the First Symposium on the Prevention of Alcohol and Other Drug Problems, Center of Alcohol Studies, Rutgers University, New Brunswick, NJ.

Hellerstein, D. J., & Meehan, B. (1987). Outpatient group therapy for schizophrenic substance abusers. *American Journal of Psychiatry, 144,* 1337-1339.

Helzer, J. E., & Pryzbeck, T. M. (1988). The co-occurrence of alcoholism with other psychiatric disorders in the general population and its impact on treatment. *Journal of Studies on Alcohol, 49,* 219-224.

Hesselbrock, M. N., Meyer, R. E., & Keener, J. (1985). Psychopathology in hospitalized alcoholics. *Archives of General Psychiatry, 42,* 1050-1055.

Holden, C. (1987). Is alcoholism treatment effective? *Science, 236,* 20-22.

Karls, J. M., & Wandrei, K. E. (1992). PIE: A new language for social work. *Social Work, 37,* 80-85.

Kaufman, E. (1989). The psychotherapy of dually diagnosed patients. *Journal of Substance Abuse Treatment, 6,* 9-18.

Kendell, R. E. (1975). *The role of diagnosis in psychiatry.* Oxford, UK: Blackwell Scientific.

Klerman, G. L., Lavori, P. W., Rice, J., Reich, T., Endicott, J., Andreasen, N. C., Keller, M. B., & Hirshfeld, R. M. (1985). Birth cohort trends in rates of major depressive disorder among relatives of patients with affective disorder. *Archives of General Psychiatry, 42,* 689-693.

Kofoed, L., Kania, J., Walsh, T., & Atkinson, R. M. (1986). Outpatient treatment of patients with substance abuse and coexisting psychiatric disorders. *American Journal of Psychiatry, 143,* 867-872.

Lehman, A. F., Myers, C. P., & Corty, E. (1989). Assessment and classification of patients with psychiatric and substance abuse syndromes. *Hospital and Community Psychiatry, 40,* 1019-1025.

Linnoila, M. I. (1989). Anxiety and alcoholism. *Journal of Clinical Psychiatry, 50,* 26-27.

Liskow, B. I., & Goodwin, D. W. (1987). Pharmacological treatment of alcohol intoxication, withdrawal and dependence: A critical review. *Journal of Studies on Alcohol, 48,* 356-370.

McLellan, A. T. (1986). "Psychiatric severity" as a predictor of outcome from substance abuse treatments. In R. E. Meyer (Ed.), *Psychopathology and addictive disorders* (pp. 97-139). New York: Guilford.

Meyer, R. E. (1989). Prospects for a rational pharmacotherapy of alcoholism. *Journal of Clinical Psychiatry, 50,* 403-412.

Miller, S. I., Frances, R. J., & Holmes, D. J. (1989). Psychotropic medications. In R. K. Hester & W. R. Miller (Eds.), *Handbook of alcoholism treatment approaches* (pp. 231-241). New York: Pergamon.

Miller, W. R., & Hester, R. K. (1986). Matching problem drinkers with optimal treatments. In W. R. Miller & N. Heather (Eds.), *Treating addictive behaviors* (pp. 175-203). New York: Plenum.

Minkoff, K. (1989). An integrated treatment model for dual diagnosis of psychosis and addiction. *Hospital and Community Psychiatry, 40,* 1031-1036.

Mirowsky, J., & Ross, C. E. (1989). Psychiatric diagnosis as reified measurement. *Journal of Health and Social Behavior, 30,* 11-25.

National Institute on Alcohol Abuse and Alcoholism (NIAAA). (1983). *Report to the U.S. Congress on alcohol and health.* Washington, DC: Government Printing Office.

National Institute on Alcohol Abuse and Alcoholism (NIAAA). (1987). *Report to the U.S. Congress on alcohol and health.* Washington, DC: Government Printing Office.

Osher, F. C., & Kofoed, L. L. (1989). Treatment of patients with psychiatric and psychoactive substance abuse disorders. *Hospital and Community Psychiatry, 40,* 1025-1030.

Othmer, E., & Othmer, S. C. (1989). *The clinical interview using DSM-III-R.* Washington, DC: American Psychiatric Press.

Othmer, E., Penick, E. C., Powell, B. J., Read, M. R., & Othmer, S. C. (1989). *The Psychiatric Diagnostic Interview—Revised (PDI-R).* Los Angeles: Western Psychological Services.

Overall, J. E., & Gorham, D. R. (1962). The Brief Psychiatric Rating Scale. *Psychological Reports, 10,* 799-812.

Penick, E. C., Nickel, E. J., Cantrell, P. F., Powell, B. J., Read, M. R., & Thomas, H. M. (1990). The emerging concept of dual diagnosis: An overview and implications. In D. F. O'Connell (Ed.), *Managing the dually diagnosed patient: Current issues and clinical approaches* (pp. 1-54). New York: Haworth.

Penick, E. C., Powell, B. J., Othmer, E., Bingham, S. F., Rice, A. S., & Liese, B. S. (1984). Subtyping alcoholics by coexisting psychiatric syndromes: Course, family history, outcome. In D. W. Goodwin, K. T. VanDusen, & S. A. Mednick (Eds.), *Longitudinal research in alcoholism* (pp. 167-196). Boston: Kluwer-Nijhoff.

Penick, E. C., Read, M. R., Lauchland, J. S., & Laybourne, P. C. (1991). Diagnosis specific psychotherapy. In B. D. Beitman & G. L. Klerman (Eds.), *Integrating pharmacotherapy and psychotherapy* (pp. 45-68). Washington DC: American Psychiatric Press.

Polcin, D. L. (1992). Issues in the treatment of dual diagnosis clients who have chronic mental illness. *Professional Psychology: Research and Practice, 23,* 30-37.

Popper, K. (1962). *Conjectures and refutations.* New York: Basic Books.

Powell, B. J., Penick, E. C., Othmer, E., Bingham, S. F., & Rice, A. S. (1983). Prevalence of additional psychiatric syndromes among male alcoholics. *Journal of Clinical Psychiatry, 43,* 404-407.

Read, M. R., Penick, E. C., Powell, B. J., Nickel, E. J., Bingham, S. F., & Campbell, J. (1990). Subtyping male alcoholics by family history of alcohol abuse and co-occurring psychiatric disorders: A bi-dimensional model. *British Journal of Addiction, 85,* 367-378.

Regier, D. A., Farmer, M. E., & Rae, D. S. (1990). Co-morbidity of mental disorders with alcohol and other drug abuse: Results from the Epidemiologic Catchment Area (ECA) study. *Journal of the American Medical Association, 264,* 2511-2518.

Reich, T., Cloninger, R., Van Eerdewegh, P., Rice, J. P., & Mullaney, J. (1988). Secular trends in the familial transmission of alcoholism. *Alcoholism: Clinical and Experimental Research, 12,* 458-464.

Ridgely, M. S., Goldman, H. H., & Willenbring, M. (1990). Barriers to the care of persons with dial diagnoses: Organizational and financing issues. *Schizophrenia Bulletin, 16,* 123-132.

Robins, L. N., Helzer, J. E., Croughan, J., & Radcliff, K. S. (1981). National Institute of Mental Health Diagnostic Interview Schedule: Its history, characteristics and validity. *Archives of General Psychiatry, 39,* 381-389.

Ross, H. E., Glaser, F. B., & Germanson, T. (1988). The prevalence of psychiatric disorders in patients with alcohol and other drug problems. *Archives of General Psychiatry, 45,* 1023-1031.

Rounsaville, B. J., & Kleber, H. D. (1985). Psychotherapy/counseling for opiate addicts: Strategies for use in different treatment settings. *International Journal of the Addictions, 20,* 869-896.

Rounsaville, B. J., Weissman, M. M., Kleber, H. D., & Wilber, C. (1982). Heterogeneity of psychiatric diagnosis in treated opiate addicts. *Archives of General Psychiatry, 39,* 161-166.

Schuckit, M. A. (1985). The clinical implications of primary diagnostic groups among alcoholics. *Archives of General Psychiatry, 42,* 1043-1049.

Schuckit, M. A. (1986). Genetic and clinical implications of alcoholism and affective disorder. *American Journal of Psychiatry, 143,* 140-147.

Schuckit, M. A. (1989). *Drug and alcohol abuse: A clinical guide to diagnosis and treatment* (3rd ed.) New York: Plenum.

Schuckit, M. A., Irwin, M., Howard, T., & Smith, T. (1988). A structured diagnostic interview for identification of primary alcoholism: A preliminary evaluation. *Journal of Studies on Alcohol, 49,* 93-99.

Schuckit, M. A., & Monteiro, M. G. (1988). Alcoholism, anxiety and depression. *British Journal of Addiction, 83,* 1373-1380.

Selzer, M. L. (1971). The Michigan Alcoholism Screening Test: The quest for a new diagnostic instrument. *American Journal of Psychiatry, 127,* 89-94.

Shapiro, S., Skinner, E. A., Kessler, L. G., Von Korff, M., German, P. S., Tishler, G. L., Leaf, P. J., Benham, L., Cottler, L., & Reiger, D. A. (1984). Utilization of health and mental health services. *Archives of General Psychiatry, 41,* 971-982.

Silverman, M. (1989). Children of psychiatrically ill parents: A prevention perspective. *Hospital and Community Psychiatry, 40,* 1257-1265.

Spitzer, R. L., Endicott, J., & Robins, E. (1978). Research diagnostic criteria: Rationale and reliability. *Archives of General Psychiatry, 35,* 773-782.

Spitzer, R. L., & Klein, D. F. (1978). *Critical issues in psychiatric diagnosis.* New York: Raven.

Spitzer, R. L., Skodol, A. E., Williams, J. B. W., Gibbon, M., & Kass, F. (1982). Supervising intake diagnosis: A psychiatric "Rashomon." *Archives of General Psychiatry, 39,* 1299-1305.

Spitzer, R. L., Williams, J. B. W., Gibbon, M., & First, M. B. (1988). *Structured Clinical Interview for DSM-III-R (SCID).* Biometrics Research Department, New York State Psychiatric Institute, 722 West 168th Street, New York, NY 10032.

Tarter, R. E., Alterman, A. I., & Edwards, K. L. (1985). Vulnerability to alcoholism in men: A behavior-genetic perspective. *Journal of Studies on Alcohol, 46,* 329-356.

Vaillant, G. E. (1983). *The natural history of alcoholism.* Cambridge, MA: Harvard University Press.

Wallace, J. (1986). The other problems of alcoholics. *Journal of Substance Abuse Treatment, 3,* 163-169.

Williams, J. B. W., & Spitzer, R. L. (1980). NIMH-sponsored field trial: Interrater reliability. In American Psychiatric Association, *Diagnostic and statistical manual of mental disorders* (3rd ed., pp. 467-469). Washington, DC: American Psychiatric Association.

Williams, J. B. W., & Spitzer, R. L. (1982). Research diagnostic criteria and DSM-III: An annotated comparison. *Archives of General Psychiatry, 39,* 1283-1289.

Woody, G. E., Luborsky, L., McLellan, A. T., & O'Brien, C. P. (1986). Psychotherapy as an adjunct to methadone treatment. In R. E. Meyer (Ed.), *Psychopathology and addictive disorders* (pp. 169-195). New York: Guilford.

Zucker, R. A. (1987). The four alcoholisms: A developmental account of the etiological process. In P. C. Rivers (Ed.), *Alcohol and addictive behavior* (pp. 27-83). (Nebraska Symposium on Motivation). Lincoln: University of Nebraska Press.

Chapter 7

THE IMPACT OF SUBSTANCE ABUSE AND POST-TRAUMATIC STRESS DISORDER

ROBERT FAHNESTOCK

Alcohol and other substance abuse is a problem of profound significance in our society. No single group is immune to the development of addiction, and some seem to be more at risk statistically than others. One such group is victims, or survivors, of traumatic events.

One of the largest groups of persons exposed to trauma who have been studied systematically are veterans of the Vietnam War. Many veterans have relied on alcohol and/or other drugs to deal with the aftermath of a unique war experience. Briggs (1984) found that the amount of alcohol consumption differentiated combat from noncombat veterans in his study. Several authors (Brancey, David, & Leiber, 1984; LaCoursiere, Godfrey, & Ruby, 1980; Wilson, 1980) reported that veterans use alcohol and/or drugs to combat anxiety, depression, and insomnia. Many veterans use substances for what has been termed *psychic numbing,* referring to the blocking or numbing of troublesome memories and emotions. Substance abuse is probably the most common factor complicating the diagnosis of post-traumatic stress disorder (PTSD) (J. Newman, 1987).

Egendorf, Kadushin, Laufer, Rothbart, and Sloan (1981) indicated in their report to Congress that exposure to combat led to an increased incidence of substance abuse in Vietnam veterans. Brancey et al. (1984) cited studies confirming that nearly a third of the Vietnam veterans surveyed had problems related to excessive drinking. Nace, O'Brien, Mintz, Ream, and Myers (1977) observed that 39% of the soldiers in their study had developed at least one alcohol-related problem and that 16% could be diagnosed as alcoholic. The Centers for Disease Control (CDC) (1987), in a random cohort study, found all-cause mortality rates to be 45% higher in Vietnam veterans than in their control group; specifically, rates of suicide, homicide, and accidental poisonings from drugs were significantly elevated.

Approximately one-third of the veterans seeking help through the nationwide Vet Center system experience substance abuse problems. Substance abuse exacerbates PTSD (Helzer, 1984). Combat veterans and other trauma survivors use substances to avoid temporarily the full impact of the emotional and cognitive aspects of previous traumatic events that are reexperienced as intrusive thoughts, memories, and, in some cases, flashbacks. This substance-enhanced avoidance delays integration of the person's experiences into a self-in-the-world view that is necessary for trauma resolution and recovery from PTSD. The consequences of the combination of PTSD and addiction can be tragic. The well-known symptoms of addiction become compounded by the symptoms of PTSD. The relationship between the two disorders is synergistic: Each complicates and exacerbates the other.

Substance abuse, when combined with PTSD, affects individuals in all aspects of their lives. For instance, *employment difficulties* include absenteeism from work, poor performance, strained work relationships, being out of step with nontraumatized peers, and secondary traumatization through the stresses of the workplace (Schnaier, 1986). *Social effects* include separation and divorce, emotionally traumatized children, alienation from significant relationships, lack of supportive relationships, insensitivity to the needs of others, and avoidance (Briggs, 1984; Brown, 1984). *Emotional effects* can involve hostility, coldness, lack of intimacy, hypervigilance, poor self-esteem, numbness, anger, resentment, and bitterness (Kormos, 1978; McCormick, 1988). In terms of *physical effects,* increased pulse rate, blood pressure, and sleep disturbance complicate the other well-known physical effects of substance abuse (Boscarino, 1981).

Those individuals with combined substance abuse problems and PTSD present a unique set of difficulties for social workers and other helping professionals. For example, McCormick (1988) pointed out a dangerous proclivity on the part of practitioners to place less emphasis on the substance-abusing behavior than appropriate, with many believing that those behaviors will diminish as a function of treating the PTSD.

In light of the seriousness of the problem of PTSD and substance abuse (co-morbidity) and the need for helping professionals to become more knowledgeable about it, this chapter traces the development of addiction in the Vietnam veteran population. It also offers an overview of the Vietnam War experience, including the etiology and effects of PTSD, and it discusses the application of practitioner roles and an ecological perspective to the task of working with this population.

THE PROCESS OF ADDICTION

In studying the development of addictions in Vietnam veterans, three groups emerge: those whose abuse began (a) prior to, (b) during, or (c) subsequent to service in Vietnam. It is estimated that 60%-70% of those veterans with PTSD also abuse alcohol and/or other drugs. Those other drugs include marijuana, opium, morphine, heroin, cocaine, and amphetamines.

Similarities exist in all three groups. For example, the theoretical basis for understanding the process of addiction can be applied equally to all three groups. In addition members of each group use substances to alter feeling states and to cope with life stressors, including stress secondary to trauma. Eventually all three groups develop the addictive life-style of abuse, followed by numerous problems and further abuse. Although these similarities exist, an awareness of differences between the groups can be equally as useful in the helping process.

For instance, veterans with a pretrauma history of substance abuse often have a pervasive life-space involvement with the substance and more pronounced substance-seeking behaviors than veterans in the other two groups. Another difference for the first group is that the abuse of substances is associated less frequently with self-medication than with groups (b) and (c). Moreover, it is reasonable to assume that a number of the veterans in the latter two categories might not have encountered substance abuse difficulties had they not served in Vietnam.

For veterans who were addicted before serving in Vietnam and for those introduced to alcohol and/or other drugs in that environment, substances were obtained easily, providing a sanctuary from stresses perceived to be otherwise unmanageable. Boettcher (1985) believed that availability alone induced many to abuse substances: "Marijuana cigarettes cost only ten cents apiece in Saigon; opium sold for a dollar per injection, morphine for five dollars per vial; a heroin habit could be supported for as little as two dollars per day" (p. 402).

Citing Defense Department studies, Boettcher (1985) noted that 25% of soldiers in 1968 used marijuana and that by 1969-1970 almost 50% were using the drug at least occasionally. Starr (1973) reported that 10%-15% of Americans used heroin in Vietnam. According to Zinberg (1972) 68% of the users of this drug were white, and over 90% of all heroin users gave up the drug on their return to the United States.

Alcohol was widely available in rear areas—base camps, staging areas, rest areas, and larger installations. My military experience demonstrated that, until the mid-1970s, alcohol use was condoned, if not enabled, by the military. Free alcohol, typically in the form of beer, was used to reward performance and to provide relief from stress. Alcohol was not, however, routinely available "in the bush," on patrols, or during missions.

Combatants rarely used psychoactive drugs or alcohol during combat. Rather it was during periods prior to hostile action or during periods of "stand down" following an engagement that substances were used by those in groups (a) and (b).

Substance Abuse Prior to Vietnam

The most accurate predictor of drinking and drug abuse problems subsequent to Vietnam service is a history of substance abuse prior to military service (Helzer, 1984). Individuals in this group typically began use during high school or earlier, learning to associate substance abuse with relaxation, peer acceptance, and pseudomaturity. Helzer (1984) found that preservice substance abuse was a predictor of assignment to combat. The reasons for this relationship remain unclear: On the one hand, it can be assumed that the use of substances during school years negatively affects good grades, test-taking performance, and motivation; on the other hand, possession of these qualities *is* necessary for selection into service schools and assignment to other than infantry occupation specialties. Veterans with prior substance abuse histories usually found no difficulty in acquiring substances. Therefore many chose to rely on use as a coping skill for relieving the stresses of military life in general and of Vietnam specifically.

Substance Abuse Beginning in Vietnam

Helzer, Robins, and Davis (1975) found that 92% of their study group of Army enlisted men had tried alcohol at least once while in Vietnam. Reports of widespread use lead to the assumption that there were few convincing sanctions against using substances to relieve tension and anxiety. Helzer (1984) found among veterans with no preservice drinking problem that 21% of noncombatants and 31% of combatants reported drinking problems or alcoholism following discharge. Similarly Boscarino (1981) found that Vietnam veterans developed a level of problem drinking not found among comparable veterans in other wars.

It is assumed that the combined factors of availability, constant tension, stress, and anxiety for which prior forms of coping were inadequate provided the catalyst for beginning and continuing abuse during and after Vietnam. Further, reinforcement in the form of substance abuse among peers in combat and in society at large was another contributing factor.

Substance Abuse Beginning After Vietnam

The smallest of the three groups of substance abusers includes veterans who managed to avoid all alcohol and drug abuse prior to or during Vietnam, only to develop later a pattern of abuse (Helzer et al., 1975). Many in this group used substances without problems during Vietnam and only later experienced substance abuse difficulties. The pattern of development of use for this group of veterans is probably similar to the group whose heavy use began in Vietnam. The major difference is that the aftermath of Vietnam became the catalyst for addictive behavior rather than the real-time stressors of combat; substance abuse in those situations was directly related to, and a symptom of, PTSD.

Underlying Theory of the Addiction Process

One useful theoretical perspective for understanding addictions in veterans who became addicted prior to, during, and after Vietnam service is the cognitive-affective-pharmacological (CAP) control theory, although other theories are also relevant. According to McCormick (1988):

> The CAP control theory of drug abuse postulates that substance abuse results from conflicts over which an individual has little or no control (cognitive component). The conflict results in anxiety (affective component) which the abuser "treats" with drugs (pharmalogical component). The use of drugs impairs the abuser's ability to learn new coping responses and drugs then become the only way to experience relief from anxiety. (p. 1312)

Responses to stress tend to become more uncomfortable as the imbalance increases between the demands on the person and his or her response capacity. As perceived stress builds, the individual responds with coping strategies such as substance abuse that may seem to work initially but that do not resolve the stress. Stress and anxiety are increased rather than decreased as the discrepancy between demands and capacity increases. This pattern of coping by using substances in response to the stress gradually becomes a problem in itself as the addiction develops.

PTSD AND ADDICTION

Characteristics of the PTSD Syndrome

PTSD is not a sign of insanity or a personality deficiency, but rather is a normal reaction to an abnormal amount of stress (Matsakis, 1989). The disorder is included in the *DSM-III-R* (American Psychiatric Association [APA], 1987) under the general heading of anxiety disorders. Steps in the development of PTSD include the following:

1. There is a history of a significant stressor (defined as an event that is outside the range of usual human experience and one that would be markedly distressing to almost anyone).
2. The traumatic event is persistently reexperienced in an intrusive manner.
3. Response takes the form of psychological numbing or reduced involvement with the external environment.
4. Stimuli associated with the event are persistently avoided.
5. Indices of increased autonomic arousal are present.
6. The duration of the symptoms exceeds 1 month.

Events recognized as significant stressors range from poverty and deprivation (Erickson, 1976), through survival of natural and human-made disasters (Blaufarb & Levine, 1972), incest (Eth & Pynoos, 1985), physical abuse (Carmen, Reicker, & Mills, 1984), and combat (Goodwin, 1987).

The symptoms observed can vary. They involve:

Reexperiencing (intrusive and unwanted thoughts or recollections of the event, recurrent dreams, and reactions to environmental reminders of the event)

Numbing or reduced involvement (marked diminished interest in one or more significant activities, feelings of detachment or estrangement from others, and constricted affect)

Hypervigilance (hyperalertness or exaggerated startle response, sleep disturbance, and memory impairment or trouble concentrating) (APA, 1987; Langley, 1982)

Estimates of the incidence of PTSD vary. Kulka et al. (1988), in their report to Congress, found that 15% of their study participants showed symptoms of PTSD (N = 8,000). Card (1983, 1987) reported that 15% of her study sample had experienced PTSD (N = 599). Ewalt (1981) cited VA hospital data showing that a slightly higher percentage of Vietnam veterans (20%) experience severe adjustment problems. Noy (1978), who studied soldiers involved in the 1973 Arab-Israeli war (one with conditions similar to Vietnam), reported 30% of those veterans are symptomatic of PTSD. Although findings differ, most authorities agree that the incidence of PTSD is strongly correlated with the intensity of combat or trauma and that the intrapsychic impact of trauma on the survivor is a highly subjective and individual phenomenon.

The Interrelationship Between Symptoms of PTSD and Addictions

The combination of immutable fear, youth, lack of identified battle lines, absence of sanctioning by the nation, lingering questions about why they were fighting, a less than heroic homecoming, rapid removal from combat and reintegration without being debriefed, and being perceived as losers all acted to facilitate development of PTSD in the Vietnam veteran. Consequently these survivors often experience guilt, depression, social alienation, irritability and elevated stress levels, nightmares, aggression or fear of aggression, exaggerated startle responses, and some report flashbacks (Langley, 1982). These symptoms or feelings, in turn, can result in employment difficulties, marital discord, mistrust and suspicion, estrangement from others, isolation, suicidal behavior, and substance abuse.

Some well-known symptoms of addiction to substances are lost time at work, drinking or drugging beyond one's intent, legal difficulties, guilt, depression, physical and psychological dependence, deleterious impact of significant others, and financial difficulties. PTSD and addictions share affective and cognitive symptoms. For example, a PTSD sufferer may drink or abuse drugs to assuage unwanted thoughts of a trauma, to lower the startle response threshold, to induce sleep, and to medicate feelings.

The following quote from LaCoursiere et al. (1980) illustrates this interplay between symptoms: "Thus, what can begin as innocent self-medication for symptoms of traumatic neurosis can lead to a vicious circle. Repetitive symptom reduction by means of alcohol leads to tolerance and an increase in alcohol consumption to maintain symptom reduction, which leads to problems from the alcohol use itself" (p. 966). Abuse of alcohol and drugs, with a known cluster of symptoms, is often an observed coping behavior in those with PTSD. Use of substances can provide temporary relief of PTSD symptoms, but it is ineffective in the long-term resolution of the condition. In addition, some unique aspects of the Vietnam war experience caused this interaction of PTSD and addiction symptoms in veterans to be more significant than in previous wars.

UNIQUE FACTORS IN THE VIETNAM WAR EXPERIENCE

The Vietnam war experience was different in many respects from any other war experience in American history. Vietnam was the first war in memory about which widely publicized opposition was voiced, creating doubt about the wisdom of the war and the veracity of the nation's leaders. The social climate of the times allowed and encouraged open nonviolent confrontation of authority. Haymen, Sommers-Flanagan, and Parsons (1987) pointed out that all wars are stressful for combatants but that certain characteristics of the Vietnam War made it even more stressful.

Characteristics of the Vietnam Combatants

The average age of combatants in Vietnam was 19.1; in Korea, 24; and in World War II, 26.3 (Jurich, 1983). While their peers at home engaged in the normal developmental tasks of late adolescence, the combatants in Vietnam were engaged in the difficult task of survival. Vietnam was the longest war in this country's history, spanning 9 years. As Ewalt (1981) pointed out, there were no stable combat units as in previous wars. A combatant typically went to the war zone alone by commercial jet and returned in the same manner—alone. Some important differences between Vietnam combatants and those in World War II are summarized in Table 7.1.

Table 7.1
Some Important Differences Between
Vietnam Combatants and Those in World War II

	Vietnam	*World War II*
Average age of combatant	19.1	26.3
Length of war	9 years	5 years
Identity of enemy	Extremely difficult	Not difficult
Gender of enemy	Men/Women/Children	Men
To combat zone	Alone	In large groups
From combat zone	Alone	In large groups
Type of warfare	Guerrilla	Conventional
Available alcohol/drugs	Yes	Rare
Public support	Ambivalent to negative	Wide public support
Public sanction	Undeclared war	Declared war
Debrief period	No	Yes
DEROS (Estimated date of rotation)	Yes	No
Homecoming	Ambivalent to negative	Positive (Hero)

Differences in the War Experience

World War II has been conceptualized as a conventional war fought by conventional methods. Vietnam was a guerrilla war, and this experience sets the Vietnam veteran apart. Brown (1984) offered the following cogent description of that war: "The unpredictable nature of guerrilla warfare, which challenged the soldiers' ideologies of right and wrong, posed an especially constant and life-threatening stress" (p. 373).

The process of identifying the enemy was dangerous and uncertain. The enemy was rarely observable by uniform as in previous wars; moreover, it was not uncommon to find women and children as combatants (Haley, 1978). The introduction of the "search and destroy" mission, the establishment of "free-fire zones," and the taking of territorial objectives to be hastily abandoned changed the face of war into one of uncertainty. Unpredictable danger was broken by periods of inactivity and boredom. A combatant seldom knew precisely when or where danger would appear, what form the danger would take, and from whom the danger would come.

Lessons poorly learned in former wars produced the concept of *date of estimated return from overseas* (DEROS) during the Vietnam War.

It was anticipated that a known departure date from the combat zone would reduce the level of stress experienced by limiting the length of time of susceptibility. Kormos (1978) and others concluded that unit morale is one of the most important protections against emotional breakdown available to the soldier, while, conversely, low unit morale adds to stress. Accordingly, under DEROS, as Goodwin (1987) suggested, unit esprit de corps was slashed as "new guys" were constantly appearing and seasoned soldiers were being rotated out at approximately the time when they had achieved proficiency.

The legitimacy of the war was questioned both at home and in Vietnam. The question of legitimacy removed from the minds of Vietnam veterans the sense of purpose, honor, and "glory" that is assumed necessary for sanction of one's aggressive acts. The absence of a sense of purpose stood out. Blank (1982), a psychiatrist who served in Vietnam, observed while in that country a sense of purposelessness in some veterans that was still evident in 1980, years after the end of America's involvement. A 1980 Lou Harris study (Harris, 1980) showed as many as 47% of Vietnam veterans thought the United States should not have entered the war. Similarly Egendorf et al. (1981) found that only 43.6% of Vietnam veterans were supportive of the war.

Racial and Gender Factors in the War

Another unique aspect of the Vietnam War was the disproportionate numbers of black Americans who served there and the type of stress they experienced. Black Americans served in Vietnam in large numbers, accounting for one-ninth of American forces in Vietnam yet constituting one-fifth of combat troops (Boettcher, 1985). Further, blacks accounted for 12.5% of all American combat deaths (Allen, 1986).

To black Americans the Vietnamese, like themselves, were people of color. Parson (1985b) believed that serving in Vietnam was particularly traumatic for black veterans who were impacted by negative stereotypes about the Vietnamese ("gook"-identification). Parson (1985a) explained this vulnerability as due to a unique type of stress that, by inference, possibly could increase vulnerability of black veterans to substances:

> Impacted stress refers to the assumption that, added to the stress of the theatre of war, many Black soldiers brought with them "cumulated stress" from psychic and social origins, related to exclusion, poverty, and cultural

> pan-suspiciousness. "Gook"-identification refers to the conscious and unconscious emotional identification with the devalued, maligned, and abused Vietnamese. (p. 175)

Estimates of the number of women who served in Vietnam range from 7,500 to 9,000 (Connelly, 1987); however, as Van Devanter (1985) pointed out, no one really knows how many women served there. It is estimated that a total of 260,000 women served in the military during the Vietnam era (Schnaier, 1986).

The incidence rate of PTSD in women equals that of men. Ironically women are unique in one regard: They are less likely than men to talk about their Vietnam experiences, and, perhaps as a consequence, their needs have been largely ignored. Schnaier (1986) reported that only 48% of female veterans have ever sought professional help for mental health problems, and for those who have sought help, only 42.9% discussed Vietnam issues. Like their male counterparts, many women who served in Vietnam continue to suffer and may turn to substances for relief.

The Vietnam Veterans' Homecoming

A final unique aspect of the Vietnam War was the lack of support at home, which made for a less than heroic homecoming experience for the vast majority of Vietnam veterans. That experience represented a key element in the "second injury" associated with blaming the victim. Fox and Scherl (1972) found that an important influence on the veterans' readjustment was the reluctance of families to listen to war stories. Hendin and Pollinger (1984) agreed: "Over and over veterans have told us that their families, including WWII veteran fathers, were too uncomfortable to listen if they talked of Vietnam" (p. 234).

EXPLANATORY THEORIES OF PTSD

In terms of PTSD, no single psychodynamic approach has surfaced that fully explains the disorder (Fairbank & Nicholson, 1982), and certainly no approach, including the CAP theory mentioned in the previous section, addresses all of the issues involved in the interplay between PTSD and substance abuse. On the other hand, a number of complementary approaches have proven to be useful. These approaches include psychoanalytic, cognitive, self-in-the-world, and developmental theories.

Past Conceptualizations of PTSD

Bleich, Garb, and Kottler (1986) pointed out that Freud, in working with World War I soldiers, observed the dynamic conflict between abreaction and repression, the fundamental shaping core of post-traumatic stress reactions. Briefly, according to psychoanalytic theory, a person who undergoes a traumatic experience feels the need to integrate the threatening event leading to a corrective experience. Because the event is in the past, he or she can only struggle with memories of events, necessitating a reexperiencing of the event through thoughts, images, and dreams. But the mental pain involved in replication of the trauma encourages the individual to repress the event rather than integrate and accept it.

Learned helplessness, or cognitive theory, offers an alternative view of how individuals cope with trauma such as combat experiences. According to Wilson (1980), learned helplessness occurs when a person is exposed to an environment in which there are aversive consequences of an uncontrollable and unpredictable nature. The person-in-situation outcome is a reduced motivation for attempting change or resolution. The person has learned that efforts in the past were ineffective, so he or she can only respond to, but not attempt to change, the situation.

Alternatively Janoff-Bulman (1985) proposed a self-in-the-world theory to explain PTSD as due largely to the shattering of three basic assumptions that victims or survivors hold about themselves and the world. These assumptions are (a) a belief in personal invulnerability, (b) a perception of the world as meaningful and comprehensible, and (c) a perception of the self as positive. Combat and other examples of trauma refute these assumptions, shattering the person's concept of self and view of the world.

Developmental theories also have been used to explain reactions to traumatic experiences. Wilson (1980) drew from Erickson's (1956) work to point out that the fifth phase of development (late adolescence) is interrupted in combat veterans. Newman and Newman (1984) explained that the individual's self-concept is crystallized during this stage. In the ideal situation, the congealing that takes place includes in that stage the review of childhood skills, goals, and values. Assuming that the tasks of the stage are mastered, the individual moves on and then is able to undergo extreme stress as an adult while managing to preserve a sense of personal motives and goals. When these developmental goals are not mastered, one possible result is a loss of the sense of self. Practice experiences indicate that a loss of self is often exemplified by comments such as "I don't know who I am anymore" and "I can't get myself together." An integration of this perspective and that of Janoff-Bulman (1985) above indicates that PTSD occurs in addicted veterans when development is already delayed by addiction and the trauma is of sufficient magnitude that the perception of invulnerability, the world as meaningful, and the positive self are dislodged.

A Proposed Conceptualization of PTSD

The developmental theoretical assumptions provide the most cogent explanation of how PTSD develops in relation to substance abuse. The resultant feelings of helplessness and impotency in affecting the environment lead to learned helplessness and abandonment of the task of integrating the traumatic stress that is being experienced.

Figure 7.1 illustrates how a trauma is cognitively filtered through a lens (one's view of the world and self) together with predisposing factors (or their absence). This process can result in the shattering of assumptions about invulnerability, the world as a "just" place, and the positive self. The trauma is then continuously reexperienced. The sufferer copes to the extent of his or her capacity and either suffers from or is rewarded by the consequences present in the environment, including addiction and the enabling behaviors of others. The goal of treatment, to be discussed in the next two sections, seeks to assist the survivor in integrating memories and experiences by improving coping effectiveness and by reducing negative environmental consequences. Improving the individual's coping patterns may consist of the elimination of the substance abuse and other ineffective modes and an increase in alternative ways of coping. Treatment should focus also on those family system factors that have been negatively affected by the combined addiction and PTSD or that have helped maintain the two conditions.

A FAMILY SYSTEMS FRAMEWORK FOR TREATMENT

Jelinek (1987) indicated that individual and group therapies usually operate from the premise that change begins within the individual. In working with Vietnam veterans and trauma survivors, it is vital that the clinician look beyond the individual to life events and the context of the family system when family ties exist or can be initiated. External

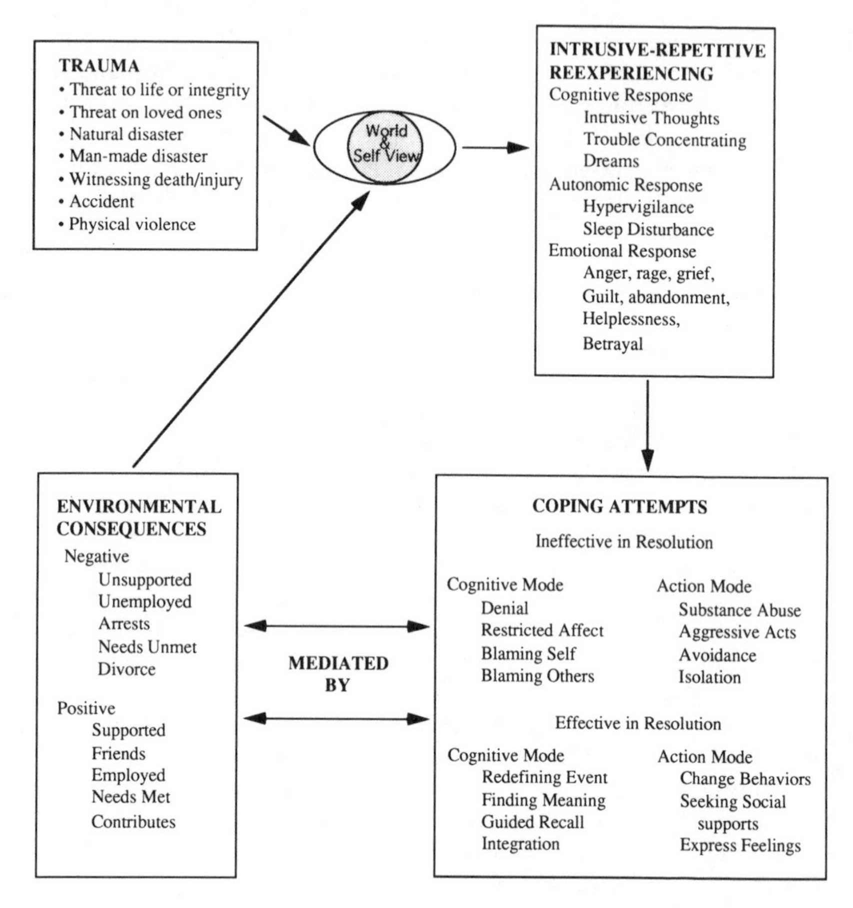

Figure 7.1. Conceptual Model of Post-Traumatic Stress Disorder

events are central and should be assessed in terms of the individual's current difficulties (Jelinek, 1987). The family can provide the context and support for the healing that must take place within the individual and between the family members. Change, however, must begin within the individual even though other forces may have contributed to or been affected by the perceived stress (Egendorf, 1985). In addition to external events and family relationships, the quality of the client-practitioner relationship is critical. The client must be confident that the social worker or other helping professional is genuine, can understand and accept him or her, and, as indicated by Blank (1982), has the unflinching ability to listen to, confront, evoke, and contain memories of trauma experiences. There must exist in the helper an ability and willingness to use self-disclosure by sharing of him- or herself sufficiently so that existing commonalities between worker and client become apparent. These and other factors are an integral part of this family systems framework of treatment, including addressing barriers to treatment, the need to build on strengths, and the creation of a "safe" environment for veterans and their families.

Addressing Barriers to Recovery

Barriers to recovery from addiction that should be addressed include chronicity, physical dependence, ignorance of the disease process, social isolation, denial, poverty and deprivation, inaccessibility to helping resources, stereotyping and second injury, coexisting disorders and psychiatric illness, and poor follow-up and aftercare. Related barriers to recovery from PTSD include lack of awareness of the disorder, exaggerated masculinity, substance abuse, coexisting psychiatric illnesses, blaming the victim, limitations and negative preconceptions of clinicians, anger and resentment against the government (the primary helping resource for veterans is the Department of Veterans Affairs), and budgetary constraints inhibiting outreach and expansion of services.

Practical experience demonstrates that it is useful to share with the client the nature of impediments to recovery and to include strategies to anticipate and counteract such barriers within the treatment contract. Some of the major barriers identified above are elaborated in the next sections.

Exaggerated Masculinity. One impediment to recovery has roots in antiquity, and is called the "John Wayne syndrome." The syndrome is a result of important differences in male and female socialization. Males are taught early in life to be more restrictive of emotions than females (Bell, 1983). The difficulty that most men experience in expressing love, tenderness, affection, kindness, and compassion is exacerbated by combat experience. Males should be given opportunities to practice expressing their feelings, along with permission and support to do so while in treatment sessions with family members, alone, or in veterans' groups. Males learn to associate nonmasculine feelings with reduced survivability. Habitual restriction of selected affect produces an interpersonal style that can be described as ultramasculine. This learned behavior inhibits working through problems in treatment and complicates family relationships, including marital, conjugal, and parent/child relationships (Figley, 1985). Perhaps the most disturbing consequence is the passing on of this interpersonal style to the next generation, the veteran's children.

Misdiagnosis. The inclusion of PTSD as a diagnosis in *DSM-III-R* (APA, 1987) corrected a deficiency that had severely negative consequences for approximately 70% of Vietnam veterans requesting help and treatment following discharge from the service. According to Erlinder (1984), mental health professionals and attorneys lacked an accepted description of symptoms. Straker (1976) reported that 77% of Vietnam veterans admitted to VA hospitals received an incorrect diagnosis of schizophrenia. Professionals tended to regard flashback experiences as acute schizophrenic episodes, according to Brende and Parson (1985).

Many clinicians were persuaded by the presence of substance abuse to look no further for the source of PTSD symptoms. This practice ill-served those veterans for whom the substance abuse was a symptom of, rather than the catalyst for, postwar psychological problems. The *DSM-III-R* is a resource for helping professionals to decrease instances of misdiagnosis when it is used appropriately.

Reluctance of Veterans to Seek Help. The last combat troops departed Vietnam in June 1972, yet many veterans remained distrustful of available mental health resources. They avoided contact with government-operated helping agencies until the creation of the Vet Centers, to be discussed later. Veterans of Vietnam often are unaware of disparities between the way they functioned prior to and subsequent to Vietnam service. An alarming number assumed the behavioral symptoms of PTSD to be normal or "just the way it is supposed to be." Many veterans were fearful of reopening old wounds.

Reluctance of Clinicians to Provide Help. Many helping professionals experience an aversion to dealing with Vietnam veterans, fearing, perhaps, their own feelings of vulnerability when confronted with a client's traumatic memories. Still others maintain a long-held bias based on stereotypical views of returning Vietnam veterans (Blair & Hildreth, 1991). Haley (1978) pointed out: "Contemplation of and confrontation of one's anxiety and vulnerability to catastrophic stress are both expected and necessary when working with combatants" (p. 265).

If practitioners have substance abuse problems themselves, this often heightens their sense of vulnerability. Countertransference issues and value conflicts frequently make the work difficult even when it proceeds. Ambivalence on the part of the practitioner is likely to be conveyed indirectly to the veteran, leading to additional feelings of rejection in the client, along with worthlessness and anger. Work on problems in such an emotional climate is likely to be difficult and ineffective.

Building on Strengths

Resolving the barriers identified in the previous section can be achieved, in part, by the active involvement of the veteran and family in the treatment. Thus, in meaningful therapeutic encounters with Vietnam veterans, it is assumed that the helping professional should not dictate the agenda. The client and the family system are full partners in determining the direction of the work. The assumption is that the client system has the ability to do the work and that the helper simply needs to facilitate the process. This assumption implies that the social worker or other helping professional is operating from a strengths perspective, in which the client system is assisted in identifying, making use of, and enhancing existing strengths. Other strengths can be developed through environmental work: enhancing family relationships, developing new community resources for physical needs, or helping a client build a new support network of other individuals who have similar problems (but varying strengths).

Providing a "Safe" Environment for Treatment: Vet Centers

Officially called the Readjustment Counseling Service, the Vet Centers are unsurpassed in effectiveness in dealing with Vietnam veterans (Brende & Parson, 1985) and enjoy an immense popularity with the veteran population. The centers were designed to provide services that include, but go beyond, individual and group methods of counseling and therapy. Family counseling and family education, vocational counseling, job search, community education, and advocacy are available, in addition to individual and group therapy and treatment (Blank, 1982). The Vet Centers provide an opportunity for social support, peer involvement, and professional assistance in a relaxed, informal atmosphere that is sensitive to veterans' needs and excoriates the unavoidable bureaucratic trappings of traditional helping approaches.

The Vet Centers are staffed by professionals and paraprofessionals whose dedication is profoundly important to the clinical services offered (Blank, 1982). Half of the personnel of these centers are Vietnam War veterans, and one-fourth are Vietnam era veterans; many are women.

In some circumstances, creating a safe environment may require inpatient treatment rather than treatment in a Vet Center. Inpatient treatment should be considered and discussed with the client when the degree of PTSD and addiction is chronic and severe (Arnold, 1985); when the client manifests ineffective control of emotions, thoughts, or behavior (Smith, 1985); or when, in the professional judgment of the clinician, the client represents a danger to him- or herself or others. Inpatient treatment is available in VA hospitals and medical centers. These units use approaches specifically designed or selected to assist combat veterans in addressing and dealing with severely disturbing memories, dreams, and behavior. Many of these units coexist with substance abuse units. Referral for substance abuse treatment prior to PTSD treatment is common, and it can enhance later treatment specific to PTSD. Referral to inpatient units is often effected through the Vet Centers.

A COMMUNICATIONS FAMILY SYSTEMS APPROACH

A communications family systems approach can be modified to address the cognitive, developmental, self-in-the-world, and systems factors identified previously as important in the development of PTSD and addiction (Jurich, 1983; Prosky, 1974). A primary goal of treatment with PTSD victims is facilitating the working through of traumatic memories within the context of the family where those symptoms have affected such relationships. This process should allow the client to reframe war memories into less threatening stimuli. Ideally the client can accept the trauma into his or her self-concept in more positive ways, while engaging the supports, such as family members and others, that are present in his or her environment. Particularly when alcohol or other drug abuse has been chronic or severe, the client's physical health should merit consideration and treatment as needed. In general, treatment with trauma survivors should include several elements: normalization, peer-group identification, social support, humor, spirituality, psychotherapy, and empowerment (Ochberg, 1989). Empowerment is achieved by building on the family's and client's strengths, providing a "safe" environment for treatment, using psychotropic drugs conservatively as needed, and applying a flexible set of treatment approaches that involve families or significant others whenever possible. The process of empowerment may occur through a combination of family treatment and/or couples therapy.

Family Treatment Sessions

Rosenheck and Thomson (1986) characterized the consequences of PTSD for the family in three basic categories; (a) emotional emptiness, (b) functional loss of the husband/father from stage-specific tasks, and (c) the emergence of "classic" interactive family patterns that augment the stress and complicate efforts to resolve it. The cumulative effect of maladaptive coping threatens marriages, family roles, and other social relationships, while recovery requires major shifts in role assignments and role performance. It is well established that good social support, particularly from the family, improves the chances for recovery from both PTSD and chemical dependency. Restoration of interpersonal relationships often requires direct and strategic intervention in family treatment sessions with the veteran, spouse or partner, children, extended family members, and other "pseudo" family members who are significant to the family though not related by blood.

Family members are co-victims; the impact of trauma and substance abuse in the life space of the family members is as equally portentous and debilitating as it is for the veteran. Matsakis (1989) observed that to the extent the veteran is perceived as "crazy," the spouse is perceived as crazy—for staying with, loving, and helping the veteran. Moreover, substance dependence is considered to be a family illness requiring major changes in the family for resolution (Weinberg, 1983); veterans normally will have abdicated power and responsibility to the spouse or partner (DeFazio & Pascucci, 1984).

Problems seen in families stem from the affect and behavior of the veteran and spouse that frustrate their attempts to interact meaningfully with the environment and with each other. On the part of the veteran, violence and rage, suspiciousness, numbing of feelings, inappropriate response to loss and grief, isolation and withdrawal, substance abuse, and controlling/demanding behavior are characteristic. Spouses often are scapegoated, shouldering the blame for marital conflicts. In turn, the spouse may experience guilt and grief over perceived losses within the marriage, and fear of aggressive behavior and violence. The spouse often lacks confidence in his or her perceptions. Both veteran and spouse frequently become overprotective and overcontrolling of their children, using unspoken rules and inconsistent limits and boundaries. This pattern, as well as the underlying family and individual issues discussed in the next sections, should be the focus of family treatment.

Numbing of Feelings. Veterans are commonly unable or unwilling to express emotions or to share feelings, finding it more comfortable and less threatening to self-isolate from their partners, families, and friends. They often respond inappropriately to loss and illness (Williams & Williams, 1985), finding it difficult to sympathize or empathize. On the surface, at least, the normal grief process is frequently absent. Education about the grief process and the application of communication exercises (to discuss the stages being experienced and their reactions, for example) during and outside of sessions are very useful to family members. These types of interventions provide an alternative to the experience of grief in combat situations that reduces survivability. More frequently the response during combat and during treatment initially is one of hostility and anger in spite of underlying true feelings.

Violence and Rage. Episodes of violence stemming from anger and rage are often the event that triggers referral for professional help. Complaints and self-reports of familial violence are not uncommon and more often than not are associated with the abuse of alcohol. Fearful of the effects of anger and rage, veterans frequently become further isolated in an effort to avoid events that stimulate these emotions. Family treatment provides an opportunity to examine such events in light of other feelings that may have remained hidden under the anger and rage. Treatment can help coach family members to respond honestly but supportively when such painful feelings (guilt, hurt, fear) are expressed by the veteran in treatment.

Women as Mainstay. Many authorities (Brown, 1984; DeFazio & Pascucci, 1984; Williams & Williams, 1985) have written of the abdication of power and responsibility by the veteran to the spouse or partner. The woman partner is often the reliable breadwinner for the family and the principle source of emotional strength. Williams and Williams (1985) cautioned clinicians to avoid confusing chronic PTSD with passivity or infantile behavior and to encourage new role assignments that realign family responsibilities as treatment helps to eliminate or make manageable the overwhelming symptoms experienced by the veteran with PTSD.

Effects on Children. As the veteran and partner disengage to a "safe" emotional distance, both frequently seek to replace the lost (though stressful) intimacy through increased intimacy with the children. As a consequence, veterans and their spouses are often overprotective and overcontrolling of their children (Jurich, 1983), holding them to exacting standards of behavior. In many cases the phenomenon of "children as parents" (Brende & Parson, 1985) is observed as children assume increased responsibility for family functioning. The unspoken rules mentioned earlier include injunctions familiar to clinicians skilled in working with children of alcoholics: don't think, don't feel, and don't talk. Helping families, including the children, identify these often unspoken rules through role playing, sculpting, and communication exercises is an important technique in this systems approach. Only then can the members be helped literally to rewrite their family rules and identify how various members may sabotage the new rules, based on past family interactional patterns.

Veterans as Identified Patients. The literature abounds with examples of the effects of one or another family member being identified as "the" problem. Williams and Williams (1985) offered the following: "If one family member is identified as a 'patient,' as is often the case with veterans, then other family members expect the veteran alone to do all the changing. Family members usually do not understand how their own behavior can perpetrate dysfunctional patterns in the family relationships" (p. 197).

Exercises designed to decode and change the many shame-and-blame messages in the family help "spread the problem." Indicators that help in decoding messages include "he/she should . . . ," "if only . . . ," "the reason . . . ," "if _______ would . . . ," then "I could . . ."

Use of Drugs in Treatment

Most pharmacological interventions used with veterans are symptomatically targeted—that is, antidepressants for depression, anxiolytics for anxiety, and neuroleptics for flashbacks and extreme agitation (Walker, 1982). In a 1985 survey of 159 VA medical centers, Atkinson, Callen, and Reaves (1985) found that only 7.1% had established medication protocols for PTSD symptoms (Reaves, Atkinson, Ponzoha, & Kofoed, 1988).

Most authorities agree with Berman, Price, and Gusman (1982), who suggested that dependence on medication may conflict with treatment when the goal is to help clients rely on individual strengths, positive family relationships, and group support to cope with stress. Drugs may help the veteran block feelings, disclosure and processing of which between family members are necessary to recovery from combat-related PTSD. Therefore drugs should be prescribed cautiously, especially when there is an existing problem of substance abuse.

In summary, family involvement in treatment sessions offers a broader data base during assessment and can be useful for enhancing follow-through and reduction of objections to treatment that require time away from the family. The family members of the trauma survivor often will need educational sessions in addition to family treatment for understanding the nature of PTSD and addictions. Twenty-five years after the cessation of hostility in Vietnam, many persons remain uninformed of the nature of the war and the differences between Vietnam and other wars that contributed to the development of traumatic stress.

Couples Therapy

It should be remembered that the center of conflicts between the veteran and the spouse derives from their fundamentally different life experiences and their efforts to adjust emotionally in light of those experiences (Rosenheck & Thomson, 1986). Issues and challenges unique to their different experiences can be worked through in couples or partners groups that have a systems focus similar to the family treatment sessions. The work in the spouse support groups can be enhanced by involvement in 12-step self-help groups such as Al-Anon and Alafam when substance abuse is occurring or has occurred. Spouses or partners need assistance in ridding themselves of feelings of guilt for behavior they may believe led to the veteran's response and behavior.

Couples work that includes an emphasis on addiction recovery and relapse prevention, restatement of marital and individual expectations, training in manifesting ownership of feelings, education in terms of linkage between the cognitive-feeling-behavior triad, and development of mutual support has proven helpful. In cases where the male partner has abdicated power and responsibility to the spouse, care should be taken in facilitating a smooth and nonthreatening transfer to a more equitable role fulfillment. The spouse group format is useful because male peers can reduce each other's possible defensiveness about these family patterns. Spouses and partners in these groups often help other women anticipate and address their reactions when the male reassumes some of the family responsibilities. Simultaneously peer "rap" groups can be used to initiate similar family role changes.

Other Aspects of Treatment

In addition to the family treatment, couples groups, and peer (rap) groups described in the previous sections, veterans may need advocacy and/or referral for other services to build on or strengthen their families and larger environments. This help may include contact with and support from organizations such as the American Legion, the VFW, Military

Order of the Purple Heart, Disabled American Veterans (DAV), and AMVETS. Such organizations articulate the concerns of veterans clearly, assist in obtaining various benefits, and aid veterans in networking among themselves. Referral and continued support for the veteran and family members to participate actively in 12-step programs and substance abuse treatment are also important. Although ongoing substance abuse by a veteran or family member should not preclude work with the PTSD, no meaningful resolution of the trauma disorder is likely to occur while the substance abuse continues. Finally it is not uncommon for such families to need and benefit from encouragement to use their informal social supports, as well as to coordinate family treatment with the members' involvement with general hospitals, probation and parole offices, child welfare services, and public welfare agencies.

CASE ILLUSTRATION: THE BROWN FAMILY

Carl Brown was referred to a Vet Center by a private psychologist for assessment and treatment of suspected PTSD. The client had self-referred to the psychologist as a result of his wife's complaints regarding his withdrawal, moodiness, anger, and violence.

Early Family History

Assessment revealed that Carl had experienced a very good early adjustment as a youngster. Socially active and popular, he played sports and graduated from high school to immediately enter a university for 4 years without attaining a degree. He married during college. His wife remembers him during college as "humorous" and "fun." To her knowledge, he was rarely, if ever, depressed or angry.

Military History

Carl received his draft notification; he was offered Officer Candidate School but elected to serve as an enlisted man to reduce the time he would be away. After routine basic and advanced infantry training, Carl was transferred to Vietnam, where he served for 1 year. Significant trauma occurred when Carl witnessed his best friend sustain the loss of an arm. On another occasion Carl ordered a newly arrived soldier to get behind a tree, suspecting the tree would offer the solder some protection. Instead the solder was killed. Carl was personally instrumental in the death of enemy troops, frequently encountered the death of fellow Americans, and witnessed much destruction. Carl vividly recalled that on the way home from Vietnam, the flight attendant on the aircraft would allow none of the returning soldiers to sit in first class. It remained empty during the flight home.

Post-Military Family History

Carl left the Army, returned home, finished college, and entered business for himself. He and his family were active in church, and they maintained close social relationships with family members and friends. His business prospered, and two male children were born over the years.

Carl began to experience bouts of anger, depression, and withdrawal. He stopped his church activities and recalled that he was frequently troubled by things that triggered memories of the war, particularly the sound of helicopters. He went to great lengths to avoid these reminders. Soon he was experiencing frequent bouts of depression and was having nightmares. He recalled that he found himself thinking about his experiences in Vietnam and experienced difficulty in concentrating on his business. He began to use alcohol and marijuana, which helped, but fearful of his wife's objections, he concealed his use of substances from her. He refused to discuss the war and what he was feeling, and he continued to withdraw from his wife and children.

There were occasions of violent outbursts that severely frightened Carl and family members. One occasion of violence found Carl striking one of his sons in the face, an act that deeply disturbed the client. That event led Carl to refer himself for treatment.

Individual, Family, and Group Treatment

Individual sessions initially provided an environment for the unfolding of Carl's story. Carl reported that this was the first occasion he had described his experience of Vietnam. Feelings and affect were solicited by the counselor, enabling Carl to identify the source of his feelings of anger and guilt and to vent those feelings.

Family treatment sessions were conducted to provide an opportunity for Carl's sons and spouse to express their feelings and concerns, to demonstrate support and caring, and to receive feedback from him. Carl was able to express his sorrow and guilt feelings surrounding the anger and violence, and the family was provided an opportunity to practice problem solving through communication exercises and homework tasks in a family context.

Carl entered a rap group with other veterans; the goals supported those of the family and individual treatment sessions: Stop all violent outbursts, improve coping skills, engage family and social supports, reduce/eliminate substance abuse, and desensitize such that reminders of Vietnam no longer elicited uncomfortable responses.

He quickly made friends in the group and began to feel accepted and understood. He said, "In group I learned how to cry. I learned to feel sad instead of angry. I had never learned to express the grief and sorrow I shut out in Vietnam." Carl attended his rap group for approximately 18 months after the family and individual sessions. The violent episodes were never repeated, nor were there further problems with substance abuse. Carl reported increased openness and sharing within the family as he has been able to remain available.

CASE ILLUSTRATION: THE STARK FAMILY

Mike Stark was referred by a community agency for help with depression and marital problems. The initial interview revealed that he had experienced multiple recent losses, including the death of his father. He indicated feeling that his marriage was collapsing around him, that his wife considered him to be too demanding and possessive, and that she was threatening to leave him. He had concerns that a divorce would destroy any chance he had of maintaining a relationship with their daughter. Mike revealed a history of substance abuse spanning the several years since he served in Vietnam.

Early Family History

Mike was raised in a small, rural community with traditional values in a two-parent family. He considered himself to be an average to better than average student and reported that he enjoyed school and his teenage years. He dated regularly, was active in sports, and involved himself in extracurricular activities.

He reported feeling close to his father and felt that his father was warmer and more supportive than most fathers. In contrast, he remembered his mother as distant and businesslike.

Military History

Mike enlisted in the Marines after high school, underwent routine basic and advanced infantry training, and was transferred to Vietnam, where he served 1 year in an infantry company. He was severely wounded, medically evacuated from Vietnam, and treated for several months at military hospitals before being released from active duty. As an infantryman, Mike was routinely exposed to dead and wounded Americans and Vietnamese. He often was required to inflict lethal violence on others, and he witnessed the death of many of his friends.

Post-Military Family History

Immediately after his release from service, Mike became listless (in his words), traveling the country in search of something that remained unidentified. The residual scarring and damage from his physical wounds remained painful, and he found it easy to obtain street drugs to combat the pain. He recalled being deeply disturbed by memories of the war, of being wounded, and recalled frequent dreams and nightmares of incidents that were either real or could be real. He used drugs to induce sleep and soon found himself unable to sleep unless under the influence of drugs.

Mike began avoiding other veterans, avoiding the constant TV news of the war, and, in fact, on numerous occasions denied that he was a veteran "so I wouldn't have to defend myself or answer questions." He was involved in several live-in relationships but found it impossible to confide in his mates or to feel trust. He remembered concluding that relationships "were not worth the hassle."

Mike's decision regarding relationships changed when he met Betty, who was well employed, busy, independent, and self-confident. After their marriage, Mike sought and secured employment. Problems began a few years later when he became increasingly possessive of Betty. A clash of wills normally excited Mike's anger and rage with more than one incidence of violence.

Couples and Individual Therapy

Both Mike and Betty began individual sessions with separate therapists. Neither of the clients was aware of PTSD or that the pattern of Mike's behavior was similar to that of other veterans. There was, however, sufficient factual evidence available to make the diagnosis of PTSD. After about 8 weeks of individual work, a couples group was recommended for Mike and Betty. The family systems focus of the group helped in addressing family issues.

For instance, Mike and Betty were able to use in-session rehearsal and role playing to improve their family's problem-solving communications. Feedback from group members provided the motivation necessary for Mike to begin sharing his Vietnam story with Betty. She responded to this "leap of trust" with increased openness and sharing, indicating to Mike that she was interested and concerned. Mike confessed that he had been fearful and ashamed to discuss his feelings and his experiences. He said to Betty, "I didn't want you to think I was a crybaby." Changes in their ability to communicate feelings and other important issues led to changes in their family relationships and roles (e.g., more tolerance of each other's views, more respect for each other). Mike was not amenable to AA or NA, electing instead to remain drug free through his own efforts. His ability to achieve abstinence on his own was evidence of his strong desire for change.

PRACTICE IMPLICATIONS

Possibly in recognition that the social work focus on the person-and-environment is consistent with the treatment of choice for this population, it is estimated that 30% of all clinical positions in the Vet Center system are filled with social workers. Practitioners from the other helping professions fulfill the remaining positions. Although clinicians in the Readjustment Counseling Service undergo specialized training, the roles performed are familiar to those of social workers and other helping professionals: educator, mediator, counselor, advocate, facilitator, networker, supporter, and liaison.

There are a few unique requirements for these roles in serving Vietnam veterans and their families. Blank (1982) stated these requirements succinctly: an unflinching ability to listen to, confront, evoke, and contain memories of a veteran's experiences of the trauma. The worker must be able to suspend judgment in reaction to the repulsion he or she might experience when informed of atrocities witnessed or committed by the client. The practitioner should have acquired experience in working with family members and other social supports of substance abusers.

It is not required that the worker be a veteran of Vietnam service, yet that qualification can heighten trust and acceptance by the client, while promoting empathy and suspension of judgment by the worker. For non-veteran helpers, extensive work with this population diminishes the shock effect of their graphic descriptions of the horror and terror of combat. This reduction can enable the worker to achieve more easily an appreciation of the client and family members' differing experiences of the world.

A potential for conflicts in the work exists for a number of reasons. For example, there can be a significant difference between the value system of the client, the family, and that of the worker. Some veterans manifest a sense of entitlement that can test a worker's or family member's understanding and acceptance. Conflicts of this nature usually are avoided by careful and explicit contracting between the helper and client system. Intra-agency and inter-agency conflicts arise when the client is unable to interact in meaningful ways with traditional helping agencies or with other members of interdisciplinary teams. Well-developed networking and mediation skills, which can be taught and modeled by the practitioner, are helpful in these situations.

CONCLUSION

The impact of substance abuse on the assessment, diagnosis, and treatment of survivors of trauma is profound. Substance abuse is being recognized increasingly as probably the most common complication in this helping process. Efforts directed toward treatment of PTSD are generally ineffectual while substance abuse continues. It is recognized that severe and chronic PTSD seriously impacts the life space of the sufferer and his or her family, but alcoholism and other drug addictions are recognized universally as life-threatening conditions that grow progressively more serious over time. For this reason, treatment of substance abuse should be considered primary until abstinence or control of the substance is achieved.

An ecological approach has proven to be consistent with the treatment of choice for this population: a family treatment approach. Treatment approaches that do not consider the family or other environmental aspects are less effective. Treatment itself should be multimodal and should address, to the extent feasible, the needs of all family members. Helping professionals, including social workers, psychologists, addiction counselors, psychiatrists, and mental health workers, need more specialized training and practice experiences to serve this clientele and their families effectively.

REFERENCES

Allen, I. M. (1986). Post-traumatic stress disorder among black Vietnam veterans. *Hospital and Community Psychiatry, 37,* 55-61.

American Psychiatric Association (APA). (1987). *Diagnostic and statistical manual of mental disorders* (3rd ed. rev.). Washington, DC: Author.

Arnold, A. L. (1985). Inpatient treatment of Vietnam veterans with post-traumatic stress disorder. In S. M. Sonnenberg, A. S. Blank, & J. A. Talbott (Eds.), *The trauma of war: Stress and recovery in Vietnam veterans* (pp. 239-261). Washington, DC: American Psychiatric Press.

Atkinson, R. M., Callen, K. E., & Reaves, M. E. (1985). VA health services for Vietnam veterans. *VA Practitioner, 2,* 72-77.

Bell, R. R. (1983). *Marriage and family interaction.* Homewood, IL: Dorsey.

Berman, S., Price, S., & Gusman, F. (1982). An inpatient program for Vietnam combat veterans in a Veterans Administration hospital. *Hospital and Community Psychiatry, 33,* 919-922.

Blair, D. T., & Hildreth, N. A. (1991). PTSD and the Vietnam veteran: The battle for treatment. *Journal of Psychosocial Nursing, 29,* 15-20.

Blank, A. S. (1982). Apocalypse terminable and interminable: Operation outreach for Vietnam veterans. *Hospital and Community Psychiatry, 33,* 913-918.

Blaufarb, H., & Levine, J. (1972). Crisis intervention in an earthquake. *Social Work, 17,* 1-4.

Bleich, A., Garb, R., & Kottler, M. (1986). Treatment of prolonged combat-reaction. *British Journal of Psychiatry, 148,* 483-496.

Boettcher, T. (1985). *Vietnam: The valor and the sorrow.* Boston: Little, Brown.

Boscarino, J. (1981). Current excessive drinking among Vietnam veterans: A comparison with other veterans and non-veterans. *International Journal of Social Psychiatry, 27,* 204-212.

Brancey, L., David, W., & Leiber, C. S. (1984). Alcoholism in Vietnam and Korea veterans: A long-term follow-up. *Alcoholism, 8,* 572-575.

Brende, J., & Parson, E. (1985). *Vietnam veterans: The road to recovery.* New York: Plenum.

Briggs, R. A. (1984). Combat level and family support: Correlates of post-Vietnam adjustment. *Dissertation Abstracts International, 45,* 1005-1013.

Brown, P. C. (1984). Legacies of a war: Treatment considerations with Vietnam veterans and their families. *Social Work, 29,* 372-379.

Card, J. (1983). *Lives after Vietnam: The personal impact of military service.* Lexington, MA: Lexington.

Card, J. (1987). Epidemiology of PTSD in a national cohort of Vietnam veterans. *Journal of Clinical Psychology, 43,* 6-17.

Carmen, E., Reicker, P. P., & Mills, T. (1984). Victims of violence and psychiatric illness. *American Journal of Psychiatry, 141,* 373-383.

Centers for Disease Control (CDC). (1987). Postservice mortality among Vietnam veterans. *Journal of the American Medical Association, 257,* 790-795.

Connelly, T. (1987). Workshop encourages women veterans to share experience. *Vet Center Voice, 9,* 5-6.

DeFazio, V., & Pascucci, N. (1984). Return to Ithaca: A perspective on marriage and love in post-traumatic stress disorder. *Journal of Contemporary Psychotherapy, 14,* 76-89.

Egendorf, A. (1985). *Healing from the war: Trauma and transformation after Vietnam.* Boston: Houghton Mifflin.

Egendorf, A., Kadushin, C., Laufer, R., Rothbart, G., & Sloan, L. (1981). *Legacies of Vietnam.* Washington, DC: Committee on Veterans' Affairs.

Erickson, E. H. (1956). *Identity, youth and crisis.* New York: Norton.

Erickson, K. T. (1976). *Everything in its path.* New York: Simon & Schuster.

Erlinder, C. P. (1984). Paying the price for Vietnam: Post-traumatic stress disorder and criminal behavior. *Boston College Law Review, 25,* 305-306.

Eth, S., & Pynoos, R. S. (1985). *Post-traumatic stress disorder in children.* Washington, DC: American Psychiatric Press.

Ewalt, J. R. (1981). What about the Vietnam veteran? *Military Medicine, 146,* 165-167.

Fairbank, J. A., & Nicholson, R. A. (1982). Theoretical and empirical issues in the treatment of post-traumatic stress disorder in Vietnam veterans. *Journal of Clinical Psychology, 43,* 44-55.

Figley, C. R. (1985). From victim to survivor: Social responsibility in the wake of catastrophe. In C. R. Figley (Ed.), *Trauma and its wake* (pp. 398-415). New York: Brunner/Mazel.

Fox, R. P., & Scherl, D. J. (1972). Crisis intervention with victims of rape. *Social Work, 17,* 37-42.

Goodwin, J. (1987). The etiology of combat-related post-traumatic stress disorders. In T. Williams (Ed.), *Post-traumatic stress disorders: A handbook for clinicians* (pp. 1-18). Cincinnati: Disabled American Veterans.

Haley, S. A. (1978). Treatment implications of post-traumatic stress syndromes for mental health professions. In C. R. Figley (Ed.), *Stress disorders among Vietnam veterans* (pp. 3-22). New York: Brunner/Mazel.

Haymen, P. M., Sommers-Flanagan, R., & Parsons, J. (1987). Aftermath of violence: Post-traumatic stress disorder among Vietnam veterans. *Journal of Counseling and Development, 65,* 363-366.

Hendin, H., & Pollinger, H. A. (1984). *The wounds of war: The psychological aftermath of combat in Vietnam.* New York: Basic Books.

Helzer, J. E. (1984). The impact of combat on later alcohol use by Vietnam veterans. *Journal of Psychoactive Drugs, 16,* 183-191.

Helzer, J. E., Robins, L. N., & Davis, D. H. (1975). Antecedents of narcotics use and addiction: A study of 898 Vietnam veterans. *Drug and Alcohol Dependence, 1,* 183-190.

Janoff-Bulman, R. (1985). The aftermath of victimization: Rebuilding shattered assumptions. In C. R. Figley (Ed.), *Trauma and its wake* (pp. 15-35). New York: Brunner/Mazel.

Jelinek, J. M. (1987). Group therapy with Vietnam veterans and other trauma victims. In T. Williams (Ed.), *Post-traumatic stress disorders: A handbook for clinicians* (pp. 209-218). Cincinnati: Disabled American Veterans.

Jurich, A. P. (1983). The Saigon of the family's mind: Family therapy with families of Vietnam veterans. *Journal of Marital and Family Therapy, 9,* 355-363.

Kormos, H. P. (1978). The nature of combat stress. In C. R. Figley (Ed.), *Stress disorders among Vietnam veterans* (pp. 3-22). New York: Brunner/Mazel.

Kulka, R. A., Schlenger, W. E., Fairbank, J. A., Hough, R. L., Jordon, B. K., Marmar, C. R., & Weiss, D. S. (1988). *Contractual report of findings from the National Vietnam Readjustment Study: Description, current status, and initial PTSD prevalence estimates.* Washington, DC: Research Triangle Institute.

LaCoursiere, R. M., Godfrey, K. E., & Ruby, L. M. (1980). Traumatic neurosis in the etiology of alcoholism: Vietnam combat and other trauma. *American Journal of Psychiatry, 137,* 966-968.

Langley, M. (1982). Post-traumatic stress disorders among Vietnam combat veterans. *Social Casework, 63,* 593-598.

Matsakis, A. (1989). The other forgotten warriors. *VFW of the U.S. Magazine, 76,* 28-34.

McCormick, N. A. (1988). Substance abuse among Vietnam veterans: A view from the CAP control perspective. *International Journal of the Addictions, 23,* 1311-1316.

Nace, E. P., O'Brien, C. P., Mintz, J., Ream, N., & Myers, A. L. (1977). Drinking problems among Vietnam veterans. In F. Seixas (Ed.), *Currents in alcoholism* (Vol. 4, pp. 315-324). New York: Grune & Stratton.

Newman, B., & Newman, P. (1984). *Development through life: A psychosocial approach* (3rd ed.). Homewood, IL: Dorsey.

Newman, J. (1987). Differential diagnosis in post-traumatic stress disorder. In T. Williams (Ed.), *Post-traumatic stress disorders* (pp. 19-33). Cincinnati: Disabled American Veterans.

Noy, S. (1978, June). *Stress and personality as factors in the causality and prognosis of combat reaction.* Paper presented at the Second Annual International Conference on Psychological Stress and Adjustment in Time of War and Peace, Jerusalem, Israel.

Ochberg, F. (1989, April). *Caring for victimized populations.* Paper presented at Mountain Empire Conference on Hostages, Prisoners of War, and Holocaust Survivors, Johnson City, TN.

Parson, E. R. (1985a). The black Vietnam veteran: His representational world in post-traumatic stress disorder. In W. E. Kelly (Ed.), *Post-traumatic stress disorder and the war veteran* (pp. 170-192). New York: Brunner/Mazel.

Parson, E. R. (1985b). The intercultural setting: Encountering black Vietnam veterans. In S. M. Sonnenberg, A. S. Blank, & J. Talbott (Eds.), *The trauma of war: Stress and recovery in Vietnam veterans* (pp. 359-388). Washington, DC: American Psychiatric Press.

Prosky, P. (1974). Family therapy: An orientation. *Clinical Social Work Journal, 2,* 45-56.

Reaves, M. E., Atkinson, R. M., Ponzoha, C. A., & Kofoed, L. L. (1988). Trends in VA mental health services for Vietnam veterans. *VA Practitioner, 8,* 93-98.

Schnaier, J. A. (1986). A study of women Vietnam veterans and their mental health adjustment. In C. R. Figley (Ed.), *Trauma and its wake* (Vol. 2, pp. 97-132). New York: Brunner/Mazel.

Smith, J. R. (1985). Individual psychotherapy with Vietnam veterans. In J. Sonnenberg, A. S. Blank, & J. Talbott (Eds.), *The trauma of war: Stress and recovery in Vietnam veterans* (pp. 125-164). Washington, DC: American Psychiatric Press.

Starr, P. (1973). *The discarded army: Veterans after Vietnam.* New York: Charterhouse.

Straker, M. (1976). The Vietnam veteran: The task of reintegration. *Diseases of the Nervous System, 37,* 75-79.

Van Devanter, L. M. (1985). The unknown warriors: Implications of the experiences of women in Vietnam. In W. E. Kelly (Ed.), *Post-traumatic stress disorder and the war veteran patient* (pp. 148-169). New York: Brunner/Mazel.

Walker, J. I. (1982). Chemotherapy of traumatic war stress. *Military Medicine, 147,* 1029-1033.

Weinberg, J. (1983). Counseling recovering alcoholics. In F. J. Turner (Ed.), *Differential diagnosis and treatment in social work* (3rd ed., pp. 193-206). New York: Free Press.

Williams, C., & Williams, T. (1985). Family therapy for Vietnam veterans. In S. Sonnenberg, A. Blank, & J. Talbott (Eds.), *The trauma of war: Stress and recovery in Vietnam veterans* (pp. 195-209). Washington, DC: American Psychiatric Press.

Wilson, J. Y. (1980). Conflict, stress and growth: Effects of war on psychosocial development. In C. Figley & S. Leventman (Eds.), *Strangers at home* (pp. 123-165). New York: Praeger.

Zinberg, N. E. (1972). Heroin use in Vietnam and the United States. *Archives of General Psychiatry, 26,* 486-488.

Chapter 8

ALCOHOL ADDICTION AND SEXUAL DYSFUNCTION

STEPHANIE COVINGTON

Four centuries ago Shakespeare stated (in *Macbeth,* Act 2, scene 3) what is still current folk wisdom about drinking: Alcohol stimulates sexual desire but makes it difficult to act upon. Clinical research in the last 20 years has affirmed the truth of that folk wisdom: Both alcoholics and nonalcoholics report that alcohol increases sexual desire, and yet alcoholics also report a greater incidence of sexual problems than do nonalcoholics. Alcohol ingestion seems to whet the appetite for sexual experience but makes the outcome of having the experience problematic. Men consistently report difficulties in getting and sustaining erections, increased time to ejaculation, and difficulties ejaculating. Women report difficulties lubricating, increased time to orgasm, difficulties in attaining orgasm, and decreased intensity of orgasm. Not only do alcoholic men and women report such sexual difficulties during active drinking, but they also report the continuation of their respective sexual dysfunctions during abstinence and recovery. Long-time chronic alcoholics—both women and men—also report a decrease in sexual desire. So it seems that as alcoholism progresses, it affects not only the sexual experience itself but also the impetus toward having the experience as well.

Van Thiel and Lester (1979) estimated that 70%-80% of chronic alcoholic men experience a decrease in sexual desire or erectile function or both. In this study of 60 alcoholic men with erectile dysfunction, only 25% spontaneously recovered their full sexual functioning after 3-6 months of sobriety. In my study of alcoholic women (Covington,

1982), 69% reported having experienced sexual dysfunction before alcoholism, 85% during alcoholism, and 74% reported continued sexual dysfunction during sobriety. The dysfunctions included lack of desire, lack of arousal, lack of lubrication, lack of orgasm, dyspareunia (painful intercourse), and vaginismus (vaginal spasms).

Sexual functioning clearly is a severe problem for both alcoholic men and women during active drinking and during sobriety. Unfortunately, however, it is the one problem area least likely to be mentioned by clients or family members during both assessment and treatment for chemical dependency. Like the culture at large, helping professionals experience discomfort in asking about sexual experiences directly and often feel incompetent in addressing clients' sexual issues and involving relevant family members in the sessions as needed.

Helen Singer Kaplan (1974), the noted sex therapist, has referred to *sexuality* as the integration of the biological, emotional, and social aspects of one's self. Sexuality thus is seen as an expression of both who one is and how one relates to others. Such a fundamental aspect of the self is closely related to how individuals experience their own self-worth. Being unable to adequately express our sexual selves can profoundly affect self-esteem and family relationships in a negative way.

Often for the alcoholic, the sexual self becomes impaired as the alcoholism progresses. This impairment then is reflected in the disruption of social and sexual relationships with others. Thus alcoholism has a primary effect on one of the most fundamental expressions of the self—one's sexuality within the context of spousal relationships and other social/peer interactions. Therefore the lack of available sexual treatment in recovery programs verges on the tragic, especially related to how the sexual issues interact with addiction to affect the family's functioning and interrelationships. Along with the importance of addressing problems of self-esteem and guilt, addressing sexual issues needs to be a priority for all chemical dependency treatment programs, as well as for counselors who provide the services.

It is widely acknowledged by treatment providers that difficult or problematic sexual experiences in sobriety are a common occasion for relapse. The connection between sexual experience and relapse makes it even more vital that clinicians learn about the relationship between sexual dysfunction and chemical dependence, as well as effective individual and family treatment strategies. This chapter addresses the following areas: (a) the connections between chemical dependency and sexual dysfunction; (b) the sexual cycle in men and women; (c) the common sexual dysfunctions;

(d) the cause of some sexual dysfunctions from family-of-origin experiences, including sexual abuse; and (e) structural family systems treatment strategies for helping resolve sexual dysfunction within chemical dependency treatment. As clinicians such as social workers, sex therapists, addiction counselors, and psychologists become more comfortable working in the sexual realm, chemically dependent persons will receive more help in confronting and resolving this aspect of their lives during recovery.

THE SOCIAL CONNECTIONS BETWEEN ALCOHOL AND SEXUAL BEHAVIOR

Alcohol as an Aphrodisiac

Alcohol use has long been associated with sexual activity in our society. In the early 20th century, one of the traditional arguments for prohibition was that it would reduce sexual promiscuity. Currently 48% of male college students and 56% of female college students (Bowker, 1977) report that they have been on a date where alcohol was used to make one of the partners more sexually willing or responsive. Beer, wine, and liquor advertisements invariably connect drinking with sexual attractiveness, flirting, dating, meeting a good-looking new partner, and romance. Drinking, if advertising is to be believed, increases virility in men and sexual attractiveness in women. And underlying the theme of increased sexual attractiveness that drinking brings is the unstated assumption that if you drink, you will have more sexual encounters with more beautiful partners and that those encounters will be both more exciting and more satisfying. This culture's deep-seated belief that alcohol is an aphrodisiac is fully exploited by liquor advertisements. Very little is heard that counters that assumption.

Much of the power of advertising is dependent on individuals having been socialized into relatively rigid male and female roles (Forward, 1986; Logan, 1992). Without the seductive siren and the superbly confident "jock" as symbols of a much greater social reality, advertising would not work. A brief look at our sexual socialization will provide insight into the interactions between alcohol and sexuality.

The Sexual Socialization of Girls and Boys

Girls and boys are socialized very differently in our culture. Behavior considered to be appropriate for a boy often appears almost in opposition to the behavior expected of girls. Boys are encouraged, even expected, to be aggressive, physically combative, inexpressive of feelings, independent, autonomous, and externally oriented. Girls are socialized to be passive, demure, expressive of feelings, dependent, interrelated, and oriented toward maintaining relationships. Since the latest phase of the women's movement in the 1970s, much has been written about male and female socialization and its restricting and pernicious effects on individual lives (Hite, 1976). Even though parents may be concerned about the effects of cultural norms and may attempt to subvert them in their individual child-rearing practices, those norms still prevail in the culture at large (Covington, 1988).

Less notice has been given to the effects of the sexual socialization system. Both males and females are socialized to have different sexual expectations of themselves and of each other. These expectations place gender above individual differences. Boys are socialized to be much more familiar with some physical aspects of their bodies; because they routinely handle their penises, they become quite familiar with their erections and when they occur. They touch their genitals often and unselfconsciously. Boys are encouraged to learn about sex as adolescents. They are expected to know about sex before they get married; after all, they are responsible for making "it" happen (Harrison & Pennell, 1989; Richmond-Abbot, 1983).

Girls, on the other hand, are actively discouraged from touching themselves and from learning about sex (Schaffer, 1981). They are reminded repeatedly to keep their hands away from "down there," and their sexual ignorance is prized. Part of the value of a virgin is her lack of sexual knowledge, her naïveté, and her utter trust in her prospective husband to awaken her sexuality. A sexually uninformed male is scorned by his peers, but a sexually informed female is considered "wild" by hers.

Males are expected to be aggressive, to be the ones who choose whom they are attracted to, to ask out possible partners, to initiate sex, to produce an erection at the appropriate moment, and to make sure their partner is sexually fulfilled. All of the responsibility in this scenario is placed on the male partner. It is not surprising that performance anxiety is reported as the male's most common reason for sexual dysfunction (Harrison & Pennell, 1989).

In contrast, the female is socialized toward powerlessness in her sexual encounters. She is expected to be passive, waiting to be approached by the male. Women who are aggressive, signaling to men their sexual interest, may be branded "sluts" and "loose women," with many agreeing that although they may be fun in bed, one should not marry them (Schaffer, 1981). So women practice giving subtle indications of their sexual interest while avoiding being direct. So much punishment is meted out to the sexually direct woman in this culture that many women have a hard time knowing when they are sexually aroused. In the sexual encounter itself, women are expected to be oriented toward the male and his needs. Even though only 30% of women experience orgasm through intercourse (Hite, 1976), it remains the most preferred sexual activity of men and is considered by many to be synonymous with "having sex." So women experience themselves as relatively passive in the sexual encounter. They wait for men to ask them out, to initiate sex, to have erections, and then to make "it" happen. Women's power in this scenario is not one of action, but only one of being able to say no (Covington, 1988).

It is becoming clearer that such sharply divided roles in the realm of sexuality create severe sexual problems for both men and women (Richmond-Abbot, 1983; Schaffer, 1981). The breakdown in communication between men and women around sexuality is a major topic on talk shows, on the best-seller lists, and in women's magazine articles. Reactions to this breakdown range from the retreat into the "new celibacy" to an increased call for sexual restrictiveness from the religious right. Regardless of the reactions elicited by this breakdown, most people are aware that the present system of socialization around sexuality is no longer working well.

Male and female socialization dovetails with beliefs about alcohol and creates different reasons for drinking behavior reported by men and women. Men, on the one hand, generally report that they drink to feel more powerful and aggressive. Men's behavior while drinking confirms this experience; men typically act more aggressive and intimidating when they are drunk. Women, on the other hand, report drinking to feel more "feminine" and less shy (Goodwin, 1981; National Institute on Alcohol Abuse and Alcoholism [NIAAA], 1986). Women tend to be introduced to alcohol and drug use by a sexual partner, whereas men first drink and use with each other. Women also tend to continue securing their alcohol and drugs from a sexual partner, as opposed to men, who purchase their own supplies. Thus women tend to be romantically involved with their drug suppliers, a strong factor influencing women's treatment and recovery (Freeman & Landesman, 1992; Wilsnack, 1984). Women's marriage partners also tend to be alcoholic and addicted far beyond the usually stated 10% norm. A picture thus emerges of the alcoholic woman as someone who has her drinking/using life merged with her love/sex relationships.

The stigma against alcoholic women, on the one hand, often is expressed in sexual terms; alcoholic women are branded as sluts, promiscuous, loose, or "looking for it." Alcoholic women are assumed to be more sexually active and less sexually selective than nondrinking women (Covington, 1982; Wilsnack, 1984). The stigma against male alcoholics, on the other hand, rarely is expressed in sexual terms. Men find themselves chastised more for problems created on their jobs, for spending money on alcohol rather than supporting their families, and for getting in trouble with the legal system. The differences in social judgments about men's and women's drinking is but another reflection of the different places that men and women occupy in our society (Harrison & Pennell, 1989; Norwood, 1985). The earliest forms of sexual socialization occur in the family, and the alcoholic family is an especially important carrier of dysfunctional sexual socialization.

Sexual Dysfunction and Growing Up in the Alcoholic Family

Sexual dysfunction is often rooted in the alcoholic family, where early sexual behavior and sexual roles are learned. Over 50% of chemically dependent men and women were raised in alcoholic families. In those families, many will have seen sexual dysfunctioning modeled by their parents (Covington, 1982; Van Thiel & Lester, 1979). The denial about drinking that pervades alcoholic homes often invades the sexual arena too. The difficulty that parents, in general, experience in talking to their children about sex usually is compounded in the alcoholic home. Many children will grow up never having had consistent and age-appropriate discussions with their parents about sex. The message that is communicated is that sex is dirty, a totally private realm that is too upsetting and too difficult even to talk about, just like the alcoholism in the family. In contrast, sexual boundaries also may be violated. Children may witness inappropriate sexual behavior between their parents during and after a drinking bout. The codependent parent may use a child as a confidant, complaining about a spouse's sexual actions. The child may be expected to protect a parent from the sexually abusive behavior of a partner (Covington, 1982, 1988, 1991).

Parents may not only model dysfunctional sexual behavior but also express inappropriate sexual behavior with their children. Some children will have experienced inappropriate sexual behavior from their parents—for example, inappropriate nudity, seductiveness, or intercourse during a parent's drunkenness. During drunken rages, other parents may have hurled sexual epithets and slanders at the children (Pilat & Boomhower-Kresser, 1992). These are just some examples of inappropriate and abusive sexual behaviors that often occur in an alcoholic family.

Clinicians who come in contact with those recovering from chemical dependency will often need to help clients and families sort out the sexual legacy of their alcoholic families. Growing up in a sexually dysfunctional environment has lasting effects on a child's sexual development. Current sexual dysfunctions in the recovering chemically dependent person sometimes reflect the impact of the family of origin, and work on family-of-origin issues may be an important part of recovery.

ALCOHOL AND THE SEXUAL CYCLE FOR FEMALES AND MALES

Physiological Mechanisms Underlying Sexual Dysfunction

Whitfield, Redmond, and Quinn (1979) outlined five physiological mechanisms by which alcohol abuse may affect sexual functioning:

1. Acute depressant effects of alcohol on physiological sexual arousal
2. Disruption of sex hormone metabolism as a result of vitamin deficiencies and liver damage
3. Interference by alcohol-induced neuropathy with the sensory pathways of sexual arousal
4. Organic brain damage resulting in decreased interpersonal and sexual interest
5. Various medical problems secondary to alcoholism that impair sexual functioning, such as diabetes, hypertension, urinary tract infections, and vaginitis

In addition to the effect of alcoholism on the physiological mechanisms that underlie sexual functioning, my research indicates that sexual difficulties may precede and contribute to the development of alcoholism, at least in some women; 79% of alcoholic women (Covington & Kohen, 1984) reported that they had sexual difficulties before the onset of alcoholism. Women may be drinking as a way to medicate their sexual dysfunctioning, seeking pleasure and relief from sexual difficulties in excessive drinking. Needless to say, this strategy does not work, and these women reported even more sexual problems during their drinking phase.

Poor sexual functioning, then, may be both the cause and the consequence of alcoholic drinking, ending in an increasingly intense spiral of sexual problems. It seems clear that sexual dysfunction may contribute to excessive drinking and that excessive drinking may cause further sexual problems to develop.

The Sexual Cycle of Females

For most women, a lack of information about their own bodies extends to the sexual response cycle. In some recovery groups for women, only one out of every eight women reports having received her primary sex education from her mother, and even then most of the information imparted was about menstruation and reproduction (Covington & Kohen, 1984). Very rarely does a woman report having been told what would actually happen to her body during a sexual encounter. Some women report having learned about the female sexual response cycle along with reproduction in sex education class, and some women report learning from friends. But most women never have talked about what really happens to their bodies during sexual arousal and experience. Women, unlike men, do not compare their sexual experiences (Covington, 1982).

Misinformation about women's sexuality is only now being corrected. The first real observational data about women's actual sexual experiences were published by Masters and Johnson (1966). Their research finally laid to rest the "myth of the vaginal orgasm," as well as supplied information about various forms of female sexual experience. Masters and Johnson (1966) found that women basically experienced the same sexual response cycle whether they were touching themselves, using a vibrator, or having sex with a partner. In all cases, the clitoris was the center of sexual pleasure, and some direct or indirect stimulation of the clitoris was required for orgasm to occur. In the 1970s, Shere Hite (1976) published the first self-reports of women about their own sexual experiences. Of the women who responded to the Hite questionnaire, only 30% reported being able to achieve orgasm through vaginal penetration alone. Most women needed additional direct clitoral stimulation to achieve orgasm.

The Excitement Phase. The first stage in the sexual response cycle is arousal or excitement. As women move from desire to actually being touched, the response of the body is heightened. Some women can experience the excitement phase without being touched. Wanting another person, reading or watching erotica or pornography, or fantasizing may all bring on the bodily sensations of the excitement phase.

As women become excited, the clitoris and its surrounding tissues fill with blood and the clitoris becomes erect, retracting under its hood. At the same time, the vagina lubricates and expands. In its nonexcited stage the vagina has a very small opening, about the diameter of a pencil, but as a woman becomes more and more excited, the vagina opens up and balloons out. The uterus also becomes engorged with blood, enlarges, and rises from its resting position. The color of the outer and inner lips, clitoris, and vaginal walls deepens and becomes darker, duskier, or rosier. Blood pressure rises, the heart rate increases, and breathing becomes faster. All of the tissues surrounding and supporting the clitoris fill with blood and become swollen. The breasts and nipples also become swollen, and the nipples become erect. Sometimes the entire body exhibits a rosy flush and the woman feels sensations of warmth and flushing. The excitement stage in women may last from a few minutes to several hours. Generally this stage lasts much longer in women than in men; women take longer from initial arousal to plateau to orgasm than men do (Covington, 1982; Masters & Johnson, 1970).

The Plateau Stage. The plateau stage refers to the period between sexual excitement and orgasm. As women become more excited, the clitoris becomes more erect, the clitoral shaft becomes quite hard, the clitoral legs that extend inside the body along the vagina continue to engorge and become rigid, and the clitoral hood enlarges. The clitoris withdraws under the clitoral hood, and the Bartholin's glands within the vagina secrete mucus (Ladas, Whipple, & Perry, 1982). The vagina continues to lubricate and gets very wet. Lubrication may moisten the inner lips. Sexual tension increases, breathing becomes rapid, muscles rigidify, and the woman may break into a sweat.

The Orgasmic Phase. Orgasm occurs when powerful, rhythmic muscle contractions begin. The clitoris shortens dramatically, and the inner lips tuck in, covering it. All of the muscles surrounding the clitoris contract involuntarily, as do the vagina and the uterus. The contractions generally occur at 0.8-second intervals and often can be felt in the vagina, clitoris, uterus, and anus.

According to Masters and Johnson (1966), all orgasms are physiologically similar and are created by stimulation of the clitoris. The source of stimulation may vary; for example, friction may be applied via her partner's tongue, by her own or her partner's finger, by a vibrator, or by vaginal penetration and thrusting of the penis. Orgasms may vary in intensity and duration and certainly in the amount of time required to produce them, but physiologically what happens is the same. They occur because of stimulation of the clitoris—direct stimulation of the glans or indirect stimulation of the hood and inner lips, the shaft, or the clitoral legs that lie internally along the sides of the vagina. However, the contractions of the orgasm occur throughout the pelvic platform and are not felt primarily in the clitoris (Masters & Johnson, 1966).

For years, reports of female ejaculation were dismissed by scientists and sexual researchers alike, but in the 1980s the possibility of female ejaculation became more accepted (Ladas et al., 1982). Female ejaculation occurs when a clear, odorless fluid, ranging from a few teaspoons to 1 cup is released from the vagina during orgasm. In the past, many women were embarrassed by this phenomenon, thinking that they were urinating. But recent studies of the female sexual response cycle show that ejaculation can occur in some women as well as men. Release of the fluid seems to be more common in women when the G-spot is stimulated (Ladas et al., 1982). In addition, the fluid release can be self-inhibited; some women report that they can stop themselves from ejaculating if they try. Perhaps more women would report experiencing ejaculation if they did not hold themselves back because of fear of urination.

According to Ladas et al., (1982), the G-spot was named after Dr. Ernst Grafenberg, who wrote about it in 1950. However, little information was available about this additional source of female pleasure until the 1980s. The spot feels like a small lump that swells when it is stimulated. It is located toward the upper front wall of the vagina about halfway back between the pubic bone and the cervix. Although it is difficult to reach by a woman herself when she is lying flat, it can be reached easily by a partner's fingers, by a dildo, or by special attachments made for some vibrators (and sometimes by a penis when the woman is in the female superior position). Some women report that their orgasms feel deeper and more pleasurable when accompanied by stimulation of the G-spot. Other women report the orgasmic expulsion of fluid, the "female ejaculation," after G-spot stimulation (Ladas et al., 1982).

In women there is no refractory period between one orgasm and continued stimulation to the next orgasm. Women may be able to have multiple orgasms if they choose to be stimulated again. After the completion of one orgasm, they can resume stimulation and become orgasmic a second or third time if they so desire (Masters & Johnson,

1966). Often the glans of the clitoris is too sensitive to be touched, but the shaft and the inner lips may be receptive. Sometimes immediate restimulation may feel uncomfortable or painful, or having one orgasm may be sufficiently satisfying and fulfilling. Women often have felt shame about their ability or inability to ejaculate or to have multiple orgasms (Masters & Johnson, 1970). There is a great deal of variation among women, and the same woman's experiences may vary radically over the course of her life.

The Resolution Phase. Resolution occurs when stimulation ceases after orgasm or after plateau without orgasm. If orgasm does not occur, resolution may take place over a number of hours. With orgasm, resolution usually takes half an hour or so. In resolution, the body returns to its unexcited state. Engorgement recedes, the glans, shaft, hood, and legs of the clitoris return to normal, and the vaginal walls collapse again to form a small opening. The uterus returns to its resting state, and the color changes recede (Masters & Johnson, 1966).

Figure 8.1 shows various courses that the sexual response pattern may take in a particular woman. In Experience A the woman is touching herself. The time from desire through sexual excitement to plateau is fairly short, and orgasm is more intense. This is typical of the masturbation experience whether by hand, other forms of pressure, water, or a vibrator (Covington, 1986a; Masters & Johnson, 1970). When women masturbate, they can provide themselves with instant and perfect feedback. In masturbation women can touch themselves wherever they need to, with appropriate pressure, and as long as they need to. If something is not working, they can change immediately to something better. Most women, when stimulating themselves, come to orgasm more quickly and more intensely than they do in partner sex, although the subjective experience may be less intense.

In Experience B the woman is having partner sex. She becomes excited to plateau, then falls back to the excitement phase, then reaches plateau again, falls back to the excitement phase, reaches plateau, and then has orgasm. Experience B is not at all atypical of women's sexuality. Women generally take much longer to achieve orgasm than men do to achieve ejaculation. It is not unusual for women to get excited to the plateau stage, then get less excited, and once again become more excited until they reach orgasm (Covington, 1986a). For example, a woman's partner may touch her breasts and stroke her inner thighs until she gets very excited; then switch to stroking around the vaginal opening, which may be less exciting; then stroke along her inner lips,

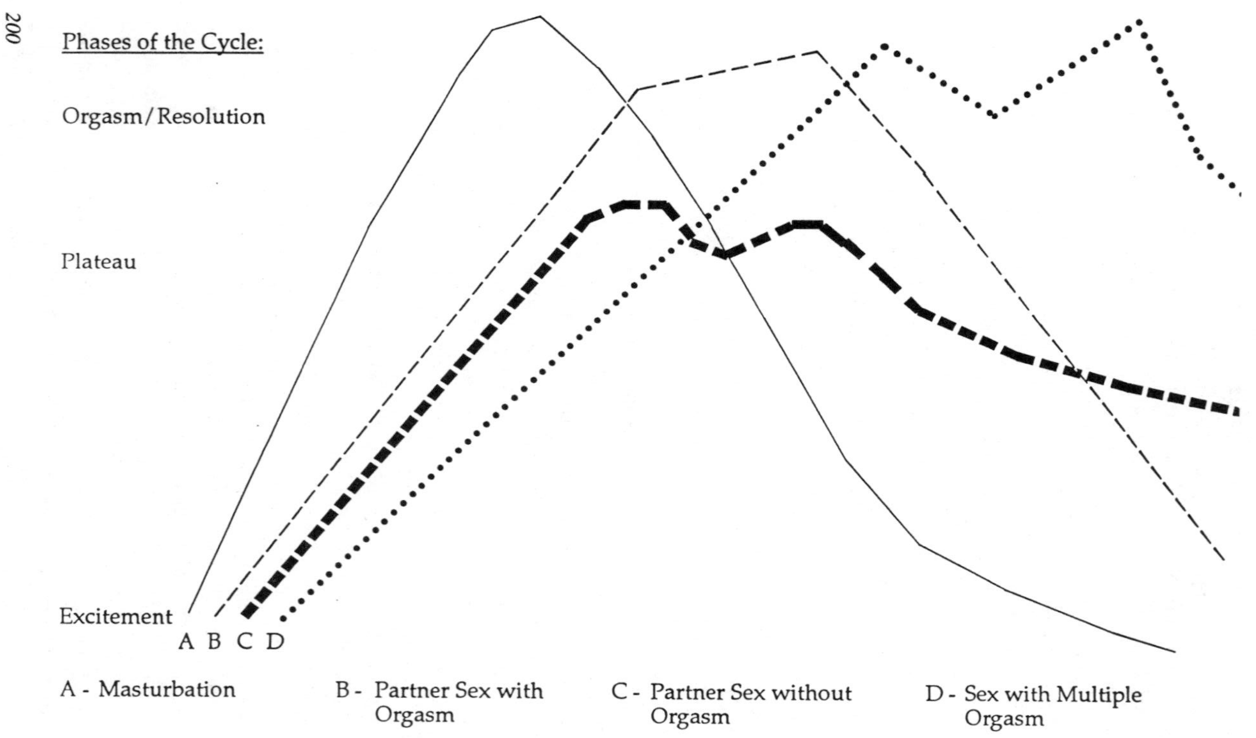

Figure 8.1. Female Sexual Response Cycle

which may be very exciting; then penetrate the vagina, which may be less exciting; and finally stroke along the clitoral shaft, which causes orgasm. Most orgasmic female sexual experiences tend to be less linear than the male experience. Rarely is there a direct line from desire through excitement to orgasm for women. Women's experience tends to lack the physiological inevitability that often characterizes male sexuality.

In Experience C the woman is having partner sex without orgasm. She gets excited, reaches plateau, and then falls back to the excitement stage again without coming to orgasm. In this case, resolution takes several hours because no orgasmic muscle spasms empty the pelvic area of blood congestion and swelling. This experience also is not unusual for women (Covington, 1986a). Some women find themselves unable to come to orgasm at all and repeatedly undergo Experience C. Some women find themselves undergoing Experience C only in certain circumstances, such as having sex when the children are still up, or only with particular partners, or with certain sexual techniques such as missionary position intercourse. Some women find themselves able to experience orgasm only when self-stimulated and not with a partner.

In Experience D the woman is stimulated to orgasm, then falls back to excitement, and then becomes stimulated to orgasm again. She is having multiple orgasms (more than one orgasm during the same sexual encounter). As mentioned previously, there is no particular period of time a woman must wait from having one orgasm until she can have the next (Masters & Johnson, 1966). For men, there is a period of time (refractory period), after the first ejaculation, during which it is physically difficult to get an erection and ejaculate again. This period lengthens with a man's age and may vary from a few minutes in a teenager to several days for a man in his 70s.

All of the above sexual experiences may occur in the life of any one woman. No experience is atypical or unusual. As women become more sexually experienced with age, they may shift from more instances of one experience to more instances of another, but it is not uncommon for women to continue to have a variety of sexual experiences throughout their lives. It is highly unlikely that women will have only one of the experiences described above.

Sexual Problems in Alcoholic Women

Experts estimate that approximately 50% of all Americans will report problems of sexual functioning during their lifetimes. That figure is even higher for alcoholics, both men and women. In my study of alcoholic women (Covington, 1982), only 55% of the recovering alcoholic women reported that they were satisfied with their sexual responsiveness at least half the time, as compared to 84% of the nonalcoholic women. Clearly difficulties with sexuality for alcoholic women extend beyond active drinking into sobriety.

The physiological effects of alcohol have a significant impact on women during their drinking phase. Alcoholic women experience more gynecological problems than nonalcoholic women. They experience more vaginitis and painful vaginal discharges. They experience more hormonal disruptions from the effects of alcohol, and they have more liver damage, which affects sexual functioning (NIAAA, 1986; Wilsnack, 1984). In addition, alcohol has a depressant effect on sexual arousal, as well as on other physiological mechanisms, creating lowered sexual desire. Alcohol inhibits vaginal lubrication, drying up the mucous membranes, making penetration less comfortable and sometimes even painful. Alcohol retards pelvic congestion, making swelling less likely to occur. With inhibited lubrication and retarded swelling, excitement to orgasm will take longer and will require more pressure, if it occurs at all. Alcohol also deadens sensory input, creating less sensitivity to touch so that these women require more stimulation to get the same effect (Covington & Kohen, 1984).

In sobriety, although these physiological factors are no longer operative, alcoholic women's sexual difficulties often continue. Alcoholic women consistently report greater sexual difficulties in sobriety than nonalcoholic women. They report lack of arousal, lack of lubrication, difficulty in coming to orgasm, lack of orgasm, painful intercourse (dyspareunia), and vaginal muscle spasms (vaginismus). Although they report fewer sexual problems in sobriety than during their drinking, they still report significant dissatisfaction with their sexual lives (Covington & Kohen, 1984).

Some of the continued sexual problems of women recovering from chemical dependency are attributable to their extensive histories of childhood sexual abuse, which is explored in more depth later in this chapter. Some problems may have existed prior to problem drinking and may have been exacerbated by the drinking. Some problems are attributable to a lack of experience with nurturing family relationships or to strict religious upbringing, lack of sexual information, lack of developing a satisfying, sober, sexual life-style before problem drinking began, and learned behavior that interferes with successful sexual experience (Covington, 1991). Alternative sexual behavior can be learned during sobriety, so women can have more satisfying sexual lives. They can acquire sexual information, become more familiar with their sexual responses, explore what kind of stimulation is effective for them, and become more assertive in asking for what they need.

The Sexual Cycle in Males

The sexual cycle in males is completely analogous to the female cycle. It is composed of the excitement, plateau, orgasmic, and resolution phases, all of which occur in the same order produced by similar biologic reflexes.

The Excitement Phase. In the male excitement phase, a vascular reflex causes the genital organs to become engorged with blood, similar to the engorgement of the pelvic structures in the female. The male experiences the engorgement as penile erection, which occurs within 3-8 seconds after direct stimulation. Males report, however, that they often have erections without any direct stimulation. Men are easily stimulated by visual and other sensory stimuli, with arousal leading to erection being fairly direct and quick. Although the time from desire to full erection in men lengthens as they age, the time is still significantly less than that for full lubrication and engorgement in women (Masters & Johnson, 1970).

In young men especially, erection may occur so easily as to be embarrassing. Men commonly report having erections from looking at erotic pictures, from touching a desirable woman, from watching others in erotic situations, and sometimes from even smelling a particular perfume. In addition to penile erection, the scrotal sac thickens, flattens, and becomes elevated, the nipples become erect, and the testicles elevate and increase in size. Other reactions reported in the description of the female excitement phase also occur: blood pressure rises, heart rate increases, and breathing becomes faster.

The Plateau Phase. As male excitement increases to the plateau phase, the penis becomes further engorged and increases in circumference. The testicles enlarge by 50%-100% and become fully elevated and rotated. Often the corona of the penis gets a purple flush, and the Cowper's glands secrete a mucous discharge. The skin becomes flushed, muscle tension increases, and hyperventilation occurs.

The Orgasmic Phase. In orgasm, contractions generally occur at 0.8-second intervals for three or four contractions, then slowing thereafter for two to four more contractions. Contractions occur in the penile urethra, the vas deferens, the seminal vesicles, the ejaculatory duct, and the prostrate. Ejaculation occurs in this phase.

The Resolution Phase. The resolution phase is characterized by loss of the penile erection, including a refractory period during which it is physically difficult for another orgasm and ejaculation to occur (Masters & Johnson, 1966, 1970). Some males have a sweating reaction during the contractions of orgasm, they may continue to hyperventilate, and the heart rate may reach 150-180 beats per minute.

Figure 8.2 shows the various experiences a man may have during the course of his sexual life. In Experience A the man is masturbating to orgasm. The line from the beginning of arousal to plateau is very steep, the plateau phase is short, and orgasm and ejaculation occur with a greater degree of physiological intensity than during partner sex.

In Experience B the man is having partner sex with orgasm and ejaculation. The excitement period is longer in duration than during masturbation, and orgasm and ejaculation occur with less physiological intensity.

In Experience C the man is having partner sex with premature ejaculation. In this case ejaculation occurs after a very short period of excitement and almost no plateau phase. Premature ejaculation is not as common a problem as retarded ejaculation for alcoholic men during their active drinking (Whitfield et al., 1979). The various physiological effects of alcohol combine to make orgasm and ejaculation more difficult to achieve. During sobriety, however, premature ejaculation again may become a common sexual problem.

In Experience D the man is having partner sex with a second orgasm and ejaculation occurring after a refractory period. In this case the man is young and the refractory period lasts less than an hour. After the refractory period ceases and before the resolution phase is complete, the man regains his erection and has another orgasm with ejaculation.

The most common difficulties experienced by men in sobriety—loss of sexual desire and erectile difficulties—are not represented on this chart. In both of these cases, erection is not achieved and penile penetration is either difficult or not possible.

Sexual Problems in Alcoholic Men

Both alcoholic and nonalcoholic men experience erectile dysfunction (impotence) with intoxication. As the alcohol level in the blood increases, males report decreased tumescence, increased latency to

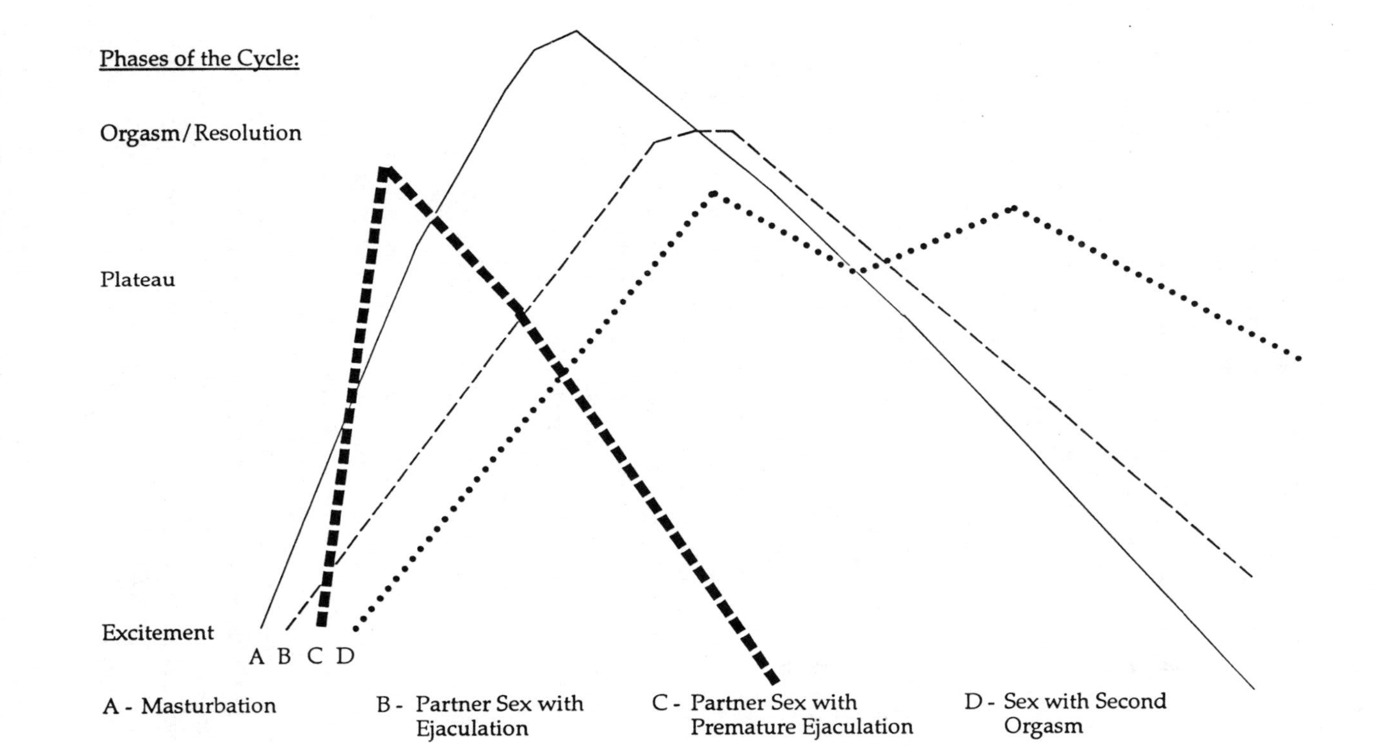

Figure 8.2. Male Sexual Response Cycle

orgasm (retarded ejaculation), and subjective reports of decreased arousal and orgasmic pleasure and intensity (Kaplan, 1979; Van Thiel & Lester, 1979; Whitfield et al., 1979). All of these physiological reactions are similar to those experienced by women. Men also report decreased sexual interest and desire as their alcoholism progresses, probably for the physiological reasons outlined above.

Like women, men do not automatically regain their full sexual functioning during early sobriety. After a year of sobriety, at least 50% of men can expect to have their ability to experience an erection restored and their tendency to retarded ejaculation ameliorated (Whitfield et al., 1979). The restoration of sexual functioning is more likely if sexual problems are talked about and sexual counseling is received so that performance anxiety is decreased (Kaplan, 1979; Masters & Johnson, 1970). It is important to reiterate that sexual behavior is learned behavior. The anxiety created by erectile dysfunction during chronic alcoholism easily carries over into sobriety, further impairing the sexual self-image.

The sexual socialization of men connects their ability to achieve an erection with power, potency, and virility. Masculine identity may be severely threatened when men are unable to attain erection consistently (Annon, 1975; Kaplan, 1974). Attaining an erection for men is analogous to lubricating in women, yet there is no similar stigma attached to women for lack of lubrication. In fact, lack of lubrication is viewed by society as a minor problem that can be resolved with a tube of lubricant from the drugstore. This is differential response to female and male sexual needs. These discrepancies must be considered as treatment strategies and planned and implemented.

A STRUCTURAL FAMILY SYSTEMS APPROACH

Chemical dependency treatment providers and counselors often avoid initiating discussions of sexual issues with their recovering clients. Just as society at large is characterized by lack of open communication around sexuality, treatment programs often leave sexual concerns unexplored. In addition, sexual issues rarely are mentioned in AA literature, and little discussion of sexuality takes place in AA meetings. This lack results in recovering clients feeling isolated with their sexual problems and unable to find a place where discussion of sexual issues is acceptable. Often clients do not realize that their problems are shared by the majority of recovering men and women. As cited earlier, most women report dissatisfaction with their sexual lives, and half of men in recovery experience difficulties in feeling sexual desire and achieving erections for at least a year after the onset of sobriety.

Many treatment programs have embraced the philosophy that work on sexual problems should be avoided during the first 6 months of recovery, when the emphasis is on maintaining sobriety. Although in-depth work on resolving long-standing sexual problems may need to be postponed until a solid foundation of sobriety has been established, other sexual tasks can be addressed by treatment programs and chemical dependency counselors (Covington, 1986b, 1991; Whitfield et al., 1979).

The PLISSIT model for handling sexual concerns, developed by Jack Annon of the University of Hawaii School of Medicine (1975), is especially appropriate for social workers and other treatment providers. P-LI-SS-IT refers to a 4-level approach for addressing sexual problems: *p*ermission, *l*imited *i*nformation, *s*pecific *s*uggestions, and *i*ntensive *t*herapy. The first three levels of the model can be used in brief therapy, in contrast to the fourth level, intensive therapy, which is a long-term process.

Theoretically each ascending level of the model requires increasing degrees of knowledge, training, and skill on the part of the clinician. Thus the model allows clinicians to match their approaches to their particular level of competence, as well as aids them in determining when referral elsewhere is appropriate (Annon, 1975). Due to the prevalence of presenting sexual problems by those in early recovery, treatment providers will want to ensure that their staff feel competent to handle at least the first two levels of the model: permission and limited information. In addition, they may want to make sure that at least one person on staff is qualified to provide specific suggestions, as well as referrals to a network of therapists who provide intensive therapy with sexual issues.

The First Level of Treatment: Permission

Sometimes people want to know that they are all right, that there is nothing wrong with them, and that their sexual behavior is not unusual. The clinician can let them know that they are not alone in their sexual concerns and that they are not unusual in their behavior. This level of treatment can be particularly effective in a group setting and is well suited for same-sex groups in chemical dependency programs in which family-of-origin and current family issues can be addressed. The peer support and relationship/boundary issues inherent in such groups then can be generalized to improved sexual relationships and family relationships outside of the groups.

In such a group, a series of sexual topics would be discussed, providing general information about the topic in a context of permission giving (Annon, 1975). For example, a women's group might discuss where women received their sex information. Permission would allow women to acknowledge that they know little about how their bodies work and the effects of early family attitudes about sexuality from socialization. That process of exploring early family experiences can reinforce that this is a common experience for women. According to Annon (1975), sometimes permission alone prevents future problems, as in the case when women then feel free to search out and read sexual information written specifically for them.

Permission can be used with clients in almost any setting as long as some form of privacy is available. In the course of reviewing a treatment plan, a client may mention that she is afraid of having sex when she is sober. The clinician can respond to that concern by saying that most alcoholic women have had the majority of their sexual experiences while drinking and that having sex sober is a common fear for women in early sobriety. Such permission giving can go beyond the acceptance of feelings to thoughts, fantasies, dreams, and even behavior.

In early sobriety one of the most common concerns will be lack of sexual interest and desire (Covington, 1986b, 1991; Kaplan, 1979). In this case the concern can be handled by giving the client permission not to engage in sexual behavior until he or she feels ready. Some work may need to be done with sexual partners who may not initially understand the need for a period of sexual abstinence. Permission can be given for clients both to engage in a wide variety of sexual behaviors and to refrain from a variety of behaviors.

It is important that clinicians be aware of their personal sexual value systems and not impose them on their clients. In addition, clinicians also need to be able to give themselves permission not to be experts and permission to refer to others with more experience. They need to be able to say they do not know the answer when they do not, a very useful modeling process for clients and family members who may be a part of the sessions at appropriate times.

The Second Level of Treatment: Limited Information

In contrast to permission, which is basically telling the client that it is all right to continue in what he or she has been doing or not doing, limited information provides the client with specific factual information directly related to his or her concerns (Annon, 1975). A typical concern that may be addressed by limited information is masturbation. For example, a woman in early recovery might come to her alcoholism counselor upset because she is no longer able to masturbate manually to orgasm in sobriety. She would express her fear that sobriety is affecting her sexuality in a negative way. Her counselor would tell her that most women are able to masturbate successfully to orgasm via vibrators due to their consistent and continuous level of stimulation. The information that the counselor would give is limited to the specific concern the client expressed, and it should be provided within a context that helps the client consider how the use of the information may affect his or her sexual partner or other family members. It is important that the counselor not launch into a general discussion of masturbation or indicate that worrying about masturbation is trivial compared to staying sober. The ability to give limited information depends on the counselor's breadth of sexual knowledge and comfort in sharing it with clients. Providing limited information is an excellent method of dispelling sexual myths. Common areas where providing limited information can be most helpful include breast and genital shape, size, and configuration, masturbation, penetration during menstruation, oral-genital contact, and sexual frequency and performance (Annon, 1975).

The Third Level of Treatment: Specific Suggestions

After giving permission and reassurance and providing limited information, some sexual problems may continue to persist. In contrast to giving permission and providing limited information, giving specific suggestions requires the clinician to have had specific training in sexual counseling. Annon (1975) noted it is also important that a sexual history be taken to guide the process of counseling. Without obtaining a history of the specific sexual problem, specific suggestions may only waste the client's time and may even compound the problem. The sexual problem history should elicit the following information: description of the current problem, its onset and course, the client's concept of the cause and maintenance of the problem, past treatment and its outcome, and current expectations of and goals for the treatment.

Specific suggestions are direct attempts to help clients change their behavior in order to reach their stated goals. It is unlikely that most counselors in a chemical dependency treatment program will have the time, knowledge, experience, and skills necessary to do sex therapy. A drug treatment program may decide to designate one staff person who attends trainings to gain skills in this area and related areas such as family-of-origin work or an intergenerational family systems approach.

The Fourth Level of Treatment: Intensive Therapy

Intensive therapy for a sexual problem begins with a comprehensive sexual history and continues with long-term individual sessions aimed at exploring and resolving problem areas in sexual experience. Although the sessions usually involve only the individual client, the Bowen's intergenerational family systems approach combined with structural is designed to help clients become more differentiated from other family members in individual sessions. This family differentiation process provides the foundation for an improved ego identity, boundary monitoring, and overall sexual functioning (Bowen, 1974). Intensive therapy generally is indicated for clients concerned with current and family-of-origin problems that have not been alleviated by previous forms of treatment. It is especially effective for problems of desire, sexually related low self-esteem, erection, ejaculation, orgasm, painful intercourse, and sexual abuse histories (Annon, 1975). Intensive therapy generally would be conducted by a therapist with special training in the sexual dysfunction. Rarely would such a person be on the staff of a chemical dependency program. It is important that treatment providers become familiar with the work of available therapists in their area and be able to provide appropriate referrals to clients and family members who require intensive therapy for their sexual problems. Follow-up coordination activities are often necessary between the referring clinician and sex therapist for consistency in goals related to sobriety, improved sexual functioning, and stronger family/social support relationships.

The PLISSIT model of treatment of sexual concerns is especially appropriate for chemical dependency programs and counselors. When put into practice, the model provides that all clients with sexual problems be given permission and reassurance. A significant portion of those clients will come back for something more and will receive limited information. A still smaller portion will return for more help and will receive specific suggestions either through the program's counselors or through a referral. Subsequently only those who really need intensive therapy will be referred for long-term structural/intergenerational family systems counseling.

Effective use of the PLISSIT model requires commitment on the part of chemical dependency programs and counselors to become knowledgeable about and comfortable with sex education, discussion of sexual difficulties, and the use of explicit sexual terms. It also requires a commitment to integrate the first level of treatment into the standard individual, family, or group process provided to such clients. Other problems, such as sexual abuse, require more specialized treatment.

SPECIAL ISSUES OF SEXUALLY ABUSED WOMEN

The high percentage of reported sexual problems among recovering alcoholic women is largely attributable to the extent of physical, emotional, and sexual abuse of women in general in our society. When compiling the results of my study that matched alcoholic and nonalcoholic women, the amount of abuse that women in this society experienced was shocking, while the survival skills and other strengths of the participants were reaffirming (Covington, 1982, 1986b).

Incidence of the Problem

Emotional abuse that included threats, verbal abuse, ridicule, degradation, harassment, yelling, jealous accusations, blame, lying, unfaithfulness, and withdrawal was reported by 71% of the alcoholic women and 44% of the nonalcoholic women in my study (Covington, 1986b). Alcoholic women reported greater frequency of emotional abuse and more chronic abuse of greater duration. Of those who emotionally abused alcoholic women, 57% were male; 64% of nonalcoholic women were abused by males. All of the emotionally abused women, both alcoholic and nonalcoholic, had experienced some instances of emotional abuse before the age of 10.

In this same study (Covington, 1986b), 51% of the alcoholic women reported physical abuse, compared to 34% of the nonalcoholic women. All of the perpetrators were known by the women, and 82% of perpetrators of abuse against alcoholic women were male, compared to 75% for nonalcoholic women. Fathers and stepfathers accounted for about 25% of the abuse against both alcoholic and nonalcoholic women. Abuse described included being hit (both with fists and with objects), slapped, thrown, spanked, and pulled by the hair. Alcoholic women also reported instances of beatings, black eyes, unwarranted surgery, fights, arm locks, drowning attempts, and police holds. Although all abuse is violent, the instances of physical abuse reported by the alcoholic women had a more violent quality about them. In the study, 74% of the alcoholic women and 82% of the nonalcoholic women had been physically abused by age 10.

At least one instance of incest, childhood molestation, attempted rape, or rape had been experienced by 50% of the nonalcoholic women. In all cases the abuse was perpetrated by a male. Alcoholic women experienced even more abuse; 74% percent had experienced some form of sexual abuse, and 93% of their abuse experiences were perpetrated by males. All of the alcoholic women who experienced sexual abuse had been violated at least once by age 10, compared to 65% of the nonalcoholic women (Covington, 1986b). Other researchers have reported similar incidence rates for women's experiences as victims of child sexual abuse and the alcohol involvement of their perpetrators (Pilat & Boomhower-Kresser, 1992).

Of the males who sexually abused alcoholic women, 86% were known by the women, 25% were male relatives, 19.6% were other known males including boyfriends, and 23.2% were unknown males. When the forms of abuse experienced by alcoholic women were compared with those experienced by nonalcoholic women, it was clear that alcoholic women have a wider variety of abuse perpetrators and that they experience more instances of abuse, more multiple incidents, and more chronic abuse of longer duration.

Clearly the emotional, physical, and sexual abuse of women is endemic in society. Even more frightening is the fact that all of the women who reported abuse in this study (Covington, 1986b) had been abused at least once by age 20. Not only is there a war on women, but that war also begins in childhood.

The amount of abuse experienced by alcoholic women has a severe impact on their sexual lives. Of the alcoholic women in the study, 71% had been emotionally abused, 51% had been physically abused, and 74% had been sexually abused. And most of the abuse had been perpetrated by family members and loved ones (Covington, 1986b). It is not surprising, then, that alcoholic women have difficulty expressing themselves sexually in intimate relationships. Clearly their intimate relationships in both childhood and adulthood have been fraught with violence and violation. Feeling desire and relaxing into arousal and orgasm require trust. Intimate relationships for alcoholic women, however, have been characterized by fear, not trust, since childhood. Treatment should be focused on addressing the fear and on the development of appropriate trust.

The Family-Focused Treatment Process

For women to be able to fully express their sexuality in a fulfilling way, they must be able to heal their abusive pasts, which often include abusive, nonnurturing family-of-origin relationships. Treatment programs and counselors both need to be aware of the extent of violence perpetrated against women, its devastating effect on intimacy and sexual expression, and the need for healing required for their eventual sexual health (Learner, 1986). Many women's drug treatment programs have started incest groups for women with 6 months or more of sobriety (Covington, 1986b; Covington & Kohen, 1984). Rape crisis centers now have groups for rape survivors who also have been addicted. Women's groups are especially important for abused women. In these groups focused on current and family-of-origin experiences, women gradually can come to recognize the extent of their own abuse, can lessen the isolation of feeling alone and/or crazy, and can learn to stop taking responsibility for abuse that was perpetrated by another. They may become empowered through these experiences and aware of the positive implications for survival. Many women choose to enter long-term therapy to continue work on their abuse issues after having been in a women's group. In this manner they are able to enhance existing strengths (such as their individual resiliency) and to develop other strengths (such as assertiveness in asking for what they need in current relationships).

The following case example illustrates this point:

Case Example

Barbara is a 29-year-old alcoholic who sought help in an alcohol treatment program after her second husband left her. Her first husband was also alcoholic. Although her second husband was physically and sexually abusive to her, she was devastated when he told her he was in love with someone else. She began missing work, and her alcohol consumption, already a problem, increased sharply. She entered an alcohol treatment program at the urging and support of her employer. In treatment, she blamed herself for the separation from her husband. She believed that her attempts to ask for more affection and support from him precipitated the separation. Although she was able to stop drinking through treatment and involvement in AA, Barbara continued to have self-esteem problems and to mourn the breakup of her second marriage, feeling that somehow she had failed. A relapse occurred after 3 months; it was frightening to Barbara, but it provided the impetus for her to share new information with the treatment counselor. Barbara mentioned that she had problems in her sexual relationships and that she had never had an orgasm. Barbara also shared reluctantly

> that she had been sexually abused by her father from the age of 10 until she was 13, when the parents divorced. She had never been able to tell her mother or anyone else about the abuse until the present time. The divorce was a bitter one, and she did not see her father after that point. He had threatened Barbara to "keep her mouth shut" because "it would kill her mother." She interpreted her mother's withdrawal after the divorce as a sign that she knew about the sexual abuse, blamed Barbara for the breakup of the marriage, and so rejected her. Much of her current behavior centered on trying to please family members: her mother, her husband, her children.

The process of treatment was used to help Barbara work through the pain of her mother's rejection and her father's sexual abuse, as well as her previously unacknowledged anger that neither had met her needs. As she gained some emotional distance from those events, she was able to begin the individuation process from her parents that was not possible in the past due to the sexual abuse by the father and the mother's rejection. A genogram was used to clarify intergenerational issues, sexual and in other areas, that encouraged Barbara to view herself as worthless. She also was helped to see that her husband's abuse and rejection repeated this cycle in her current life. A referral was made to a practitioner who was skilled in the area of intensive and long-term sex therapy, while the intergenerational family systems work was continued by the referring counselor. Barbara's alcohol treatment was considered to be effective when in aftercare she was able to maintain sobriety and admit that she had the right to ask for more than she had been getting in her second marriage (Beck, 1988).

Working through abuse issues is absolutely critical for the recovering alcoholic woman. Without coming to some form of sexual and family relationship healing, it is likely that she will return to self-medicating her pain, if not through drugs and alcohol, then through eating disorders, addictive relationships, and other forms of compulsive behavior often substituted for alcohol and drug abuse during sobriety. The extent of female sexual abuse makes it imperative that it be addressed openly in treatment programs. Just as issues that were first associated with male alcoholics, such as low self-esteem, have been incorporated into treatment programs, the inclusion of this most important issue for women is vital.

CONCLUSION

Throughout this chapter various roles have been discussed for social workers, sex therapists, and counselors in chemical dependency programs to better meet the needs of their sexually dysfunctional clients in recovery. The steps that need to be taken as part of these roles designed to enhance clients' strengths are summarized below:

1. Become aware of the interconnections and relationships around issues of chemical dependency, sexuality and sexual dysfunction, and nonnurturing, abusive family relationships.
2. Incorporate sexual issues into family treatment and group therapy sessions to enhance natural helping tendencies of family members and peers and in individual counseling programs.
3. Become aware of one's own sexual attitudes and beliefs and the need to refrain from imposing them on clients.
4. Create a referral network for sexual issues that goes beyond each practitioner's level of experience based on the model presented in this chapter.
5. Become aware of the special sexual issues of women, including the influence of female sexual socialization and the extent of sexual abuse.
6. Create women's groups that provide a safe place for women to begin to explore the connections between their addictions, family relationships, sexual abuse, and sexual dysfunctions.

Sexuality as a fundamental aspect of being is profoundly affected by alcoholism, but the spontaneous recovery of sexual health is not ensured by sobriety. It is up to treatment programs, chemical dependency counselors, social workers, and sex therapists to ensure that sexual issues are addressed during each client's recovery. The process can help develop a life-long pattern of viewing themselves and other women as resources to one another, thus enhancing their individual strengths and their family and peer support networks.

REFERENCES

Annon, J. (1975). *The behavioral treatment of sexual problems: Vol. I. Brief therapy.* New York: Harper & Row.

Beck, A. T. (1988). *Love is never enough.* New York: Harper & Row.

Bowen, M. (1974). Alcoholism as viewed through family systems theory and family psychotherapy. *Annals of the New York Academy of Science, 233,* 115-122.

Bowker, L. H. (1977). *Drug use among American women old and young: Sexual oppression and other themes.* San Francisco: R & E Research Associates.

Covington, S. S. (1982). *Sexual experience, dysfunction, and abuse: A comparative study of alcoholic and nonalcoholic women.* Doctoral dissertation, Union College Graduate School, Schenectady, NY.

Covington, S. S. (1986a, March/April). Misconceptions about women's sexuality: Understanding the influence of alcoholism. *Focus on Family, 6,* 43-44.

Covington, S. S. (1986b, May/June). Facing the clinical challenges of women alcoholics: Physical, emotional and sexual abuse. *Focus on Family, 10,* 37-44.

Covington, S. S. (1988). *Leaving the enchanted forest: The path from relationship addiction to intimacy.* San Francisco: HarperCollins.

Covington, S. S. (1991). *Awakening your sexuality: A guide for recovering women and their partners.* San Francisco: HarperCollins.

Covington, S. S., & Kohen, J. (1984). Women, alcohol and sexuality, In B. Stimmel (Ed.), *Cultural and sociological aspects of alcoholism and substance abuse* (pp. 41-56). New York: Haworth.

Forward, S. (1986). *Men who hate women and the women who love them.* New York: Bantam.

Freeman, E. M., & Landesman, T. (1992). Differential diagnosis and the least restrictive alcohol treatment. In E. M. Freeman (Ed.), *The addiction process: Effective social work approaches* (pp. 27-42). New York: Longman.

Goodwin, D. W. (1981). *Alcoholism: The facts.* New York: Oxford University Press.

Harrison, D. F., & Pennell, C. R. (1989). Contemporary sex roles for adolescents: New options or confusion? *Journal of Social Work and Human Sexuality, 8,* 27-46.

Hite, S. (1976). *The Hite report.* New York: Macmillan.

Kaplan, H. S. (1974). *The new sex therapy: Active treatment of sexual dysfunctions.* New York: Brunner/Mazel.

Kaplan, H. S. (1979). *Disorders of sexual desire and other new concepts and techniques in sex therapy.* New York: Simon & Schuster.

Ladas, A., Whipple, B., & Perry, J. (1982). *The G spot and other recent discoveries about human sexuality.* New York: McGraw-Hill.

Lerner, H. G. (1986). *The dance of anger.* New York: Harper & Row.

Logan, S. M. L. (1992). Overcoming sex and love addiction: An expanded perspective. In E. M. Freeman (Ed.), *The addiction process: Effective social work approaches* (pp. 207-221). New York: Longman.

Masters, W., & Johnson, V. (1966). *Human sexual response.* Boston: Little, Brown.

Masters, W., & Johnson, V. (1970). *Human sexual inadequacy.* Boston: Little, Brown.

National Institute on Alcohol Abuse and Alcoholism (NIAAA). (1986). *Women and alcohol: Health-related issues* (Research Monograph 16, DHHS Publication No. ADM 86-1139). Washington, DC: Government Printing Office.

Norwood, R. (1985). *Women who love too much.* New York: Pocket Books.

Pilat, J., & Boomhower-Kresser, S. (1992). Dynamics of alcoholism and child sexual abuse: Implications for interdisciplinary treatment. In E. M. Freeman (Ed.), *The addiction process: Effective social work approaches* (pp. 65-78). New York: Longman.

Richmond-Abbot, M. (1983). *Masculine and feminine sex roles over the life cycle.* Reading, MA: Addison-Wesley.

Schaffer, K. (1981). *Sex roles and human behavior.* Cambridge, MA: Withrop.

Van Thiel, D. H., & Lester, R. (1979). The effect of chronic alcohol abuse on sexual function. *Clinics in Endocrinology and Metabolism, 8,* 499-510.

Whitfield, C. L., Redmond, A. C., & Quinn, S. J. (1979). *Alcohol use, alcoholism and sexual functioning.* Unpublished manuscript. Baltimore: University of Maryland School of Medicine.

Wilsnack, S. C. (1984). Drinking, sexuality, and sexual dysfunction in women. In S. C. Wilsnack & L. J. Beckman (Eds.), *Alcohol problems in women* (pp. 189-227). New York: Guilford.

Chapter 9

SELF-MEDICATION AND THE ELDERLY

BRENDA CRAWLEY

Substance abuse among the elderly can be classified in several ways, ranging from cigarette use, alcohol abuse, use of illegal drugs, misuse or abuse of prescription medication/drugs, and/or misuse of over-the-counter (OTC) medications/drugs. Some authors even include caffeine or sugar addiction under the substance abuse umbrella. These latter substances, along with tobacco, are not addressed in this chapter. The use of illegal drugs by the elderly has received very limited attention in the literature and in research. Therefore not much is known about the use of those substances by the elderly, and for that reason they are not included in this chapter (Abrams & Alexopoulos, 1988; Gfroerer, 1987). Alcoholism among the elderly *is* included in the discussion due to a pattern in this population of combining alcohol with other substances or medications. Unlike many of the substances identified above, alcoholism among the elderly has received the greatest amount of attention in the research and treatment literature (Adams, Garry, Rhyne, Hunt, & Goodwin, 1990; Dupree, 1989; Gurnack & Thomas, 1989; Maypole, 1989).

This chapter examines why medication/drug misuse and abuse is an important problem in the elderly, distinguishes misuse from abuse including prescription and OTC medications, and then relates how those drugs are used by older adults for self-medication purposes. Alcohol misuse and abuse is addressed in terms of typical patterns of problem usage among the elderly. The role of physicians and other health care professionals is included in the discussion. I identify later-life family structures, dynamics, and interactions as they relate to medication/drug misuse and abuse and the role of the older person and family members when intergenerational family systems treatment is provided. Finally the implications for practice by helping professionals are summarized.

OVERVIEW OF ELDERLY DRUG MISUSE/ABUSE

Substance abuse among the elderly is unique when compared with abuse in other age categories because frequently abuse and/or misuse by the elderly is related to medications taken for a range of health conditions that surface in the later years of life. Cicirelli (1990) underscored the point that the health conditions that surface during later life are not necessarily *caused* by older age itself. Over a decade ago it was estimated that about "forty percent of older adults require at least one drug/medication a day to carry out the basic activities of daily living" (Chenitz, Salisbury, & Stone, 1990, p. 1). Cooper, Love, and Raffoul (1982) found that their aged respondents used an average of three medications per person. Thus benzodiazepines, antihypertensive agents, gastrointestinal medications, metabolic drugs, cardiovascular drugs, anti-inflammatory agents, sleep-inducing medications, and the like are high-use agents by older adults (Bernstein, Folkman, & Lazarus, 1989; Smart & Adlaf, 1988). In addition, older abusers frequently misuse and abuse OTC drugs for a variety of ailments. In contrast, young and midlife substance abusers' drugs of choice include marijuana, cocaine and its derivatives, and PCP. All ages are subject to abuse cigarettes and alcohol.

Why the Problem Is an Important One

There are several important reasons for concern regarding elder drug abuse and misuse. The obvious reason is that a person's quality of and satisfaction with life are considerably lowered by the ravages of any type of substance abuse or misuse, including medications, alcohol, and/or illegal substances. It is also the case that as individuals age, the loss of spouses, family members, friends, co-workers, and others of significance occurs and places additional stress on adjustment to the normal declines of aging. In addition, it is critical to consider the demographic trends that project that older people will increase from their current 12% of the population (approximately 27 million) to 32 million by the year 2000 and to approximately 17% by the year 2020 (Gurnack & Thomas, 1989; Raffoul, 1986). This increase means there simply will be many thousands more elderly persons needing programs and services—in short, a greater strain on resources.

Also, there are generally severe, persistent, and complicating reactions to medication/drug misuse and abuse (Bernstein et al., 1989; Weiss & Greenfield, 1986). Thus normative stress on the physical and mental health of the elderly is exacerbated when drug abuse/misuse is involved (Speer, O'Sullivan, & Schonfeld, 1991). Side effects of misuse and abuse create diagnostic and treatment difficulties for the medical profession and, in some cases, prolong the ill health of the misuser or abuser, with an accompanying strain on family members and their resources (Bernstein et al., 1989; Raffoul, 1986).

For all these reasons—quality of life, projected demographic increases, adverse reactions and side effects, and the human and financial costs of providing programs and services—society has a significant stake in dealing with medication/drug misuse and abuse among the elderly. In addition the toll on families and their members weakens the overall well-being of society as fewer citizens are functioning at healthy or optimum capacity (Banaszynski, 1992; Gurnack & Thomas, 1989). Restoring abusers and family members to more functional levels should be the overall goal of all treatment efforts.

Misuse/Abuse of Prescription Medications

A review of the literature and research reveals general consensus about the purpose of appropriate medication use and the characteristics of medication/drug misuse and abuse. Several sources initially address the purpose of drugs and proper medication/drug use as a forerunner to identifying patterns of abuse and misuse. It is necessary to recognize the former in order to identify and assess the severity of the latter. Chenitz et al. (1990) identified the general purpose of drugs as "to improve function, decrease discomfort and pain, and improve quality of life. In addition, drugs are used to manage illness or reduce the effect of an illness on the individual" (p. 1). When properly prescribed medications/drugs are taken according to instructions, then issues of abuse or misuse are moot.

If, however, there is intentional or unintentional underuse, overuse, improper use, or inappropriate prescribing by physicians, drug misuse has occurred (Chenitz et al., 1990; Raffoul, 1986). The concern for drug misuse among the elderly is heightened when the following sober statistics are considered (Bernstein et al., 1989; Chenitz et al., 1990; Raffoul, 1986):

Over 75% of today's 7,000+ drugs were developed within the last two decades.

Elderly persons use, on the average, about 10 drugs, while nonelderly persons use, on the average, about 3.4 drugs.

The elderly constitute only about 12% of the population yet account for 25% of all prescriptions for drugs.

The most prevalent type of drug misuse involves *underuse* of drugs, when the individual fails to take prescribed products or takes less than the quantity indicated, as illustrated by Table 9.1. *Overuse* is simply that—the person takes more than is prescribed, on the basis of his or her assessment of how much is needed, or doubles or triples the amount prescribed to make up for forgetting to take the medication at the designated time intervals (Bernstein et al., 1989; Gurwitz & Avorn, 1991). *Erratic use* involves bypassing the physician's prescribed schedule by time or day(s) and using the medication out of sync with the schedule. The dangers and consequences inherent in any form of misuse are as varied as the medication/drug side effects and individual reactions that are possible (Gurwitz & Avorn, 1991).

It is known that family members cannot always be present to monitor the schedule of the elderly person's medication needs. Family members are likely to notice the symptoms of drug misuse only when there are related emotional, intellectual, physical, behavioral, or other changes in the older person. Numerous authors recommend educating family members on how to recognize and monitor drug misuse and abuse among older family members and relatives (Schonfeld & Dupree, 1991; Weiss & Greenfield, 1986).

In contrast to the above definitions of *drug misuse,* "drug abuse is the use of a drug for other than the intended purpose, and in the elderly, may constitute extreme cases of drug misuse" (Chenitz et al., 1990, p. 1). Drug abuse by the elderly frequently revolves around legal, not illegal, drugs, but as Chenitz et al. (1990) pointed out, legal drug abuse is a serious problem for older people (see Table 9.1). Raffoul (1986) detailed the physiological, psychological, social, and socioeconomic factors leading to drug abuse and misuse by elders. Those factors include an increasingly high-risk health status and a decreasing ability

Table 9.1

Characteristics of Drug Misuse/Abuse Among the Elderly

	Patterns of Misuse and Abuse	*Potential Health Provider Influences*	*Potential Family Influences*
Drug Misuse			
Prescribed Drugs	*Underuse:* reduction of recommended amount due to side effects *Overuse:* doubling or tripling the amount to make up for failure to use at proper intervals *Erratic use*: changing the medication schedule (by day or times)	Inappropriate prescribing by physicians (not considering the use patterns, combined effects, or side effects of drugs for a particular individual) Failure to explore and monitor the regimen for a client by other health and interdisciplinary practitioners	Failure to monitor the purchase, medication schedule, or symptoms of drug misuse in a family member
OTC Drugs	Protracted use beyond amount or duration recommended	Failure to explore patterns in the use of OTC drugs, especially re combined effects	Same as above
Drug Abuse			
OTC Drugs	Combining contraindicated prescription and OTC drugs or substituting the latter for prescription drugs	Same as above	Failure to monitor the purchase, medication schedule, or symptoms of drug abuse in a family member
Legal and Illegal Drugs	Compulsive use of legal drugs for other than intended use or compulsive use of illegal drugs involving in both instances a physical and psychological addictive pattern to which all other functions and needs become secondary (e.g., alcohol or methamphetamines)	Failure to take a drinking or drugging history to determine the presence and severity of substance abuse problems and an appropriate medication regimen or contraindications	Same as above

to budget finances, keep bills paid on a current basis, and purchase basic resources such as an adequate supply of food.

Misuse/Abuse of Over-the-Counter (OTC) Drugs

Misuse and abuse of substances by older adults includes not only prescribed drugs but also OTC drugs and medications. Abrams and Alexopoulos (1988) reported that OTC drug use increases with age, particularly for women. In fact, due to economic factors, lack of trust in the medical profession, lack of transportation, and a need to maintain as much independence and control over their lives as possible, the elderly are very likely to seek out and use nonprescription medications to treat numerous health problems (Weiss & Greenfield, 1986). Use of aspirin, laxatives, digestive aids, cold remedies, and antihistamines is common. Protracted use in general becomes misuse with some serious consequences; this is even more true for OTC products whose combined use with certain prescription drugs is contraindicated. Examples of serious consequences include the following (Abrams & Alexopoulos, 1988; Kofoed, 1985):

Extended use of laxatives has been implicated in digitalis toxicity.

Prolonged use of aspirin involves difficulties such as aspirin-induced hypothermia.

A range of toxicities can occur from drug interactions with OTC medications and products.

Drug misuse from OTC products is especially difficult for family members to identify unless a member is responsible for purchasing and/or administering the products. Otherwise the elderly family member tends to use these medications in private and without assistance. The elderly will reveal their OTC misuse only as a last resort because so much is at stake in having or maintaining control over their health and finances. Some misuse occurs when older adults use OTC medications/drugs instead of prescribed medications and physician-rendered health care for financial reasons (Abrams & Alexopoulos, 1988; Weiss & Greenfield, 1986).

The Self-Medication Process

In addition to the factors above that can influence medication/drug abuse and misuse, older adults increasingly may begin to self-medicate with substances as a means of coping with the varying types of losses that confront them. Those losses include decreased functioning from their own aging processes; the deaths of spouses, friends, and sometimes children; economic stresses and decreased resources; involuntary or unanticipated early retirement; and possible reduction in physical and leisure-time activities (Abrams & Alexopoulos, 1988; Kofoed, 1985). Self-medication is also a way to gain control or to feel in control because the individual self-diagnoses, evaluates, and determines (prescribes) the ailment and its remedy.

During these times of later-life ongoing changes and, in some instances, personal crises in familial and interpersonal relationships and financial and business affairs, others are often the doers, the analyzers, and the prescribers. Thus the older adult seeks a domain of control along with a financially manageable means of coping with and adapting to the current stage in the life cycle (Kofoed, 1985). Also, the self-medication process may create an illusion that the individual is presently as functional as he or she was at a younger age in other important areas affected by the losses—for example, in the areas of physical activity and decision making (Abrams & Alexopoulos, 1988).

Family treatment for situations involving self-medication should be focused on helping the elderly person acknowledge, grieve, and cope more effectively with the losses, as well as find alternative sources of control that are less likely to impede healthy functioning (e.g., control over leisure-time activities or selection of peer supports). Schonfeld and Dupree (1991) recommended helping other family members understand the effects of losses and the need for control over some important aspects of their lives by older adults. Certainly encouraging the family and the older person to collaborate in finding some balance in the area of control can do much to open up and facilitate communication between them. It can help also to eliminate the complex reasons for self-medication and to enhance recovery in the elderly person (Maypole, 1989).

ALCOHOL ABUSE AND MISUSE

In addition to the problems of medication/drug abuse and misuse discussed in the previous section, alcohol abuse and misuse is a serious problem for some older adults. Alcohol abuse can involve self-medication as a way of coping with losses and other traumatic changes in later life, similar to the pattern of abuse that occurs with other drugs at that stage. "Roughly two-thirds of older alcoholics are early-onset drinkers, while one-third are late-onset drinkers" (Robertson, 1992, p. 28). Persons in the former group have abused alcohol for an extended period of their lives and oftentimes are cited as poor or high-risk candidates for successful treatment, while the latter are seen as having "an excellent chance for recovery" (Robertson, 1992, p. 28). Exact figures are not available for elderly alcohol abusers. It is known, however, that there is a lower rate of alcohol abuse among older adults relative to the rates for young or midlife adult alcohol abusers (rates for the latter have been estimated at 10%) (Graham, 1986).

Similarities and Differences in the Types of Abuse

Alcohol abuse among the elderly is serious whether it is early or late onset. In both types of alcohol abuse, the danger is exacerbated by the pattern of combining alcohol with other drugs and medications. Another factor is the difficulty involved in providing effective, age-appropriate alcohol treatment for two types of abuse that often have different consequences (Abrams & Alexopoulos, 1988; Schonfeld & Dupree, 1991; Smart & Adlaf, 1988; Speer et al., 1991). Schonfeld and Dupree (1991) noted, for instance, that their "early-onset subjects demonstrated the effects of a long-standing problem. They were intoxicated more frequently, experienced more severe emotional problems and experienced physical withdrawal symptoms more frequently" (p. 591).

In contrast, late-onset older adults tend to be stabler in terms of residence and have less severe emotional problems, although significant others perceive them as having *more* severe problems than early-onset abusers. Both types of abusers report similar stresses (e.g., cumulative losses and feelings of loneliness and depression), but the reduction of supports for late-onset abusers may be from recent losses that contribute to the abuse, while decreases in this area for early-onset abusers tends to be from others becoming alienated in reaction to the drinking over the years (Schonfeld & Dupree, 1991). The process of reestablishing social supports during family treatment may need to be addressed differently for the two types of abusers. For late-onset abusers, identifying new sources of support may be indicated. In comparison, early-onset older adults may need help in "mending" the ties with former supports (Schonfeld & Dupree, 1991).

Current and Future Consequences of Elderly Alcohol Abuse

A number of here-and-now consequences occur when older adults abuse alcohol. Family members are certainly more aware of alcohol abuse than they may be of medication/drug misuse or abuse (unless health symptoms are immediately revealed). Thus there are usually more opportunities for observing the elderly person's drinking behavior, especially in social situations involving family gatherings, peer interactions, church events, and other leisure-time activities. Family members and others who are in contact with older adults on a regular basis can observe more readily the effects of mood and behavioral changes induced by alcohol. But "closet drinkers" are more difficult to detect at any age (Adams et al., 1990; Maypole, 1989). Frequent falls, more than the usual forgetfulness, unexplained expenditures, and decreased appetite may be consequences of hidden drinking, as well as other conditions related to aging. The symptoms can signal the need for family members to explore the situation to determine what should be done in spite of the range of possible causes.

In addition to these current consequences for older adults and their families are some future consequences related to elderly alcohol abuse in general. Gurnack and Thomas (1989) identified five reasons for concern about "problem drinking in later life" (p. 642). First, the demographic trends point to increasing numbers of older persons. Second, it is expected that older persons in the future are much more likely to use social services than previous older cohorts, so there will be greater demand for services than currently. Third, trends among younger cohorts suggest there will be "fewer abstainers and more heavy drinkers," which indicates there will be larger future cohorts of elderly alcohol abusers. Fourth, there will be a need to develop more precise diagnoses of geriatric alcohol abuse. Fifth, the costs of treatment and intervention resources are extremely high and are expected to escalate in the future (Gurnack & Thomas, 1989, pp. 642-643).

THE ROLE OF PHYSICIANS AND OTHER HEALTH CARE PROFESSIONALS

Just as family members can have difficulties identifying the symptoms and consequences of an older person's medication or substance abuse, physicians frequently acknowledge similar difficulties in diagnosing such conditions. Kofoed (1985) indicated that doctors must have an "index of suspicion" in order to diagnose OTC abuse or misuse (p. 55). And Chenitz et al. (1990) suggested that prescription drug misuse or abuse among the elderly may stem at least in part from the physician's and other health professionals' behaviors, such as "(a) inaccurate diagnosis, (b) inaccuracies in drug treatment, (c) polypharmacy, including failure to consider drug interactions, and (d) deliberate overmedication, particularly in elderly institutionalized, psychiatric patients" (p. 6). In the same vein, Lamy (1983) identified similar contributory factors on the health provider's part, including the following (pp. 658-659):

Failure to consider and use other (nondrug) patient management procedures such as drug education or an external support person to administer medication as needed for health and safety

The use of inaccurate and inflexible diagnoses

The related use of inaccurate treatment(s)

Prescribing without consideration of drug interactions

Overmedication without monitoring drug effects

Failure to consider patient characteristics such as attitude and extent of available social supports

Failure to consider the patient's life-style and quality of life

Failure to give clear patient instructions

Family members, as much as the elderly abuser, bear the consequences of the health care professional's intentional or unintentional contributory behaviors. Even when family members accompany the elderly patient to the doctor's office or health care facility, they may or may not be able to elicit sufficient information from physicians and other medical personnel to assist the older family member in following the prescription. It certainly has been pointed out that physicians spend very little time in discussions with patients in general (Weiss & Greenfield, 1986). Increasingly medical schools are seeking ways to train doctors in how to spend productive time attending to and discussing patients' concerns and their questions regarding their health, medical condition, and care (Kail, 1989). Other helping professionals such as social workers, psychologists, and gerontologists can assist family members in eliciting needed medical and social information for preventing and resolving substance abuse among the elderly. An understanding of the important dynamics and roles among family members and older adults is essential for facilitating this process and addressing other high-risk conditions that confront individuals at this stage of the life cycle.

LATER LIFE FAMILY DYNAMICS AND ROLES

Later Life Dynamics

In later life, older adults face many positive as well as negative experiences. Positive later life experiences may include (a) launching the last child from the home nest, (b) finding work or career plans unfolding as anticipated (these may involve either upward, lateral, or downward activities—whichever is desired), (c) maintaining or improving a functional marriage, (d) having sufficient friendships and social relationships, (e) having adequate or better financial status, and (f) possessing good or better health based on the individual's definition of *health*. Negative or distressful experiences may include the opposite of those listed above—for example, (a) adult children can remain in the home longer than is desired by the older parents; (b) work and career plans may not be realized if involuntary or forced early retirement is necessary; (c) the spouse, relatives, kin, friends, and co-workers may die, thereby shrinking the valued relationship pool that was anticipated while growing older; (d) there may be financial downturns or not as much money for the retirement years as anticipated; and finally (e) the diminishment or loss of physical or mental health can signal potential or actual loss of autonomy and possible lowered self-esteem.

Intergenerational Family Dynamics and Roles

In addition to the above later life dynamics associated with diminished physical and mental health, older persons encounter the health care system and health care professionals who provide diagnoses and treatment that significantly impact and shift the nature and dynamics of family life (Brubaker, 1990). Cicirelli (1990) emphasized that a great part of the impact and shift occurs as spouses and family members assume some or most measures of responsibility for care and for monitoring the health needs of the older family member. Certainly level and type of care will vary by the nature and severity of the health and medical needs of the older adult. But whatever the illness, condition, or disease, in response to drug misuse or abuse, the spouse, family members, kin, or other caretakers may need to employ similar types of assistance to the older person. By understanding some important intergenerational dynamics in later life families, the appropriate type and level of caregiver assistance can be identified more readily.

Brubaker (1990), Cicirelli (1990), and Kail (1989) identified several common elements of intergenerational family relationships and dynamics in later life that can affect the family's role, as well as the assistance that is provided for addressing the older person's drug abuse or misuse. First, families with elderly members share lengthy family histories (Brubaker, 1990). Out of these experiences, they usually have determined the family roles that govern their interactions and behaviors: These include primary roles such as scapegoat, mascot, helper, mediator, and placater. They have developed various ways and styles of handling or not handling conflict, anxiety, stress, and emergencies. Moreover, later life families have, to some extent, worked out a family support network. This network means that family members often "look out after each other's welfare," such as "when an elderly family member engages in self-destructive behaviors, for example, smoking, poor diet, or lack of exercise, others in the family typically urge the individual to modify the behavior in question. They may exhort the older person to watch his or her diet, . . . get a medical check-up, and/or take prescribed medication" (Cicirelli, 1990, pp. 213-214).

A third common dynamic is that later life families have both worked out and continue to work on providing psychological support for and to family members. In these families, communication patterns (for good or ill) have been well established. Such patterns can facilitate or hinder the older family member's correction of medication/drug abuse or misuse. On the one hand, in some families, adult children do listen to elderly parents' "symptoms and complaints and show concern" (Cicirelli, 1990, p. 215). On the other hand, in other later life families, parents are not comfortable discussing these health concerns or they fear a loss of self-esteem and maybe even autonomy if they share those concerns with their adult children (Rathbone-McCuan & Hashimi, 1982).

In speaking directly to ways in which families with elderly members can provide support, Cicirelli (1990) identified the following kinds of support (which could be expanded and applied in family treatment sessions involving psychoeducation and assigned homework tasks for various members):

Preventive and anticipatory care
Lay consultation
Mediation when conflicts or a lack of clarity exists
Psychological support

Crisis response and acute care

Long-term care

Bereavement and grief sharing

Attention to indicators of the need to vary family support due to changes that occur over time

Support from among different family members

Kail and Litwak (1989) identified four key areas in which family, friends, and neighbors can play a role in preventing the misuse of drugs and in assisting in patient compliance with physician's instructions:

1. Ensuring the elderly person's understanding of the doctor's directions
2. Making certain the medications are purchased
3. Encouraging the person to follow the regimen
4. Helping the person handle side effects as appropriate

The types and levels of helping vary among the four primary sources of support identified by Kail and Litwak (1989): spouse, kin (sons and daughters, grandchildren, nieces and nephews), friends, and neighbors. Because the relationship of the older person varies among these groups, each will provide assistance in the four areas above on the basis of the structure and dynamics of the specific type of relationship. For example, for providing assistance in the elderly person's understanding of the physician's directions, Kail and Litwak (1989) suggested that because of age proximity, a spouse may be functioning at a similar level of communication and comprehension as the patient and thus may be *somewhat helpful* in this area. In contrast, a son or daughter may be *especially helpful* because he or she is not as likely as a spouse to be impaired. One result might be that, when possible, the son or daughter would take the parent to the doctor's office or medical facility and assist in helping him or her to understand the medication directions.

Kail and Litwak (1989) saw all but the friend category as being *very helpful* in ensuring that medicine was purchased, whether the assistance was in the form of actually purchasing and/or paying for the products. Friends certainly can provide *low to moderately helpful* assistance, depending on several factors, including time availability. Monitoring the regimen can be easier for a spouse who is nearby than for kin who live far away. Although telephone contact can bring a level of monitoring, neighbors can assist with on-the-spot, short-term monitoring, whereas friends, depending on the length and nature of the friendship plus their proximity, can provide either long- or short-term assistance to help the older person follow his or her regimen.

Kail and Litwak (1989) further identified whether the spouse, kin, neighbor, or friend has observed directly the side effects as the criterion that determines whether they will be helpful to the older person in handling those side effects. These are some very specific ways in which family structure, support networks, and members' roles can assist older substance misusers or abusers in taking preventive or corrective action to end inappropriate behaviors. Others in the support network, such as kin, friends, or neighbors, also have roles to play in helping correct medication/drug misuse or abuse in the older person. An additional advantage in using these resources during treatment is that they will continue to be present in the environment after treatment ends to provide supports to older adults and their families

CASE ILLUSTRATION: LATER LIFE SUBSTANCE ABUSE

The later life family dynamics identified in the previous section suggest that some substance abusers could benefit greatly from a combined intergenerational and strategic family systems approach to behavior change. Understanding the dynamics of the later life family developmental cycle, social workers and other helping professionals can use as part of treatment the shared family history, family rules governing interactions and behavior, established functional roles between and among members (particularly the cross-generational roles), and the established functional patterns of handling conflict, anxiety, stress, and crises (Hartman & Laird, 1983).

Overview of the Case Example

The case example below illustrates how some of the above factors can be useful to helping professionals in assessing and intervening with an intergenerational and strategic family treatment approach.

Case Example

A 72-year-old woman, Lillian Scott, was being treated for a severe case of hypertension. Her 43-year-old daughter, Pat Dillard, usually took her to the doctor's office. She also called and checked on her parents every other day by telephone; she usually visited them about once every 2 weeks. During the last 2 months, she had noticed that her mother had seemed lethargic, appeared to have difficulty following conversations, complained of headaches, and was losing weight. She initially attributed most of these things to what she considered to be normal signs of aging, but on her last visit, she noticed an unopened bottle of her mother's prescribed medication for hypertension with the previous month's date. At first she had simply thought that her mother may have purchased a new bottle while finishing up an old one. When she visited a few weeks later, she found the bottle still only partially used. She spoke with her mother about her medicine regimen. Ms. Scott explained that because she had made some dietary changes, she believed she could take less of her medicine, which often made her dizzy. The daughter became alarmed because she knew hypertension could be a silent killer. Ms. Dillard spoke with her father, Earl Scott, and asked whether he knew about the mother reducing the prescribed dosage of her medicine. He indicated that he did not know about it. He responded by saying, "You know your mother will do the right thing as she always does. She's just trying to figure out how to take the medicine." While Ms. Scott appreciated her daughter's concern, she was confident that the side effects she was feeling were temporary and that as her diet improved, they would disappear. She told her daughter, "I am an adult and know what's best for me, and besides, the doctors don't know everything!"

Although the daughter acknowledged to herself that she and her mother had disagreed in the past about values and ways to problem-solve, they had not had previous conflicts over the mother's medical care. Recently, however, the mother had seemed more "defensive" about what was best for her and Mr. Scott in terms of their overall health. The daughter knew that her mother attended some of the activities at a neighborhood senior center on Tuesdays and Thursdays. She called and asked whether anyone at the center could assist her in convincing her mother to see the doctor about this matter. A social worker returned her call later that day. Ms. Dillard explained the situation and made an appointment to see the worker.

The Assessment and Family Treatment Process

When they met, the worker and the daughter scheduled a time for the mother to meet with them on the following Tuesday. The worker validated the daughter's concerns and encouraged her to call the doctor's office and inform the doctor of the situation. The doctor's nurse agreed that it was important for Ms. Scott to come in for a reevaluation. Then the daughter and social worker role-played three possible scenarios that might be used by the daughter to convince Ms. Scott to go for a medical appointment (here the worker used the family treatment strategies of role rehearsal and homework assignments). The three scenarios grew out of the worker's exploration of the cross-generational communication patterns between the mother and daughter. The practitioner also explored with Ms. Dillard the family dynamics usually involved in dealing with conflict and stress between the parents and between them and the daughter, especially the mother. Ms. Scott often would argue or seem not to listen to her daughter's suggestions. Sometimes she later would follow the suggestions, but she tended also to do the opposite if she was sufficiently angry with the daughter.

The three role-play scenarios were designed to illustrate how those family dynamics might affect the present issue. The scenarios were role-played in the following sequence: (a) The daughter spoke to the mother and directly asked her permission to schedule an appointment with the doctor, (b) the daughter informed the mother that she had spoken with the nurse and that the nurse would call the mother on a certain date and time to schedule an appointment, and (c) the daughter told her mother that she had scheduled an appointment for her on Tuesday at the time she normally goes to the senior center (as this meant the mother would be available) and would pick up and take her to the doctor's office. The worker role-played the mother in each scenario while Ms. Dillard played herself.

During their discussion following the role plays, the worker and Ms. Dillard analyzed the different levels of freedom and control involved in each scenario for Ms. Scott. The homework assignment that Ms. Dillard agreed to included deciding which strategy she judged to be the most effective, based on her family's rules for interaction, acceptable behaviors, and appropriate support. Then she was to use whichever strategy she selected to gain her mother's agreement to schedule a medical appointment. By assigning these homework tasks to the daughter and by not assuming any course of action to be more or less desirable than the other, the practitioner demonstrated respect not only for the client's right to self-determination but also for the family's history of interactions and supportive behaviors as addressed in the previous section.

In addition, Ms. Dillard is working on what Cicirelli (1990) identified as providing temporal changes in family support to facilitate greater assistance as may be needed over time. This latter point underscores the intergenerational concerns and issues that now confront this family. Issues include (a) what will be the appropriate role for the adult daughter to assume in relation to her aging mother's medication abuse and to the father's diminished ability to monitor both his and the mother's medical regimen, (b) what information the daughter must gain regarding the aging process in order to effectively assist her mother and perhaps eventually her father in these areas, and (c) what should be the appropriate configuration of support among immediate/extended family members and other social networks?

The doctor's tests and diagnosis revealed that the dietary changes had not sufficiently altered the mother's hypertension condition to reduce or eliminate the medication. Ms. Dillard explained to him how adamant the mother was to use the diet as part of her "cure." The doctor explained to her that he could only provide the facts and underscore the importance of the prescription being followed. The visit with the doctor was followed by a joint visit to the practitioner's office a few days later. During the discussion with Ms. Scott and Ms. Dillard, the worker acknowledged the mother's need to regain control of her life, specifically her health. She pointed out it was clear that Ms. Scott had always enjoyed excellent health, had eaten nutritious meals, and exercised in moderation.

Ms. Scott said she could hardly believe her medical condition; she even thought the doctor could be exaggerating the seriousness of her condition. She always had control in this matter—she had even continued coming to the senior center. She was not going to submit to just growing old, getting in a rocking chair, and dying. She expected her daughter to understand this and to help her remain independent. Ms. Dillard was quite surprised to hear her mother's experience and view of the situation. To her it had been a simple matter of following the doctor's orders.

The practitioner worked with the daughter to help her become more knowledgeable about the losses and the family dynamics involved in handling the mother's aging processes. She also helped Ms. Dillard identify the cross-generational and paradoxical role she could have as an adult child to the mother in this noncompliant situation—that is, helped Ms. Dillard see that she could refrain from controlling the situation by facilitating the mother remaining in control. This role might mean enhancing her mother's understanding of the doctor's directions, making certain the medication is purchased, encouraging her to follow the regimen, and/or helping her handle the side effects. Discussion with the mother resulted in an agreement to follow the prescription for 4 months while still engaging in the dietary modifications (the strategy of reframing based on the strategic family systems approach). This approach supported the doctor's recommendation that the mother continue the good changes she had initiated. The mother agreed to let the practitioner know on Tuesdays and Thursday, while she was at the center, whether she had followed the prescription. Ms. Scott reluctantly agreed to let her daughter ask her about whether she was taking the medicine daily (this could be done through telephone calls every other day) if and only if the daughter did not nag or hassle the mother. Again the mother reiterated that she was an adult and could take care of herself.

The practitioner asked how her husband and grandchildren might "help" her. She occasionally saw her 24-year-old grandson and saw her 21-year-old granddaughter every Sunday afternoon, as she always stopped by for an hour or two to visit after church. Ms. Scott indicated that because Earl, her husband, was at home daily, he could check on her taking the medicine. She decided that she did not want her grandchildren burdened with her problem and wanted to keep those relationships conflict-free. Both grandchildren were currently supportive, and she did not want to lose their voluntary involvement with their grandparents.

The worker thought that the agreed-on plan likely would work. She contracted to see Ms. Dillard for several additional sessions, as the latter wanted to know more about the aging process as well as how to appropriately shift her interactions and role with her parents in their later years. The daughter also wanted help in handling unfinished family issues between her and the mother, who she hoped would accompany her to a few sessions with the practitioner. She was concerned about not putting her son and daughter, with whom her mother had a good relationship, in the middle of her conflicts with Ms. Scott over the medication abuse and control issues.

The Role of the Older Adult

Although a number of family members were involved in this case example, the key role is that of Ms. Scott as the older adult. Both she and her husband use alcohol moderately. Increasing the couple's and daughter's understanding of substance abuse and eliminating Ms. Scott's medication misuse can prevent the likelihood that either parent might become vulnerable to late-onset alcoholism as aging leads to additional losses for them. However, as Chenitz et al. (1990) and Lamy (1983) pointed out, medication/drug misuse and abuse is not the sole responsibility of the older person. On the one hand, if inadequate or inappropriate instructions are provided or if the health provider is not patient in answering questions and ensuring that the older person understands, the provider bears responsibility for any failures in carrying out the regimen.

On the other hand, though, are some areas of responsibility that the older person must be educated about by helping professionals, as Ms. Scott was in this case situation. These responsibilities include asking for additional information when the health provider's instructions are not clear, monitoring and reporting side effects, following the recommended schedule and amount in taking the medicine, avoiding the use of outdated drugs, and reporting the use of OTC products so that these can be considered in the diagnosis and recommended treatment.

The amount and frequency of alcohol use should be shared also with the physician at the time medications are being prescribed, as well as any changes in the pattern use. In this way the physician can decide whether there is any danger of the alcohol use interacting with or hindering the effects of the prescribed drugs. Moreover, there is a need to avoid the use of multiple physicians and pharmacies, except as recommended, because this multiplicity makes it more likely that incompatible and dangerous combinations of drugs will be prescribed. Finally, when more than one physician is involved, the older adult and the family members should keep each physician informed of the medication/drug products being prescribed by other sources (Chenitz et al., 1990; Kail, 1989; Lamy, 1983).

CONCLUSION

A number of implications can be inferred for helping professionals from this discussion about substance abuse among the elderly. As stated, there are several reasons why abuse in this population group is important. These reasons include quality-of-life factors, projected demographic increases in the population, adverse reactions and side effects, and the costs to society of providing programs and services to address the problem. In some practice settings, helping professionals can be effective in the work to correct medication and drug abuse. For example, the settings include general and VA hospitals, family programs that serve older adults, home health care and support programs, senior centers, and institutional programs such as nursing and retirement homes. One implication is that helping professionals in those settings should possess sufficient knowledge and skills related to systems theory, the aging process, and substance abuse to intervene with older adults, their families, and other helping professionals.

Another implication is the need for those professionals to assume a variety of roles, including that of outreach worker, broker, advocate, teacher, behavior change agent, consultant, and administrator (Johnson, 1986). In the *outreach* role, social workers and gerontologists can help identify older persons in the community who are either at risk or potentially at risk for noncompliance in medicine intake and other forms of substance abuse. As *brokers,* helping professionals can connect the older person who is experiencing difficulties in compliance to other health providers who then can assist in developing plans for self-monitoring their medication compliance. Whether targeting outpatient or inpatient services, the practitioner as an *advocate* must strive to help the elderly abuser gain adequate information and educational services about substances.

In the role of *teacher,* the practitioner could, after proper orientation and training and in conjunction with other health professionals, teach older adults and family or social supports the importance of following the medicine regimen and skills in obtaining appropriate information regarding medical care. The *behavior change agent* role might involve engaging the client and family in family treatment focused on behavioral changes necessary to support recovery. As a *consultant,* the helping professional can work with a multidisciplinary team to ensure that each understands the issues of substance misuse and abuse among the elderly, along with the concerns of family members and other caregivers. Finally, as *administrators* of programs that directly or indirectly impinge on the lives of older persons, another implication is that such programs will need to be modified at a policy level to reduce the problem of elderly substance abuse. This type of structural change is as necessary as the intergenerational and strategic change strategies that have been discussed in this chapter in regard to families. Support for both types of change activities and the practitioner roles identified above can be found in the growing literature that underscores the seriousness of this problem (Kail, 1989; Raffoul, 1986; Rathbone-McCuan & Hashimi, 1982).

REFERENCES

Abrams, A. C., & Alexopoulos, G. S. (1988). Substance abuse in the elderly: Over-the-counter and illegal drugs. *Hospital and Community Psychiatry, 39,* 822-823, 829.

Adams, W. L., Garry, P. J., Rhyne, R., Hunt, W. C., & Goodwin, J. S. (1990). Alcohol intake in the healthy elderly: Changes with age in a cross-sectional and longitudinal study. *Journal of the American Geriatrics Society, 38,* 211-216.

Banaszynski, J. (1992). Ties that blind: Facing up to the family secret. *Modern Maturity, 35,* 32-36, 64.

Bernstein, L. R., Folkman, S., & Lazarus, R. S. (1989). Characterization of the use and misuse of medications by an elderly, ambulatory population. *Medical Care, 27,* 654-659.

Brubaker, T. H. (1990). An overview of family relationships in later life. In T. H. Brubaker (Ed.), *Family relationships in later life* (pp. 13-26). Newbury Park, CA: Sage.

Chenitz, W. C., Salisbury, S., & Stone, J. T. (1990). Drug misuse and abuse in the elderly. *Mental Health Nursing, 11,* 1-16.

Cicirelli, V. (1990). Family support in relation to health problems of the elderly. In T. H. Brubaker (Ed.), *Family relationships in later life* (pp. 212-228). Newbury Park, CA: Sage.

Cooper, J. K., Love, D. W., & Raffoul, P. R. (1982). Intentional prescription nonadherence (noncompliance) by the elderly. *Journal of the American Geriatrics Society, 30,* 329-333.

Dupree, L. W. (1989). Comparison of three case-finding strategies relative to elderly alcohol abusers. *Journal of Applied Gerontology, 8,* 502-511.

Gfroerer, J. (1987). Correlation between drug use by teenagers and drug use by older family members. *American Journal of Drug Alcohol Abuse, 13,* 95-108.

Graham, K. (1986). Identifying and measuring alcohol abuse among the elderly: Serious problems with existing instrumentation. *Journal of Studies on Alcohol, 47,* 322-326.

Gurnack, A. M., & Thomas, J. L. (1989). Behavioral factors related to elderly alcohol abuse: Research and policy issues. *International Journal of the Addictions, 24,* 641-654.

Gurwitz, J. H., & Avorn, J. (1991). The ambiguous relation between aging and adverse drug reactions. *Annals of Internal Medicine, 114,* 952-965.

Hartman, A., & Laird, J. (1983). *Family-centered social work practice.* New York: Free Press.

Johnson, L. C. (1986). *Social work practice: A generalist approach* (2nd ed.). Boston: Allyn & Bacon.

Kail, B. L. (1989). Drugs, gender and ethnicity: Is the older minority woman at risk? *Journal of Drug Issues, 19,* 171-189.

Kail, B. L., & Litwak, E. (1989). Family, friends, and neighbors: The role of primary groups in preventing the misuse of drugs. *Journal of Drug Issues, 19,* 261-281.

Kofoed, L. L. (1985). OTC drug overuse in the elderly: What to watch for. *Geriatrics, 40,* 55-58, 60.

Lamy, P. P. (1983). Drug abuse by older adults—Who is responsible? *Drug Intelligence and Clinical Pharmacy, 17,* 657-659.

Maypole, D. E. (1989). Alcoholism and the elderly: Review of theories, treatment, and prevention. *Activities, Adaptation and Aging, 13,* 43-54.

Raffoul, P. R. (1986). Drug misuse among elderly people: Focus for interdisciplinary efforts. *Health and Social Work, 11,* 197-203.

Rathbone-McCuan, E., & Hashimi, J. (1982). *Isolated elders.* Rockville, MD: Aspen.

Robertson, N. (1992). The intimate enemy: Will that friendly drink betray you? *Modern Maturity, 35,* 27-28, 30, 65.

Schonfeld, L., & Dupree, L. W. (1991). Antecedents of drinking for early- and late-onset elderly alcohol abusers. *Journal of Studies on Alcohol, 52,* 587-592.

Smart, R. G., & Adlaf, E. M. (1988). Alcohol and drug use among the elderly: Trends in use and characteristics of users. *Canadian Journal of Public Health, 79,* 236-242.

Speer, D. C., O'Sullivan, M., & Schonfeld, L. (1991). Dual diagnosis among older adults: A new array of policy and planning problems. *Journal of Mental Health Administration, 18,* 43-50.

Weiss, K. J., & Greenfield, D. P. (1986). Prescription drug abuse. *Psychiatric Clinics of North America, 9,* 475-490.

Part II

RESEARCH AND EVALUATION OF SUBSTANCE ABUSE SERVICES FROM A FAMILY SYSTEMS PERSPECTIVE

EDITH M. FREEMAN

Practice and research or evaluation have been traditionally separate areas within the substance abuse treatment field. Not only has a separate cadre of experts developed in each of these areas, but also, until recent years, seldom have individual researchers or practitioners developed expertise in both areas. This emerging trend of blending practice and research is being reflected gradually in the current substance abuse literature. The logical place to begin this integration process, which can benefit families, helping professionals, and program administrators, is in the areas of individual and program evaluations of family-focused services (perhaps the more rigorous area of outcome/practice effectiveness research soon will follow in this integration process).

Part 2 of this book is focused on the areas of individual and program evaluation for family-focused services. The two chapters in this section reflect the same family systems perspective found in the chapters in Part 1. Chapter 10 addresses single system evaluation with addicted families, using an empowerment approach and describing the process and how-to steps involved from intake (baseline) to the treatment phase to posttreatment follow-up. Chapter 11 provides both the philosophical assumptions and steps necessary for effective practitioner- and family-involved program evaluation activities. That chapter's discussion focuses also on how to conduct program evaluations consistent with the continuum of care proposed in Chapter 1 for family prevention, intervention, and treatment services. Both chapters creatively use case and program examples from the chapters in Part 1 to illustrate how practitioners and administrators can apply the respective methodologies at the level of the individual family or program.

Chapter 10

SINGLE SYSTEM RESEARCH IN FAMILY-FOCUSED ALCOHOL TREATMENT

EDITH M. FREEMAN

One of the main benefits of using single system research in alcohol treatment programs with individual families is the opportunity to help those families regain control over their lives and to empower themselves. The alcoholic is compulsively focused on securing, maintaining, and consuming a supply of alcohol, while family members struggle to maintain the social and economic equilibrium of the alcoholic member for the survival of the unit (Freeman, 1992; Greenleaf, 1981). The resulting loss of control, family relationships, intimacy, social supports, identity, and financial resources often involves a series of disempowerment experiences that may be exacerbated initially when the family and the addicted member enter treatment. Consequently the process of treatment can reinforce the sense of disempowerment if administrators, program developers, evaluators, and clinicians do not understand the unique and common experiences and needs of families with an addicted member.

A 37-year-old widowed Hispanic woman with several teenagers and a grandchild in her household addressed this issue while being interviewed during an ethnographic study of her multicultural community, designed to help the residents identify their strengths, concerns, and needs. In discussing her concerns, she pointed out what many people need in order to become self-sufficient and empowered during treatment:

> Many times I've had problems, and I couldn't figure out how to deal with the problems. I've looked to the people at ____ (social agency) for answers. . . . They give me advice, and the problems go away, but it's also within the person to have to understand the problem and get your mind cleared up. (Freeman & O'Dell, in press)

This woman indicated that empowerment not only is a result of effective problem-solving but also involves personal growth and development from gaining an understanding of the problem internally and being able to "move on" once this understanding has been achieved. Her definition implies that treatment programs should encourage families to become actively involved in the work and to experience both the problem-solving and the personal growth aspects in order to empower themselves. One benefit of the use of single system research is that it provides an opportunity and a set of practical but individualized procedures that are useful for achieving this important treatment goal.

Simon (1990) indicated a second benefit from using single system research is that it helps practitioners integrate practice and research so that the major focus remains on the client systems' service needs. This integration is particularly important in the addictions field, where the development of relevant and appropriate research strategies for practitioners has been difficult (Bratter & Forrest, 1985; Freeman, 1985; Meyer, 1984). A third benefit in using such research is given often as the main rationale—that it provides documentation of the process and outcomes of the work. This last point addresses the issue of accountability, which is gaining importance in a number of related areas, including the addictions, family treatment, and community development fields (Freeman & O'Dell, in press; Hartman & Laird, 1983; Valle, 1981).

This chapter highlights the connection between family empowerment and the use of single system research in alcohol treatment. The process and procedures necessary for actively involving and helping to empower families in identifying, implementing, and documenting the work toward recovery then is summarized. Finally case vignettes from previous chapters are used to illustrate how these procedures can be applied to individual families in ways that help the practitioner blend practice and research activities. The chapter is relevant to clinicians such as addiction counselors, social workers, psychologists, psychiatrists, and family therapists, as well as administrators and program developers and evaluators. In terms of the latter, the discussion in this chapter lays a foundation for Chapter 11, which addresses program evaluations of family-focused alcohol treatment services.

LINKING EMPOWERMENT WITH THE USE OF SINGLE SYSTEM RESEARCH

Defining the Concept of Empowerment

As a currently popular term, *empowerment* has a seductive quality for practitioners, especially those working with addicted clients and their families. Current use of this term implies that the clinician does something significant to the client, and thus the focus is on the clinician's power. The difficult nature of alcohol treatment and the lack of clarity about what treatments work best with particular clients can lead clinicians to devalue their work and themselves. This sense of devaluation and disempowerment may make them more vulnerable, at an unconscious level, to concepts that imply they are powerful. However, there is a negative consequence for clients who are in treatment with those clinicians, because an implicit emphasis on the clinician's power is likely to impede recovery and to decrease the family's sense of efficacy.

A more useful definition of *empowerment* centers on this concept of *client efficacy and power.* Although it is clear that one person cannot empower another (Freeman, 1992), according to Simon (1990), one person can contribute to the conditions under which individuals, families, and communities empower themselves. This definition indicates that empowerment is both a process and an outcome: a process of acting effectively and positively to change one's environment in meaningful ways and a sense of competence and value that are the result of such actions (Freeman, 1992).

Figure 10.1 contains an empowerment pyramid that illustrates how clients' goals can result in different levels of empowerment. Although a particular sequence may seem to be implied by this pyramid, the levels of empowerment do not always occur in a linear progression. A client or family can move from one level to any other level; for example, knowledge about addictions can be gained through alcohol education and can lead to an awareness of the consequences and severity of an individual's addiction. At the top of the pyramid, the *awareness level* refers to the development of insight about oneself or a particular issue and a beginning positive attitude shift that can result in low levels of

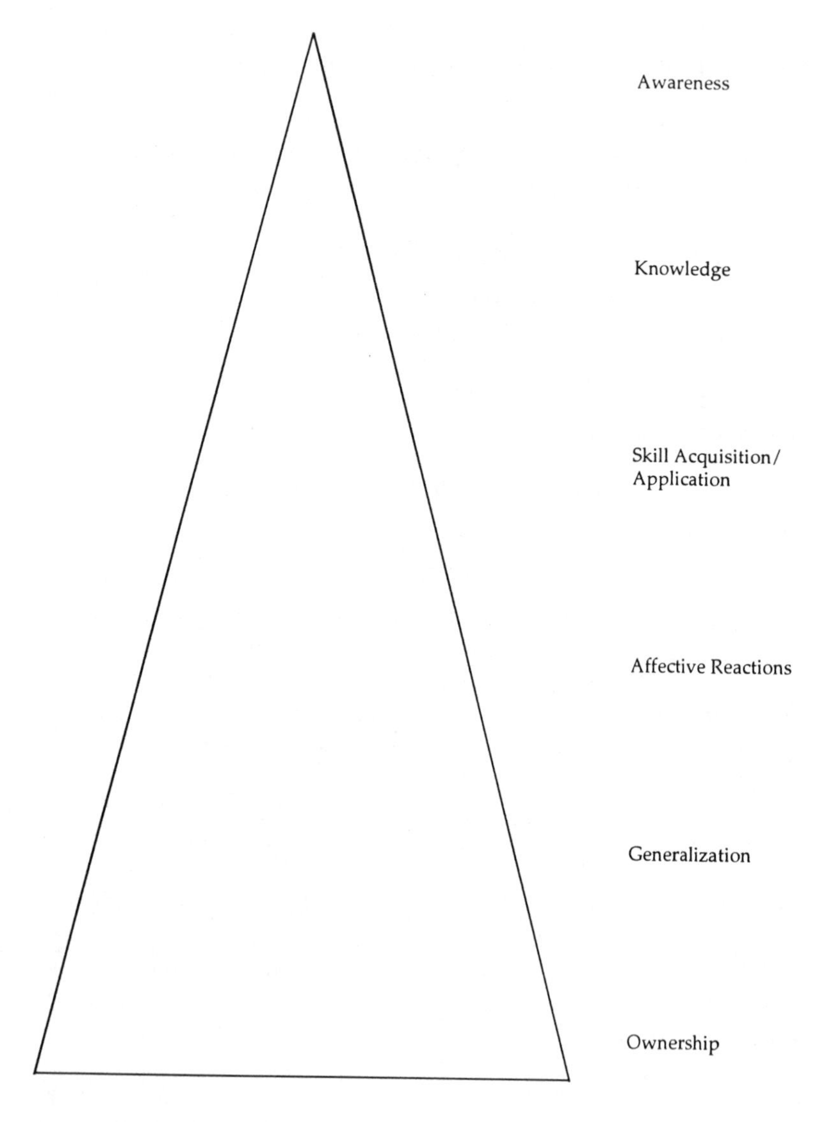

Figure 10.1. Family Empowerment Pyramid

empowerment for a client. The *knowledge level* implies acquiring and understanding a defined area of culturally relevant and useful information; the *skill level* focuses on the effective application of such knowledge by the individual in significant life situations.

Experiencing *affective reactions* helps anchor the sense of being valuable that comes from applying knowledge effectively. Moreover, it is related to a person's hope for continued mastery and competence in the future—in the area of relapse prevention, for example. *Generalization* is the process of applying knowledge to new problems and situations and the use of positive risk taking without giving blame/shame messages to oneself and others. Moving down the pyramid implies more in-depth involvement and growth on the part of the client to the ownership level. At the *ownership level* is an acknowledgement of the person's own significant role in changing some aspect of the environment and a sense of efficacy and satisfaction with that role (Freeman, 1991).

The Role of Single System Research

The above definition and empowerment pyramid imply that addicted individuals and their families will seek their optimal level of functioning based on whether there is a "goodness of fit" between their needs and environmental resources (consistent with theories of self-actualization, ego psychology, the life model, and general systems) (Germain & Gitterman, 1980; Maluccio, 1979; Maslow, 1967; Towle, 1965; Turner, 1986). Client empowerment is more possible when a goodness of fit exists. It is less likely when most of the family resources are directed toward meeting one need: the addicted member's compulsive need for alcohol and for protection from the consequences of the abuse through the system's denial and enabling behaviors. Single system research clarifies and documents if and to what extent the alcohol addiction of one member has disrupted the typical day-to-day patterns of living within a family and what may be needed to restore and enhance those patterns.

This type of research consists of a variety of user-friendly methods for ensuring systematic problem identification, problem-solving data collection, and evaluation of the effectiveness of a particular treatment with one client or client system (Corcoran, 1985; Levy, 1987). Because this type of research requires the active involvement of the unit at each step during treatment and monitoring, it provides the family with those elements of empowerment identified previously: the resources for problem solving and the growth and development derived from understanding the problem and then moving on. For instance, letting go of blame/shame messages about negative family experiences associated with the addiction becomes possible when the members are able to recognize through the use of simple measurement tools that they are giving these messages to each other and their impact on the family's recovery process. The positive feedback provided by these single system research tools can lead to empowerment at higher levels, such as the skill or ownership level, along with supplying the means for documenting the work.

SINGLE SYSTEM RESEARCH: DOCUMENTATION OF PROCESS AND OUTCOMES

Intake and assessment with addicted clients and their families begins with history taking and observation. The use of simple measurement tools associated with single system research assists in this collaborative process of assessing the client system and its problem situation (Kinney & Leaton, 1978). Nelson (1985) noted that single system research methodology allows social workers and other clinicians to specify what is observed in a defined way and defined time period during phases of assessment or baseline activities, treatment, and follow-up services in which practice and research are blended.

The Assessment or Baseline Phase

The assessment or baseline phase, the initial phase of practice and single system research in family-focused treatment for alcohol addiction, involves several tasks (Bloom & Fischer, 1982; Campbell, 1988; Nelson, 1985):

1. Problem definition and clarification
2. Data collection
3. Data presentation related to the system's likely denial of the addiction problem
4. Goal setting and contracting with the family system
5. Treatment specification
6. Research design specification

Bloom and Fischer (1982) emphasized that problems must be defined clearly in concrete, specific, and behavioral terms so that they are observable and measurable. Clarity in this initial phase ensures later opportunities to determine progress, regression, or achievement of objectives. In family-focused alcohol treatment, it is important not to limit the problem definition and clarification to the addiction or to the addicted family member's behavior. A systems perspective requires that all factors and circumstances affecting and affected by the addiction be included as part of the problem definition (Freeman & Landesman, 1992; Shaffer & Kauffman, 1985).

For example, low self-esteem in an alcohol abuser often precedes his or her addiction. If it is not included as a part of the problem definition and thus as a target for treatment, the low self-esteem may be a major barrier to the person's recovery. In many situations a family's concentrated focus on the addiction may restrict the problem-solving experiences and skills of all of the members. The problem definition should include those deficits because they are often the basis for a family's fears and resistance to change. Family members may assume that only the addicted member will have to change; making their related needs part of the problem definition can emphasize the requirement for *system* change during initial baseline activities.

The process of problem definition and clarification is facilitated through data collection, which may take a number of forms: (a) direct observation of the family dynamics during intake, while the members present their problems to, and discuss their problems with, the clinician; (b) the psychosocial history taking, along with completion of a drinking/drugging history; (c) the use of questionnaires, scales, and checklists designed to assess the presence and severity of alcohol addiction and related health and mental health problems; and (d) the use of retroactive or concurrent baseline data collection procedures. The latter procedures are designed to help clients and families collect data concurrently with the intake/assessment process (Hudson, 1982).

Client logs, self-anchored scales, and home observation forms are examples of procedures that can be used by the client and other family members to identify the incidence, frequency, and context of the problems either retroactively based on recall or concurrently (Freeman & Pennekamp, 1988). For instance, a client who insists that he or she can control the drinking and therefore is not addicted might be asked to keep a log to count the amount and frequency of alcohol used during a brief period.

From a systems perspective, a family member could be encouraged to rate his or her anger with the addicted person on a self-anchored scale during typical problem situations in which the latter avoids communicating. It can be assumed that this data collection procedure could help illustrate the circularity of the family's problems related to the addiction, the purpose it serves for the unit, and family members' reactions to the addiction. Another family member might use a simple home observation form constructed during intake to record instances when the other members blame their dysfunctional behavior on the addicted person. Concurrent baseline data collection should be maintained for at least seven data points (representing weeks, days, or briefer periods), depending on the severity of the problem and the difficulty in data collection. The usefulness of the data being collected to the family and clinician also determines how long the baseline phase should last (its relevance and predictability) (Bloom & Fischer, 1982).

Data presentation involves organizing and summarizing the baseline data in ways that invite the family to help interpret the results and to decide what ought to be done about them. The goal is also to further clarify the system's problems. The presentation can be accomplished through the use of graphs and/or verbal summaries of the data. As the discussion precedes, the clinician should ensure that all members' points of view are heard and respected, while at the same time disagreements are acknowledged and accepted (Prosky, 1983). Freeman and Landesman (1992) noted there should be a balance between members sharing how they have experienced the addiction and other problems and not placing blame for all of the system's problems on the addicted member. Often the family's denial system about the existence or severity of the addiction is challenged in this process. In those situations, the use of single system procedures as a part of data presentation and assessment is actually an intervention. (See Chapter 1 for a more detailed discussion about clinician-guided family interventions.) By diminishing the system's denial during the intervention, the process also may enhance a family's commitment to treatment and recovery.

Goal setting and contracting are a natural result of the sifting and rank ordering that occurs during data presentation. Just as there are many facets to one problem and several problems may be identified during baseline, a balance between these different dimensions should be considered in developing the goals and objectives between (a) the addiction problem, as well as other important problems, (b) various levels of empowerment needed by each member (based on the empowerment pyramid), (c) conflicting individual and family system needs, (d) short- versus long-term needs/outcomes, and (e) focus on positive and negative behaviors.

Furthermore the use of single system procedures requires that the objectives be as observable and measurable as the problem definition

(Bloom & Fischer, 1982). It is often useful to identify indicators of change related to each objective so that progress toward the objectives can be measured. For example, identifying situations where problem-solving communication is needed, developing and practicing strategies of effective communication, and applying those strategies in family meetings represent incremental indicators for monitoring movement toward an increased skill in communication between family members. It is likely that increased communication and coping skills can enhance recovery by teaching alternatives to drinking and by reducing family stressors that can precipitate a relapse. Campbell (1988) summarized the purpose in setting measurable objectives: specifying the desired changes over time and the amount of change expected to occur as a minimum.

Treatment and research design specification are related activities that should be discussed between the clinician and the family in treatment. The clinician is usually an expert in the use of particular treatment approaches, but the family is the expert in what is likely to work with their system and how an approach could be used. In addition, encouraging the family to speculate on what will not work helps decrease potential sabotage activities by various members and strengthens the connection between how they view the problem and the relevance of the selected treatment approach for addressing the problem. Specifying the treatment includes identifying the overall treatment model—for example, a family systems problem-solving approach—as well as the types of strategies or components that might be used. Examples of strategies involved in the above approach include identifying the steps in problem solving, role playing, and doing homework assignments to resolve family dilemmas and issues (Prosky, 1983; Turner, 1986).

The research design specification helps the clinician and the family members grapple with what data should be collected, by whom, with what measures, and how often before, during, and after treatment. Measures are available for monitoring the frequency, duration, intervals (combining frequency and duration), or intensity (or magnitude) of a behavior. Some of these procedures are simple write-in or tally forms that can be adapted to the specific client or family (Tripodi & Epstein, 1982). Others consist of standardized rapid assessment instruments (RAIS) such as the Clinical Measurement Package, which produces global ratings of seven characteristics including self-esteem, family relationships, and depression (Hudson, 1982). Generally these measures can be organized into quantitative and qualitative methods. The former are useful primarily for quantifying behaviors, thoughts, and

Table 10.1
Examples of Single System Designs for Family-Focused Alcohol Treatment

Type of Design	*Experimental Phases or Conditions*
Basic Time Series Design	
(Variation of Basic Design: Extended follow-up phase after termination to monitor maintenance)	A-B A-B-A
Reversal or Withdrawal Design	
(Return target behavior to pretreatment levels and reintroduction of same or new treatment)	A-B-A-B
Multiple Element Designs	
Alternating Treatments Design (Counterbalance two different treatments, vary their order)	A-B/C-B or A-B/C-C or A-BCD
Successive Treatments Design (Application of treatments in sequence)	A-B-C or A-B-A-C
Multiple Target Design (Application of different treatments to different target behaviors)	A_1B_1 A_2B_2 A_3B_3
Multiple Baseline Design	
(Application across behaviors [same client], across different clients [same problem], or across settings [same client and same problem])	A_1B_1 A_2B_2 A_3B_3

NOTE: Key: A = stable baseline condition or phase without treatment
B = first treatment phase
C = second treatment phase involving a different treatment approach

feelings (RAIS), while the latter focus more on descriptions of those factors, often in conjunction with some minimal quantifying activities (a log with a self-anchored scale) (Freeman & Pennekamp, 1988).

The selection of measures should be based on their ease of administration and the willingness of the family to complete them at the regular time intervals required by the particular design. Table 10.1 presents some of the most common single system research designs, ranging from the simplest A-B design involving one baseline and one intervention period, to the more complex designs. Nesbitt (1989), Nelson (1985), and other researchers indicated that the A-B design's simplicity makes it especially useful with addiction, relationship, and communication problems.

The Treatment Phase

In using any single system design, a plan is needed for answering questions from family members and the clinician that are bound to come up during the treatment phase. This phase is designed to clarify the following common questions and issues (Bloom & Fischer, 1982; Freeman & Pennekamp, 1988; Nelson, 1985; Valle, 1981):

- Whether the intervention is being implemented as planned
- The pattern of change and whether it is in the problem areas (including the addiction), direction, and magnitude desired, based on the family's multi-dimensional objectives
- The usefulness of the selected measures in providing meaningful and timely feedback about these changes
- The effectiveness of the treatment approach and strategies in causing these changes
- Whether the family is empowering itself via the change experience and what it believes is the source of this empowerment or the barriers to it

Specifying and agreeing during the baseline phase what treatment will be used lays a good foundation for deciding how to monitor whether the treatment is being implemented as planned. Family members can complete session summaries at regular intervals to describe what took place in family, group, and individual sessions from their perspective. This reporting not only helps monitor the treatment's implementation but also provides feedback on the effects of treatment and when it may need to be changed (discontinued, modified, or supplemented with other treatment approaches) (Nelson, 1985).

Because of the variety of problems experienced by families with an addicted member, the treatment phase often may consist of several subphases rather than one continuous phase. When feedback indicates that the pattern of change is too slow or too fast, the clinician can help the family members discuss their fears and ambivalent feelings about change. At times the addicted family system may regress in an effort to maintain the status quo even though individual members are attempting to work toward identified objectives. Open discussions about their fears and ambivalences can normalize those feelings and help clarify whether the research design needs to be changed—that is, whether other treatment approaches (or subphases) need to be added.

For example, a clinician might begin the treatment phase with an intergenerational family systems approach to address cross-generational addiction problems in the family described at the beginning of this chapter: the 47-year-old Hispanic widow who lived with her teenage children and a grandchild. Family problems included the oldest son being addicted and conflicts between the head of the household and her teenage daughter about how to parent the grandchild. If the mother and daughter conflicts escalate and create stress that encourages the son to return to drinking, another treatment approach may need to be used simultaneously with the current one. Rational emotive therapy or some other cognitive approach might be useful for clarifying and modifying the mother's and daughter's shoulds/oughts for each other and their individual negative self-talk statements (Turner, 1986). This addition would result in a change in the research design: from an A-B design to an A-B-BC design to represent the two combined treatment approaches.

This process of monitoring the pattern of change is useful for another reason: It can indicate when progress is being made toward objectives, when objectives should be revised due to achievement, or when objectives need to be split into smaller goals (in terms of more short-term objectives or a different level on the empowerment pyramid). Monitoring also may help determine whether the procedures or measures being used are appropriate or inappropriate and in what specific ways. This monitoring includes (a) whether the feedback from using a particular procedure or measure is specific enough, (b) whether it measures the behavior it was selected to measure, and (c) whether the feedback is received in a timely enough manner to be useful to family members.

For instance, in the first circumstance, (a) above, a log may need to be used in conjunction with RAIS or self-anchored scales to provide more specific information about the family or individual situations that affect the members' ratings of their feelings on those instruments. In the second circumstance, (b) above, a client-monitoring form may reveal that rather than measuring problem-solving efforts by a couple, it is measuring their passive/aggressive behaviors. This problem could require the clinician and family to revise either the problem definition and objectives, the monitoring procedure, and/or the treatment approach during this phase. The third circumstance, (c) above, might involve a treatment session summary form completed by the recovering member. If summaries indicate that the client needs feedback from family members on his or her communication skills daily rather than every other day for reinforcement, the feedback process should be modified.

This monitoring process also can reveal whether the selected treatment approach is causing important changes consistent with the objectives. In the last example above, monitoring could help determine whether the communication exercises during treatment are effectively increasing the individual's skills in that area or some external factor, such as a week-long seminar at work, has influenced the changes.

Finally, monitoring during the treatment phase helps clarify how the family is experiencing this process in terms of empowerment. If single system procedures are implemented inadequately and without the members' involvement, their sense of disempowerment from previous losses, including the loss of control, is likely to increase. When such procedures are implemented effectively, however, family members will be able to identify their level of involvement in the change process, based on visible, accumulated data they have helped collect. They can help decide when data collection procedures and treatment approaches need to be changed, when various members seem to be ready to generalize new skills (generalizing conflict negotiation skills or refusal skills from family interactions to the work setting or to a peer network), and what aspects of the treatment process facilitate or hinder whether empowerment occurs and at what level. It is the clinician's ethical responsibility to ensure, through careful and mutual monitoring of the treatment phase, that the treatment and single system research procedures are effective and that they are "doing no harm" by making a family's situation worse.

The Posttreatment or Follow-Up Phase

The posttreatment or follow-up phase consists of the period of aftercare that follows treatment and the period when aftercare has been completed. Wodarski's (1981) conclusion is that this phase provides the opportunity to determine whether the changes in the problem situation are lasting. However, the focus is on both maintaining the gains that have occurred during treatment and addressing issues related to lifelong recovery that could not be addressed until after treatment or that the family was unable to address at that time. The issues emphasized during this phase related to continued recovery and single system research include the following:

- Whether the recovering person and family members are able to maintain the positive changes in recovery and related areas that were noted during treatment and during aftercare

- Whether relapse prevention strategies that were not needed during treatment are being implemented effectively during aftercare and later by the family
- The extent to which the family is able to work on "buried issues" that, if left unresolved, could threaten lifelong recovery and continued empowerment opportunities

During aftercare and at specified intervals for at least 2 years following aftercare, single system procedures can be used in two ways to monitor whether the gains made during treatment are being maintained. First, the family members will have learned some methods for monitoring their situation that they should be expected to continue after treatment ends. A part of the posttreatment contract or the contract developed during aftercare with families should focus on what periodic monitoring procedures they will continue to use for their own feedback and reinforcement. The results of those monitoring procedures and how to interpret and apply them to the process of recovery and family healing are appropriate topics for aftercare sessions.

Second, the clinician should use simple follow-up procedures that he or she can administer for monitoring the family's continued posttreatment progress. Many families are able to use combined aftercare services and a 12-step program to maintain the progress made during treatment. Findings from the clinician's monitoring procedures can be used to support those from the family's self-monitoring procedures or to draw attention to important differences. The need for this type of support is even more significant for the period following aftercare, when many of the early environmental supports provided for families in recovery may no longer be available (Freeman & Landesman, 1992). A telephone survey, a written questionnaire, or an unstructured face-to-face interview can be used every 6 months for the 2-year follow-up period to determine whether the family is still in recovery (whether the treatment is still effective) or additional services are needed.

Determining the need for additional services is the most important benefit of this follow-up phase. The family will have learned some relapse prevention strategies during treatment and aftercare that they are not required to use until a later part of the recovery process. Single system research procedures can determine where in the problem-solving chain the family is having difficulties with relapse prevention. They might be referred for a few "booster" treatment sessions in relapse prevention or another related area, a specialized treatment program designed for codependents or incest survivors, or a specialized 12-step program for same-sex or ethnic minority clients as the need indicates (Blume, 1985; McRoy & Shorkey, 1985; McRoy, Shorkey, & Garcia, 1985; Smith, 1988).

"Buried" issues such as incest, early parental rejection and abandonment, identity conflicts related to sexual preference, or cultural conflicts from racism and discrimination may surface only during the posttreatment phase. What initially appears to be regression in family functioning based on feedback from monitoring actually may be the result of unresolved issues that were not addressed during treatment. Such feedback during and following aftercare simply means that additional or more specialized treatment such as the examples in the previous paragraph are needed. Analysis of the feedback with the family and the clinician's sensitivity toward the possible existence of these and other unresolved issues are necessary before it can be assumed that the previous treatment was ineffective.

CASE ILLUSTRATIONS: INTEGRATION OF PRACTICE AND RESEARCH

The preceding discussion on the use of single system research in alcohol treatment has highlighted both the process involved in using this methodology and some of the practice/research issues that must be addressed from a systems perspective. The case illustrations that follow build on that discussion by providing examples of how this methodology can be applied in a manner that helps practitioners blend practice and research effectively. These cases are useful also for illustrating how empowerment opportunities can be used with families and family issues during this monitoring process.

Case Illustration: The Jones Family

The Jones family from Chapter 2 is appropriate for illustrating the A-BCD single system design and procedures. That African-American family consists of Esther Jones (late 30s), David Jones (late 40s), and their children, Karla (13), Aaron (12), and Gina (4). Ms. Jones is a dental assistant who is both physically and verbally abused by her husband, an alcoholic who at times also verbally abuses the children. Mr. Jones is a supervisor in a department store. Gina was referred to the social worker at a community center by her pediatrician because of depression. Mr. Jones is unwilling to be involved in treatment and does not want anyone to know about his alcohol abuse.

In using single system research methodology, the clinician could have involved Ms. Jones in completing the ecomap (Germain, 1979), Hudson's Index of Marital Relations (IMR) (Hudson, 1982), and a psychosocial assessment to begin to define the problem. Direct observation of Gina in the play therapy room and the CAST (Pilat & Jones, 1985), a screening instrument for children of alcoholics, could augment data obtained from Ms. Jones. This process would have produced concurrent baseline data on the family's strengths and problems: Ms. Jones's awareness and skill in using social supports and the unit's sources of stress, the frequency and severity of family conflicts and violence, Gina's depressive symptoms, and the severity of the father's alcohol abuse from Ms. Jones's and Gina's perspectives. Ms. Jones might have agreed to keep a log describing and counting Gina's depressive symptoms, including nightmares, reduced food intake, and being quiet and withdrawn at school. The log could have included events and family interactions that occurred before, during, and after the occurrence of those symptoms to identify the circular nature of problems within the family.

Baseline data from the log and these other sources might have been useful not only for developing an observable and measurable definition of the problem but also for helping Ms. Jones see more clearly the severity and consequences of Mr. Jones's addiction for all of the members. The knowledge and awareness obtained from her baseline data collection efforts could have resulted in her growing sense of empowerment. Her intervention with Mr. Jones might have occurred earlier in the helping process as a result. Objectives could have included increasing Gina's appropriate expression of feelings about the father's drinking and abusive behavior in a safe environment, decreasing the number of nightmares, increasing her daily food intake to _______ (depending on her baseline rates), increasing the mother's understanding of alcohol addiction and her ability to be supportive to Gina, and increasing the family's social supports.

Treatment in this case involved a combined expressive play therapy for Gina and family treatment for the mother-daughter dyad with eventual referrals for the other two children to age-appropriate 12-step and divorce peer groups. In addition to the combined communication and problem-solving family systems strategies described in Chapter 2, the clinician used bibliotherapy to increase Ms. Jones's understanding of alcohol addiction and her ability to be supportive to Gina (by reassuring Gina of her love and helping her express her fears verbally rather than through the depressive symptoms). Gina's target behaviors and the very appropriate involvement of her siblings in productive activities outside the home could have been monitored during treatment to ensure that their strengths were maintained and that the treatment or other environmental factors did not worsen the situation. The clinician and Ms. Jones could have continued to use the baseline measurement procedures during treatment for feedback at regular intervals about the progress being made (the client log, ecomap, IMR, CAST, and direct observation of Gina).

Treatment outcomes included concrete evidence of Ms. Jones's movement from awareness of her social supports (via the ecomap) to her increased skill in using those supports (attendance at an interracial Al-Anon group; asking for/receiving child care, financial help, and verbal encouragement from her extended family; and discussing her concerns about divorce with her minister). Other outcomes were decreases in Gina's nightmares and increases in her appropriate expression of feelings during treatment related to her father's abusive behaviors. If single system research procedures had been used in this case, it might have been possible to determine patterns in Gina's changes; the relationship between her appropriate expression of feelings and the number of nightmares is not clear. Equally important, it was not clear what aspects of the treatment approaches resulted in which specific changes—for example, what aspects helped Ms. Jones in her decision making about the divorce.

Follow-up monitoring procedures could have been used also during the posttreatment phase to monitor whether the family was able to maintain the treatment outcomes described above. For instance, Ms. Jones might have been encouraged to continue her use of the log for several months during the posttreatment phase in order to document whether Gina's progress in reducing the depressive symptoms was maintained. In addition, if family meetings had been used during the treatment phase to improve the family's communication skills, those meetings could be continued during the posttreatment phase. Hawkins, Catalano, Brown, and Vadasy (1988) strongly support the role of family meetings in helping parents reduce the addiction risk factors their children are exposed to in both the home and community.

Freeman and Gordon (1992) developed a Check List for Family Meetings and A Family Meeting Rating Form to help families structure

Date ____________
Recorder ____________

This check list should be completed at the end of each family meeting by the member identified as the recorder. It may be helpful to have other family members review the completed check list for accuracy. Write NA for any item on the list that does not apply for the particular meeting.

_______ 1. An agenda was planned before or at the beginning of the meeting to clarify the meeting's purpose.

_______ 2. If this was the first family meeting or one involving behavior related to a ground rule, ground rules were developed, revised, or reviewed based on suggestions from family members.

_______ 3. A "Fun Things" list was developed together and/or was used to select an activity for family members to do during the meeting or at another time.

_______ 4. If the activity selected by the family was for another time, a written plan was completed for the activity (i.e., indicating a specific time, day, and place).

_______ 5. Each child or youth in the family was given a specific role in the meeting or for an activity that was planned for another time.

_______ 6. The content and interactions that occurred during the meeting were reviewed with the members at some point before the meeting ended.

_______ 7. The meeting ended with a positive interaction between family members (e.g., a game, refreshments, verbal or nonverbal expressions of caring, a family gram complementing each member).

_______ 8. A specific plan was made for getting back to unfinished topics identified by any family member at a later date.

_______ 9. A family gram was written to include anything family members needed to remember about the meeting for the future.

_______ 10. A date and time were set for the next family meeting.

_______ 11. If this was a "stock taking" family meeting (every fourth meeting or sooner if requested by any family members), each member rated and discussed his/her ideas about the quality of the meetings.

Figure 10.2. Checklist for Family Meetings

and monitor their meetings (see Figures 10.2 and 10.3). These monitoring forms could assist the Jones family in creating empowerment experiences for each other during their meetings. In the process, the members might set new objectives to decrease their codependent behaviors and other "buried" risk factors that could heighten their vulnerability to addictions (e.g., if

Please circle the number for each of the 3 rating topics that captures your point of view about the family meetings. Date ____________

Family Members Ratings

Family Member's Initials	I feel comfortable sharing my ideas and feelings with the family.					I feel important & good about myself during our meetings.					Our family meetings are valuable					Comments
	Hardly Ever		Sometimes		Almost Always	Hardly Ever		Sometimes		Almost Always	Hardly Ever		Sometimes		Almost Always	
____	1	2	3	4	5	1	2	3	4	5	1	2	3	4	5	____
____	1	2	3	4	5	1	2	3	4	5	1	2	3	4	5	____
____	1	2	3	4	5	1	2	3	4	5	1	2	3	4	5	____
____	1	2	3	4	5	1	2	3	4	5	1	2	3	4	5	____
____	1	2	3	4	5	1	2	3	4	5	1	2	3	4	5	____
____	1	2	3	4	5	1	2	3	4	5	1	2	3	4	5	____
____	1	2	3	4	5	1	2	3	4	5	1	2	3	4	5	____
____	1	2	3	4	5	1	2	3	4	5	1	2	3	4	5	____
____	1	2	3	4	5	1	2	3	4	5	1	2	3	4	5	____
____	1	2	3	4	5	1	2	3	4	5	1	2	3	4	5	____
____	1	2	3	4	5	1	2	3	4	5	1	2	3	4	5	____
____	1	2	3	4	5	1	2	3	4	5	1	2	3	4	5	____
____	1	2	3	4	5	1	2	3	4	5	1	2	3	4	5	____
____	1	2	3	4	5	1	2	3	4	5	1	2	3	4	5	____
____	1	2	3	4	5	1	2	3	4	5	1	2	3	4	5	____
____	1	2	3	4	5	1	2	3	4	5	1	2	3	4	5	____

Figure 10.3. Family Meeting Rating Form (For Stock-Taking Meetings)

the older children's involvement in activities and jobs outside the home escalated to workaholism as they grow older). The two forms for monitoring family meetings and the log could provide ongoing feedback to the family about their progress during this follow-up phase and could supplement any data collected simultaneously by the clinician.

Case Illustration: The Brown Family

Carl Brown and his family were described in Chapter 7. The combined treatment provided to them can be represented by the following single system research design: A-BC-BCD-D. In that design, A is the baseline phase; BC is the combined individual and family sessions involving a communications family systems approach; BCD is the combined individual, family, and group approaches; and D is the group approach alone. The family members involved in the treatment sessions included Carl, his wife, and their two latency-age sons. Carl was referred to a Vets Center after a private psychologist he had initiated treatment with suspected that Carl suffered from PTSD. Carl initially had sought treatment because of his wife's complaints about his withdrawal, moodiness, anger, and violence toward her and the children. These problems did not develop until several years after his service in Vietnam; at that time, Carl began using alcohol and marijuana to cope with his flashbacks and fears.

The practitioner could have assisted the family in developing baseline data on Carl's substance abuse, the source and severity of his anger and violence, and the family's communication problems. That information also would have been useful in developing a clear definition of the problem. For instance, the severity and consequences of Carl's substance abuse could have been measured by using the MAST (Michigan Alcohol Screening Test) with Carl and the CAST with his sons (Pilat & Jones, 1985; Selzer, 1971).

In addition, Hudson's (1982) Generalized Contentment Scale (GCS) could have rated Carl's level of depression as the possible source of his anger at intake (concurrently) and for two or three significant periods prior to intake (retroactively). The emotional distance and barriers to communication might have been clarified by having the couple complete a client self-monitoring form either together or separately for comparison purposes (Tripodi & Epstein, 1982). A simple form could have been designed by the couple to reflect the following data about the family's communication patterns:

Date ______________

Recorder(s) ______________

We will list below each situation where communication was a problem.

	Situations	Who Was Involved	What Happened
1.			
2.			
3.			
4.			

Because Carl's problem involves withholding and hiding his feelings except the anger, it might have been premature to have the couple include their feelings on this self-monitoring form. Encouraging that type of sharing too soon might cause Carl to close off his feelings even more. Instead Carl might be willing to describe his feelings about those typical family situations *and* his Vietnam flashbacks in a log that only he would read until he was ready for the clinician and his family to read it.

If Carl agreed to use the log during baseline, he also could be asked to rate the identified feelings on a self-anchored scale. The feedback from his scale could be analyzed with data from a comparable rating scale that his wife and/or sons would complete (Bloom & Fischer, 1982). Data presentation during baseline could be enhanced by this feedback; that is, it could assist in clarifying the problem and specifying the treatment and research design. Examples of the self-anchored and rating scales that might be used with the Brown family are as follows:

Mr. Brown's Self-Anchored Scale

Date ______________

Situation:

Extent to which I expressed my feelings:

1	2	3	4	5	6	7
Didn't express feelings at all or did through violence			Expressed feelings nonverbally but without violence			Expressed feelings verbally and non-verbally without violence

Ms. Brown's Rating Scale

Date ________________

Situation:

Amount of anxiety I felt about my husband's expressed or unexpressed feelings:

____

1	2	3	4	5	6	7
Little or no anxiety			Moderate anxiety			Intense anxiety

The use of the log and these scales, as well as the other measures that have been described, would be continued for both the baseline and the treatment phases. Objectives based on the family issues included in the problem definition (e.g., Carl identifying his inner feelings after each situation involving communication problems, flashbacks, or anger/violence) would guide the focus of treatment and monitoring. The awareness and affective levels of empowerment are important dimensions of objectives to be developed with Carl; PTSD causes individuals to repress their feelings, presenting barriers to growth in that area. Objectives for Ms. Brown and the sons might emphasize the skill level where monitoring would focus on their use of alternatives that could help protect them from Carl's violence.

The measures identified previously could have provided feedback on the effectiveness of the communications family systems treatment approach in achieving the above objectives. For example, as indicated in Chapter 7, the following treatment outcomes were achieved in this case: improved family communication patterns through members expressing their feelings and concerns, the elimination of all violent episodes, improved family coping skills with elimination of Carl's substance abuse as a key factor, improved family and social supports, and Carl's decreased sensitivity to reminders of Vietnam. First, the log could have improved these outcomes by documenting what aspects of treatment facilitated the very slow process of healing that is typical of PTSD (e.g., Carl sharing one feeling or event that he had experienced in Vietnam as a result of a family sculpting exercise that reflected the emotional climate of the family).

Second, the simple self-monitoring form could have helped family members analyze, after the fact, which of the communication and coping skills that they were learning in treatment could have been used in the problem situations listed. This process could have documented and strengthened the effects of the treatment approach. The experience of sharing this task also might satisfy her need for emotional involvement and his need for controlling how much he shared with others.

Third, documentation of treatment could have been enhanced by using the GCS (Hudson, 1982) to help Carl identify the triggers for his depression and the patterns (thus documenting how he was applying the knowledge about depression and addiction he had gained from treatment). Also, such feedback is evidence of the relevance and utility of the treatment (by helping him gain control over symptoms he was concerned about and perhaps a sense of empowerment).

In the follow-up phase of monitoring, Carl could have continued his log entries until he decided whether his reactions to the Vietnam experience had been exorcised or made manageable. If he still had low levels of depression periodically, intermittent administration of the GCS (Hudson, 1982) might reassure him that the depression remains at those low levels (that his progress is being maintained). The clinician might use a telephone or face-to-face family interview every 6 months or so to collect data on maintenance of positive changes, relapse prevention, and the emergence of any unresolved issues during and after the group counseling (aftercare) phase.

CONCLUSION

A commitment to focus assessment and treatment on the total ecology of the addicted family and its environment is difficult to implement. Many factors can impede this goal, including the strong denial system of families, their many losses and disempowerment experiences, a tendency by service providers to define problem solving narrowly without attention to the internal growth aspects, the lack of extensive research exploring how family systems approaches can be applied to addictions treatment, and the lack of relevant and appropriate research strategies for clinicians in the addictions field. Although all of these factors are important, appropriate and relevant research strategies offer a means for exploring how many of the other factors can be addressed.

Therefore in this chapter the discussion on single system research was designed to clarify how this methodology can enhance and document the recovery, personal growth, and empowerment opportunities of families in a way that blends practice and research. The emphasis in planning and implementing these procedures has been on issues of utility, effectiveness, and professional ethics. The benefits also have been highlighted. Clinicians can become more self-aware and self-correcting by analyzing the meaningful feedback that develops out of their mutually planned work with addicted families. Program planners, evaluators, and administrators can be more client-centered in the policy decisions that they make on the basis of these systematic findings. And finally, families can strengthen and empower themselves from their active involvement throughout this process.

REFERENCES

Bloom, M., & Fischer, J. (1982). *Evaluating practice: Guidelines for the accountable professional.* Englewood Cliffs, NJ: Prentice-Hall.

Blume, S. (1985). Women and alcohol. In T. E. Bratter & G. G. Forrest (Eds.), *Alcoholism and substance abuse* (pp. 623-638). New York: Free Press.

Bratter, T. E., & Forrest, G. G. (Eds.). (1985). *Alcoholism and substance abuse.* New York: Free Press.

Campbell, J. (1988). Client acceptance of single system evaluation procedures. *Social Work Research and Abstracts, 24,* 21-25.

Corcoran, K. (1985). Aggregating the idiographic data of single-subject research. *Social Work Research and Abstracts, 21,* 8-12.

Freeman, E. M. (1985). Toward improving treatment effectiveness with alcohol problems. In E. M. Freeman (Ed.), *Social work practice with clients who have alcohol problems* (pp. 83-105). Springfield, IL: Charles C Thomas.

Freeman, E. M. (1991, October). *Facilitating client empowerment.* Unpublished paper presented for Staff Training Institute, Kansas City, KS.

Freeman, E. M. (1992). Empowerment opportunities for black adolescent fathers and their nonparenting peers. In J. T. Gordon & R. Majors (Eds.), *America's black male: His present status and his future* (pp. 266-279). Chicago: Nelson-Hall.

Freeman, E. M., & Gordon, J. T. (1992). *A family-centered evaluation of the Kansas Family Initiative.* Unpublished manuscript, Institute for Community Development and Research, Lawrence, KS.

Freeman, E. M., & Landesman, T. (1992). Differential diagnosis and the least restrictive treatment. In E. M. Freeman (Ed.), *The addiction process: Effective social work approaches* (pp. 27-42). New York: Longman.

Freeman, E. M., & O'Dell, K. (in press). Helping communities redefine self-sufficiency from the person-in-environment perspective. *Social Work.*

Freeman, E. M., & Pennekamp, M. (1988). The search for patterns: Linking cases and programs. *Social work practice: Toward a child, family, school, community perspective* (pp. 164-186). Springfield, IL: Charles C Thomas.

Germain, C. B. (1979). Space, an ecological variable in social work practice. *Social Casework, 59,* 515-522.

Germain, C. B., & Gitterman, A. (1980). *The life model of social work practice.* New York: Columbia University Press.

Greenleaf, J. (1981). *Co-alcoholic, para-alcoholic: Who's who and what's the difference?* New Orleans: 361 Foundation.

Hartman, A., & Laird, J. (1983). *Family-centered social work practice.* New York: Free Press.

Hawkins, J. O., Catalano, R. F., Brown, E. O., & Vadasy, P. F. (1988). *Preparing for the drug free years: A family activity book.* Seattle: Developmental Research and Programs.

Hudson, W. (1982). *The clinical measurement package: A field manual.* Chicago: Dorsey.

Kinney, J., & Leaton, G. (1978). *A handbook of alcohol information.* St. Louis: C. V. Mosby.

Levy, R. (1987). Single subject research designs. In *Encyclopedia of social work* (Vol. II, pp. 588-593). Silver Spring, MD: National Association of Social Workers.

Maluccio, A. N. (1979). Promoting competence through life experiences. In C. B. Germain (Ed.), *Social work practice: People and environments* (pp. 282-301). New York: Columbia University Press.

Maslow, C. H. (1967). Self-actualization and beyond. In J. F. Bugental (Ed.), *Challenges of humanistic psychology* (pp. 265-276). New York: McGraw-Hill.

McRoy, R. G., & Shorkey, C. T. (1985). Alcohol use and abuse among blacks. In E. M. Freeman (Ed.), *Social work practice with clients who have alcohol problems* (pp. 202-213). Springfield, IL: Charles C Thomas.

McRoy, R. G., Shorkey, C. T., & Garcia, E. (1985). Alcohol use and abuse among Mexican Americans. In E. M. Freeman (Ed.), *Social work practice with clients who have alcohol problems* (pp. 229-241). Springfield, IL: Charles C Thomas.

Meyer, C. (1984). Integrating research and practice. *Social Work, 29,* 232-239.

Nelson, J. (1985). Verifying the independent variable in single-subject research. *Social Work Research and Abstracts, 21,* 3-8.

Nesbitt, S. (1989). *Single subject research in a family service agency.* Unpublished doctoral dissertation, University of Illinois at Chicago, Chicago.

Pilat, J. M., & Jones, J. W. (1985). A comprehensive treatment program for children of alcoholics. In E. M. Freeman (Ed.), *Social work practice with clients who have alcohol problems* (pp. 141-159). Springfield, IL: Charles C Thomas.

Prosky, P. (1983). Family therapy: An orientation. In F. J. Turner (Ed.), *Differential diagnosis and treatment in social work* (pp. 106-118). New York: Free Press.

Selzer, M. L. (1971). The Michigan Alcoholism Screening Test: The quest for a new diagnostic instrument. *American Journal of Psychiatry, 127,* 89-94.

Shaffer, H., & Kauffman, J. (1985). The clinical assessment and diagnosis of addiction. In T. E. Bratter & G. G. Forrest (Eds.), *Alcoholism and substance abuse* (pp. 225-251). New York: Free Press.

Simon, B. (1990, June). *Women's empowerment: Past and future.* Paper presented at the conference Building on Women's Strengths: A Social Work Agenda for the 21st Century, University of Kansas School of Social Welfare, Lawrence, KS.

Smith, A. W. (1988). *Grandchildren of alcoholics: Another generation of co-dependency.* Deerfield Beach, FL: Health Communications.

Towle, C. (1965). *Common human needs.* New York: National Association of Social Workers.

Tripodi, T., & Epstein, I. (1982). The use of forms for client self-monitoring. In *Research techniques for clinical social workers* (pp. 121-133). New York: Columbia University Press.

Turner, F. J. (1986). A multitheory perspective for practice. In F. J. Turner (Ed.), *Social work treatment: Interlocking theoretical approaches* (pp. 645-659). New York: Free Press.

Valle, S. (1981). Interpersonal functioning of alcoholism counselors and treatment outcomes. *Journal of Studies on Alcohol, 42*, 783-790.

Wodarski, J. S. (1981). *The role of research in clinical practice: A practical approach for the human services.* Baltimore: University Park Press.

Chapter 11

EVALUATING ALCOHOL AND OTHER DRUG ABUSE PROGRAMS

MICHAEL S. CUNNINGHAM

Research findings indicate that family-oriented programs offer tremendous promise for alcohol and other drug abuse prevention (Office of Substance Abuse Prevention [OSAP], 1991). A number of family system strategies and approaches to prevention and treatment have been described in chapters throughout this book. During the past decade, a number of new and innovative programs have emerged. Presently, however, the need to identify new strategies and approaches is not the most critical need facing the field. Instead the pressing need is to identify the programs that, through careful and consistent implementation, have demonstrated effectiveness in achieving desired outcomes (National Institute on Drug Abuse [NIDA], 1991). This accomplishment will require that those programs be evaluated by systematically applying precise field-based methodologies.

The purpose of this chapter is twofold. The first is to provide an overview of significant issues related to evaluating AOD programs using family-focused approaches. The second is to furnish some concrete examples of questions, strategies, and considerations in evaluating family-focused AOD programs. The program examples that are used in this chapter to illustrate these strategies are drawn from two of the chapters included in Part 1 of this book.

The emphasis in this chapter is on *program* evaluation, not on case or research evaluation. The chapter addresses issues related to evaluating family-focused AOD programs, not to the specific strategies and services provided to families or in support of families. It is oriented for policy and program decision makers and practitioners, not for researchers and evaluators. The focus is on implementing program evaluations that provide useful and appropriate information for individuals responsible for the development and implementation of family-focused AOD programs.

The chapter is not a how-to of program evaluation, and it is not designed to train the reader to conduct evaluations. Instead the goals are (a) to increase knowledge and understanding of family-focused program evaluation to assist decision makers and practitioners to become better consumers and producers of family-focused program evaluation and (b) to encourage the initiation and continued enhancement of evaluation in programs. In doing so, the different types of program evaluation are discussed, and some practical tips on when and how to use each of them effectively are provided.

The chapter begins with a discussion of the philosophical and conceptual tenets of program evaluation in celebration of the importance, strengths, diversity, and social context of family life. The role and purposes of program evaluations also are described, including those relevant to family-focused AOD programs. Following that are sections on the different types of evaluation, theory related to evaluation, and critical evaluation issues for decision makers. A multistep evaluation process is described. The chapter concludes with suggestions about how one might design and implement evaluations to address programs serving drug-addicted runaway youth and codependent adults.

PHILOSOPHICAL TENETS

Five interconnected philosophical tenets are woven throughout this chapter. The first is that the family and family services are fundamental to effective AOD programming. The family unit must be the essential building block to design and implement programs that are effective at reducing the incidence, prevalence, and consequences of alcohol and other drug problems.

The second is that the family must be viewed as being capable of fostering growth and health and that it is a system of interrelated, interdependent, and interacting parts. The system is dynamic in nature, and effective programs must address the interactions, relatedness, and dependence of the system as a whole.

The third tenet is that there are different types of family configurations and no one type is inherently better or worse than the others. The purpose of sound program evaluation is to document and quantify the effectiveness of the family-focused programs. Family-focused programs build on the strengths, and support the different types, of families as they seek to provide nurturing, guidance, healing, and recovery to the family unit and individual members.

The fourth tenet is that ethnicity and culture must crosscut all phases of program evaluation, design, planning, implementation, and analysis. Culturally appropriate evaluation designs, procedures, and measures must be included. Issues such as validity and reliability must be addressed from a cultural perspective. Evaluation methodologies must be developed that are sensitive to the cultures and ethnicities of the families who are the focus of the program. The cultural competence of the evaluation staff is critical to effective program evaluations (Cunningham, 1992).

The fifth tenet is that alcohol and other drug problems are complex and are intimately woven into the very fabric of our society. Family-focused programs must take into account the relationships between the individual family members, their peer group, the family as a whole, the community, the overall environment, and the type, potency, and availability of alcohol and other drugs. The similarities and differences in beliefs, norms, attitudes, behaviors, and policies existing within and between the above-mentioned groups must be addressed. Evaluations must recognize such complexity and establish procedures to either include or control for the impact of these factors.

ROLE AND PURPOSE OF PROGRAM EVALUATION

For Programs in General

Program evaluation, in general, is the systematic collection, analysis, and interpretation of program-related data (Weiss & Jacobs, 1988). The overall purpose of program evaluation is to provide answers to questions such as the following:

- What is the need or aspiration we are seeking to address?
- What do we want to accomplish?
- Why do we think we can accomplish it?
- What are we doing to accomplish it?

- What have we accomplished?
- How did we accomplish it?
- What has been the impact of our accomplishments?
- What do we want to accomplish next?

In addition to providing answers to the above questions, program evaluation provides structure to programs that might not be spelled out as clearly otherwise. More specifically, program evaluation provides a structured framework to specify and explicitly state:

The assumptions and beliefs on which the program is based
The goals and objectives of the program
The effectiveness of the program in implementing the processes and activities and achieving the goals and objectives

This type of evaluation is distinguished from research evaluation, which is oriented primarily to identifying and measuring the long-term impact of the methodology and strategies employed.

Program evaluation is designed mainly for an internal audience, although it is not uncommon for the findings to be disseminated to other interested persons and organizations. It is used generally to guide program planning, implementation, improvement, and responsiveness to community needs and aspirations (Littell, 1986). Evaluation research is more externally oriented and is intended to provide information to contribute to advancing the state of the art, theory, practice, and evaluation (Weiss & Jacobs, 1988).

Program evaluation also is distinguished from case or individual evaluation. *Case or individual evaluation* is concerned mostly with assessing the changes in the specific individual, group, or family receiving a specified array of services or activities. Chapter 10 addresses this type of single system documentation of family-focused services in alcohol and other drug treatment programs. Program evaluation, although it may assess the outcomes of the one unit receiving the services, is from the perspective of the individuals, groups, or families as a *whole*.

For Family-Focused Programs

Program evaluation of family-focused programs should be both useful and usable. The purpose of this type of evaluation is to provide information to assist in accomplishing the following tasks and goals:

Accountability. Family-focused AOD programs are a fairly recent phenomenon. They do not have a long history and are not available in large numbers. As such, they do not have a sustained base of support and political clout. They also tend to be focused more on prevention, which is also a relatively new and difficult-to-evaluate technology. Therefore funders and policy makers are skeptical of their effectiveness and require close scrutiny of those programs. Furthermore communities with scarce resources need to be assured that their investment is being used in the most cost-effective manner possible.

Guiding Program Development. Program evaluation is designed to provide programmatic decision makers with information they need to know to plan, implement, enhance, and sustain these relatively new family-focused AOD programs. Evaluation in this context is an ongoing and evolving process that looks at what the program is doing, what services are being provided, what services are needed, and what changes or improvements are necessary. This information allows practitioners to base decisions on systematically collected and analyzed data, as opposed to intuition and informal, sporadic observations.

Measuring Effectiveness. Program evaluation of family-focused AOD services can provide answers to the following questions related to effectiveness:

- Is the program working?
- Are we being effective?
- Who is benefiting and how?
- When are they benefiting?
- What are they benefiting from?

This measurement allows programs to continually assess the achievement of their objectives and to identify areas for program enhancement and improvement.

Determining Future Needs. Family-focused programs exist in an environment in which the needs and aspirations of families are often supported and reinforced by a range of community systems and services. The evaluation design should include collecting information on the needs and gaps in this diverse network of services and resources. This collection will allow the program to continually receive and disseminate feedback from both the participants and the community to guide future program development.

Theory and Model Development. Although most program evaluations of family-focused services are not focused on theory and model development, they can provide a basis for more research-oriented program design and evaluation as a secondary purpose. The experiences of such programs can suggest areas for more concentrated exploration and the use of more rigorous methodologies and measures. Family-focused efforts are designed to help families and communities grow and develop. They are based on providing and maximizing family resources and support intended to strengthen families. Program evaluation can provide information to determine whether the services truly are supporting families and are benefiting those they were implemented to serve (rather than meeting the needs of science).

DIFFERENT LEVELS AND TYPES OF EVALUATION

Factors to Be Considered

The level and type of evaluation selected is affected by the resources available and the stage of development the program is in. Sophisticated and complex evaluations require major commitments of program staff, time, and resources. In some cases the evaluations can cost more than the services being delivered. In addition, programs that are fairly young or that do not have a consistent, formalized, and well-documented process are inappropriate for sophisticated research and impact-oriented evaluations. They would best benefit from formative or process-oriented evaluations. The determination of the level and type of evaluation that a program should use is based on the following factors:

Who the audience is
What they need to know
What type of evaluation will provide the necessary information

The Range of Evaluation Approaches

A number of authors have categorized the levels and types of evaluation approaches (Jacobs 1984; Littell, 1986; Office of Substance Abuse Prevention [OSAP], 1990; Springer, 1990). Jacobs (1988) suggested a 5-tiered approach to evaluation of family-focused programs beginning with the *preimplementation tier,* which emphasizes doing a needs assessment. The second tier is the *accountability tier,* which involves the systematic collection of client-specific and service utilization data. This tier is often called "program monitoring." The third tier is the *progress clarification tier,* which features using the information collected in the previous two tiers to improve program operations. It asks and answers the question "How can we do better?" The fourth tier is the *progress toward objective tier,* which evaluates the program effectiveness and measures the achievement of outcome objectives. The fifth tier is the *program impact tier.* This tier is based on the use of experimental and quasi-experimental designs and measures the program impact (Jacobs, 1988, pp. 50-61). A program's stage of development in this evaluation approach determines which of the five tiers of evaluation is most appropriate. For instance, a new program may need only to begin with a needs assessment as the foundation for evaluation. A program at a more advanced stage of development may need to implement the progress toward objectives tier, which builds on evaluation efforts completed on the previous three tiers.

Other evaluators have used a formative and summative categorization, with formative evaluation encompassing needs assessments and process analysis, while summative evaluation includes outcome and impact evaluation and a cost-effectiveness analysis (Littell, 1986). Springer (1990) used a different framework; he identified three approaches to evaluation:

1. Formal research that is designed to produce generalized information on effective strategies
2. Monitoring and accountability that provide standard numerical information to document the amount of work done by the program
3. Program self-assessment that is a process of constant self-questioning to identify information to be used for ongoing program improvement

Evaluation in the above context is viewed as an ongoing, formative, and flexible process to help improve program efforts and address the ever-changing needs of the community (Springer, 1990). Finally other researchers have advocated the use of a scheme based on evaluating the program's process (steps and procedures), evaluating program outcomes (immediate objectives), and evaluating program impacts (changes in the ultimate areas the program would like to affect—reduction in family addiction risk factors) (OSAP, 1991).

To summarize, most of these models are predicated on the same common and basic process:

Identifying goals and desired outcomes
Describing the activities to accomplish goals and outcomes
Describing what changes have taken place, whether the goals and outcomes have been achieved (OSAP, 1991)

To implement this common evaluation process requires that evaluators verify, document, and quantify the program activities and their effects. This common evaluation model can be integrated with a basic program development process consisting of the following steps: (a) conditions to be addressed, (b) activities to address each condition, (c) outcomes or changes, and (d) impact on the community. As noted previously, the selection of the appropriate type and level of evaluation should be based on analysis of a program's needs, the resources available, the stage of program development, and information availability. Selecting the appropriate type will be a tremendous help to program development. Premature or inappropriate selection of an evaluation approach can have long-lasting negative consequences for the participants, program, staff, and community.

LINKING FAMILY THEORY AND EVALUATION

Current Programmatic Efforts

A review of effective human services interventions by Schorr and Schorr (1988) identified seven attributes that effective family-focused interventions have in common:

1. Broad spectrum of services
2. Cross-traditional boundaries
3. Context of family, environment, community
4. Services coherent and easy to use
5. Professionals redefine their roles
6. Skilled, well-trained, committed staff
7. Comprehensive, flexible services

These systems-related attributes support the implementation and continued development of family-focused programs in AOD treatment and prevention. Dunst, Trivette, & Deal (1988) identified four similar principles that have been shown to be both necessary and sufficient for guiding the design, planning, and implementation of programs using family-focused strategies and approaches:

1. Promote positive child, parent, and family functioning; base intervention efforts on family-identified needs, aspirations, and personal projects.
2. Enhance successful efforts toward meeting needs; use existing family functioning styles (strengths and capabilities) as a basis for promoting the family's ability to mobilize resources.
3. Ensure the availability and adequacy of resources for meeting needs; place major emphasis on strengthening the family's personal social network; promise use of untapped but potential sources of informal aid and assistance.
4. Enhance a family's ability to become more self-sustaining with respect to meeting its needs; employ helping behaviors that promote the family's acquisition and use of competencies and skills necessary to mobilize and secure resources (Dunst et al., 1988, pp. 48-49).

These principles provide the bridge to link theory and research in family functioning to program practice and thus to program evaluation.

The theoretical link also must be made between family functioning and alcohol and other drug abuse treatment, intervention, and prevention. Family involvement has long been recognized as important to successful intervention and treatment outcomes. (The relationship between intervention and treatment with families is discussed in Chapter 1.) In addition to the role of the family in intervention and treatment, recent research has focused on the critical role of the family in preventing AOD problems. Research has identified four family factors that can increase the risk of AOD problems:

1. Family alcohol and drug behavior and attitudes
2. Poor and inconsistent family management practices
3. Family conflict
4. Low bonding to family (Hawkins, Catalano, & Miller, 1992)

The identification of these family factors suggests that programs that promote, support, and reinforce healthy family growth and functioning will reduce risk and increase individual and family resiliency to AOD problems.

However, the relationship between increasing family functioning and decreasing AOD use has not yet been evaluated (OSAP, 1991).

Evaluations *have* identified a number of problems in traditional alcohol and other drug programs that are not family focused:

Inadequate use of theory
Failure to consider differences in the causes or use of different substances
Failure to consider community and target population differences in program development
Failure to reach youth in high-risk environments
Interventions that are inherently weak or narrow in focus
Weak implementation
Weak program assessments (OSAP, 1991)

The effective implementation of appropriate and precise evaluations can be used as the basis for providing the necessary information to address these problem areas.

Unfortunately the existing quantity and quality of theoretically explicit AOD family-focused program evaluations is limited (NIDA, 1991; OSAP, 1991; Weiss & Jacobs, 1988). In most cases, the programs have been in existence for too brief a period to undergo major outcome and impact evaluations. In other cases, evaluation was thought to be too costly an endeavor or the conceptual/theoretical assumptions of the program were unclear. The complexity of AOD problems requires long-term, sustained, systemic and multidimensional programs. The fear is that unrealistic expectations of showing immediate reductions in AOD use and problems will not be fulfilled and will result in programs not being funded. There has also been a failure on behalf of policy and programmatic decision makers to use theory-based evaluation findings as a basis for making policy and program decisions. They have tended to rely on other measures, such as intuition, political clout, informal feedback, and observations to base their decisions.

In addition to these factors, which are mostly external to the actual evaluation methodology and process, are a number of other factors that limit the effective application and use of existing evaluation efforts:

- The use of inappropriate and inadequate measures: Measures that are appropriate for measuring individual effects are inappropriate for program evaluation and family systems assessments. There is a general lack of psychometrically proven methods (Sigafoos, Reiss, Rich, & Douglas, 1985; Walker & Crocker, 1988; Weiss & Jacobs, 1988).

- The use of experimental or quasi-experimental evaluation designs: Research-oriented designs are inappropriate for evaluating most service delivery programs, especially those that are relatively new in their developmental cycle (Jacobs, 1988).
- A failure to design evaluations that are sensitive to and based on the ethnicity and culture of the community and program participants: Most evaluations were designed by, based on, and reflective of Anglo culture (Slaughter, 1988).
- Evaluations have not included client system input or environmental and contextual issues in methodology, design, measures, procedures, and analysis (Cunningham, 1992; Walker & Crocker, 1988; Weiss, 1983).
- A lack of clarity and understanding of the theoretical and conceptual basis for the program and strategies selected to be implemented: In addition, there is a failure to link theory and research findings with programmatic practice and evaluation (Dunst et al., 1988).
- A lack of effective methods to disseminate findings, build evaluation capability, and transfer technology: At best, most of our learnings are in fugitive literature and not professional journals (Cronbach, 1982; Jacobs, 1984).

Future Directions

Culturally sensitive and specific evaluation designs must be used in future evaluation efforts. Most evaluation designs have been based on methodology derived from experience in evaluating programs that have been designed for, managed by, and based on the needs, values, priorities, and resources of male Anglo Americans. Evaluations must be designed intentionally to include the values, needs, resources, and priorities of the ethnicity and culture being served by the program. Gender issues, too, must be considered so that programs and evaluations become more sensitive to the needs and priorities of women. Measures, data collection instruments, and techniques must be culturally sensitive. The evaluators must be culturally competent (Cunningham, 1992).

Environmentally oriented evaluation designs are needed. Effective AOD family-focused programs use a framework that views the individual and family within a larger environment, taking into account the conditions and context within which the family lives and functions. Walker and Crocker (1988) emphasized that the interrelatedness, interdependence, and interaction of all of these elements must be included in the design, implementation, and interpretation of the evaluation findings.

Risk-focused programs and evaluations are critical to the continued development of the AOD field. Evaluations of programs that employ risk- and protective-factor research and approaches are necessary. The efficacy of these programs must be documented and analyzed to serve as a basis for continued program development in this promising area (Hawkins et al., 1992).

CRITICAL EVALUATION ISSUES FOR PROGRAM DECISION MAKERS

As previously stated, program evaluations provide the means for policy and programmatic decision makers to (a) identify goals and objectives, (b) describe the activities implemented to achieve the objectives, (c) measure whether any changes have taken place, and (d) determine whether the goals or objectives have been accomplished. Evaluation is designed to verify, document, and quantify process or treatment activities and their effects (OSAP, 1991). In addition, evaluation should be integral to both program planning and decision making for continued program enhancement and development. The most important use of evaluation is to guide program development and to ensure responsiveness to community and program needs (Littell, 1986). Therefore evaluation must be based on the questions that the program needs answers to, the developmental stage of the program, and what information may be required by external sources. As mentioned above, the answer to the question "When to evaluate?" is at the planning stage and is involved all the way through the developmental life cycle of the program.

A critical question to address is "What type of evaluation should be done?" The 6-step model of program assessment described below will help determine what questions a program seeks to answer and thus what levels of evaluation are related to each set of questions. Based on the stage of program development, a program may need to answer questions at only one level or at multiple levels of evaluation:

1. Needs Assessment: *Is there a need for a program? If so, what type and for whom?* Needs assessments determine the extent, type, and parameters of AOD problems faced by families in a community. They determine how the community defines AOD problems and where these problems fall on the hierarchy of needs, values, or goals within the community. They also look at the relationships between AOD problems

and other health and social issues in the community, what resources are available to address the problems, needs, and aspirations, and the varying expectations of community members about how the problems will be resolved. The needs assessment provides important information for understanding a community and the problem of AOD; it also helps guide program planning and implementation.

2. Specify Goals and Objectives: *What are the goals and objectives? What do we want to accomplish?* This step will identify the primary goals and objectives of the program, who the target groups are (e.g., African-American families in a public housing project), and state what outcomes are being sought. Critical to this step are clear and specific objectives that are realistic, attainable, and measurable. The objectives are useful for clarifying the aims and outcomes of the program, while also providing the foundation for the other three levels of evaluation.

3. Process Evaluation: *What did we do, and how did we do it?* The process evaluation describes the activities, steps, and procedures implemented to accomplish the objectives. It will describe both the service delivery process and document the related program activities. The process evaluation will provide information about how the program is functioning and will make any underlying assumptions explicit. In addition, it will serve a program-monitoring function to help ensure that parts of the program are not neglected and that resources are allocated on the basis of identified needs. A good process evaluation will provide information on why the program did or did not work, information critical for program management and development, as well as for determining whether the program is now ready for outcome evaluation.

4. Outcome Evaluation: *What were the specific accomplishments?* The outcome evaluation will assess changes in the indicators selected to measure a program's objectives. It will determine the direct effect of the program by assessing whether the objectives specified in Step 2 have been achieved. Outcome evaluation is concerned primarily with program effectiveness. It should be employed only after the program is operating with satisfactory efficiency across all of the processes deemed to be required for successful implementation.

5. Impact Evaluation: *What were the ultimate effects of the program?* Impact evaluation assesses the generalized effects of the program on the incidence and prevalence of AOD problems in the target population and/or community. It also measures whether there has been a reduction

in the risk factors related to AOD use and an increase in protective factors. Impact evaluation is a long-term, intensive process that requires a significant commitment of time and resources. It also requires extremely sophisticated evaluation designs and should be undertaken only when a program has achieved successful implementation (which has been well documented), consistent accomplishment of objectives, and a sufficient magnitude of delivery to achieve more short-term, generalized effects.

6. Interpretation and Decision Making: *What do the evaluation findings mean for ongoing policy, programmatic, and theory development?* The evaluation data must be reviewed and assessed critically to determine the implications for program operations, community needs, conditions, resources, and aspirations. In addition, program evaluation can provide information to support ongoing theory building and strategy development for family-focused AOD programs. The findings also must be assessed in light of the experiences of other programs using similar strategies and focusing on similar problems, needs, communities, and target populations. Although often neglected, the legal, moral, cultural, and ethical implications of the findings must be considered for policy and programmatic decision-making purposes.

7. Dissemination and Technology Transfer: *How can we share the results? How can they be used by others?* This step is focused on making the evaluation findings available and accessible to others. It is concerned also with making the information useful and usable. In addition, this step emphasizes how to translate and transfer the findings to multiple audiences with different needs and different levels of knowledge and understanding.

The use of this 7-step process will enable program staff and administrators to select, design, and implement evaluations consistent with the needs of their programs and communities. In addition, it provides the basis for advancing the body of knowledge on effective family-focused AOD programs and strategies.

THE FAMILY-FOCUSED CONTINUUM OF CARE

The multistep evaluation process in the previous section helps assess the effectiveness of AOD programs in providing family-focused services.

Such services should be consistent with the AOD continuum of family services described in Chapter 1. The general questions listed for each step in this evaluation process can be translated into more specific evaluation questions for prevention, intervention, and treatment continuum of services. Table 11.1 provides examples of evaluation questions appropriate for each step in the evaluation process for the prevention segment of the continuum.

Similar questions have been developed to guide the 5-step evaluation process for family-focused intervention and treatment services. Again, the stage of program development and the existence of various resources help determine which level of questions is relevant to a particular program and which level of evaluation is therefore appropriate. Table 11.2 contains questions for the different evaluation levels/steps related to intervention services, while Table 11.3 contains the questions related to evaluation of family-focused treatment programs.

KEY PRINCIPLES TO GUIDE FAMILY-FOCUSED PROGRAM EVALUATION

From the information discussed in previous sections of the chapter, a number of key principles for effective family-focused program evaluation have emerged:

- A thorough understanding of family systems theory, the ecology of human development, addictions theory and practice, and risk- and protective-factor research is crucial. The linkages and dynamic relationship between each element must be understood.
- The research basis for family systems approaches, risk-focused approaches, and the strategies identified along the continuum of care in Chapter 1 must be understood.
- Program evaluation must assess the linkages within the family system and the context and environment in which the family operates.
- The type of evaluation selected should be based on the stage of development of the program and the program's developmental needs relevant to that stage.
- The primary purpose of program evaluations is to guide program development. The evaluations should be management focused to support policy and programmatic decision making.
- The evaluation design and measures must fit the program rather than the program fitting the design. Standardized instruments and measures should

text continued on page 285

Table 11.1

Alcohol and Other Drug Services Continuum of Family Services Prevention

Evaluation Steps	*Questions to Be Considered*
Step I: Needs Assessment	1. What are the types and extent of risk factors existing in your community? 2. What resources are currently available for families? 3. What types of families are most at risk for AOD problems in your community? 4. Does your community see family-related prevention services as a high priority? 5. What are the differences in prevention needs and priorities among the different ethnicities and cultures in your community?
Step II: Goals or Objectives	1. Do the objectives target families? Do the objectives target contextual issues impacting families? 2. Do the objectives identify family risk or protective factors to be reduced or strengthened? 3. Do the objectives specify the number and type of families to be reached? 4. Are the objectives realistic, attainable, and based on sound family systems and prevention theory and practice?
Step III: Process Evaluation	1. Did the implemented activities target and involve families? 2. Did the activities focus on reducing and strengthening risk and protective factors? 3. Were the implemented activities consistent with the objectives and program design? 4. Were the targeted families reached? 5. How well did the program implement the program design and plan?
Step IV: Outcome Evaluation	1. Were the family-focused objectives achieved? 2. What type and number of families benefitted from the program? 3. Which activities displayed more or less effectiveness for what type of families? 4. What was the relationship between the type, intensity, and frequency of services and achievement of the objectives? 5. What changes have taken place in the linkages and interaction between families and other systems in the community?
Step V: Impact Evaluation	1. Were there reductions in risk factors and increases in protective factors that can be attributed to the strategies used? 2. Were there changes in the incidence of AOD problems that can be attributed to the strategies used? 3. What combination of programs, services, and activities is necessary to create a measurable change in AOD problems and risk factors? 4. What changes in conditions that impact family AOD use and problems can be attributed to the strategies used?

Table 11.2
Alcohol and Other Drug Services Continuum of Family Services Intervention

Evaluation Steps	*Questions to Be Considered*
Step I: Needs Assessment	1. What are the existing intervention services and resources available in your community? 2. What is the demand for intervention services? 3. How are the intervention and treatment services structured and coordinated? 4. What is the relationship between those experiencing AOD problems and those entering treatment? 5. How many and what type of the existing services and resources focus on the family unit? 6. What's missing from the family-focused intervention services and resources in your community?
Step II: Goals or Objectives	1. Do the outcomes specify both moving the family into treatment and reducing family resistance to change? 2. Do the objectives specify the number and types of families to receive intervention services? 3. Are the objectives realistic, attainable, and based on strategic and intergenerational family system theories? 4. Are the objectives quantifiable and measurable? 5. Do the objectives target both the families and the contextual issues impacting families?
Step III: Process Evaluation	1. Were intervention services provided to families? What services? 2. How were the services planned, organized, and implemented? 3. Were the implemented activities consistent with the goals and objectives? 4. How well did the program implement the program design and plan? 5. What were the supports, barriers, and steps undertaken to maximize program delivery?
Step IV: Outcome Evaluation	1. Were the objectives achieved? 2. Was there an increase in families entering treatment and a decrease in families resistant to change? 3. What type and number of families benefited from the program? 4. What was the relationship between the type, intensity, availability, and frequency of services and the achievement of the objectives? 5. What changes have taken place in the linkages and interactions between families and intervention-related systems in the community?
Step V: Impact Evaluation	1. Were there increases in attitudes toward treatment and families entering treatment which can be attributed to the strategies used? 2. Are families in the community more responsive to making changes? 3. Do the community services and systems support and facilitate identifying and involving the families in treatment? 4. What level and linkages among resources and services are necessary to measurably increase the number and involvement of families entering treatment?

Table 11.3
Alcohol and Other Drug Services Continuum of Family Services
Treatment

Evaluation Steps	*Questions to Be Considered*
Step I: Needs Assessment	1. What are the number, type, and location of families experiencing AOD problems? 2. What are the number, type, and location of family-focused treatment services? 3. How are the services structured and coordinated? 4. Is there community support for family-focused treatment services—for what services? 5. What are the gaps and what's missing in the treatment system?
Step II: Goals or Objectives	1. Do the objectives focus on families? 2. Do the outcomes specify changes in families and AOD related problems experienced by families? 3. Do the objectives specify the strategy to be used, the services to be provided, and the outcomes anticipated? 4. Are the objectives realistic, attainable, and based on family systems theories? 5. Are the objectives quantifiable and measurable?
Step III: Process Evaluation	1. Were treatment services provided to families? What services were provided? Who received the services? 2. How were the services planned, organized, and implemented? 3. Were the implemented activities consistent with the goals and objectives? 4. How well did the program implement the program design and plan? 5. What were the supports, barriers, and steps undertaken to maximize program delivery? 6. How were the services coordinated and linked with other community services?
Step IV: Outcome Evaluation	1. Were the family-focused objectives achieved? 2. What type and number of families benefited from the programs? 3. Which services showed positive outcomes? How about combinations of services? 4. What was the relationship between the type, intensity, availability, and frequency of services and the achievement of the objectives? 5. How many families needed relapse services? 6. Are there differences in the effectiveness of services based on types of services and extent of problems?
Step V: Impact Evaluation	1. Did the provision of services decrease the prevalence of AOD problems among families in the community? 2. Are families in the community more responsive to making changes? 3. Are services linked and well coordinated? 4. Are families aware of services and willing to use them if needed? 5. Is the system responsive to the needs of families and the community?

be employed only if they are consistent with the design and objectives of the program.

- Culturally and gender-appropriate designs and evaluation procedures must be employed with input being encouraged from the different ethnic groups being served. Culturally competent evaluation staff are essential.
- Evaluating the process in addition to the outcomes of programs must be a high priority.
- Program staff must be involved in the evaluation process, and evaluation must be seen as a key component of the program from the earliest stage of program planning and development.
- Evaluation findings must be analyzed and presented in a manner to facilitate ease of understanding and usefulness to program decision makers and practitioners, not researchers or evaluators.
- The evaluation design and the data collected should be assessed to determine whether there have been any unintended negative side effects of the program. The guiding principle should be "do no harm."
- The ethical and moral implications inherent in the use of control and comparison groups should be discussed and considered in the selection of an appropriate program and evaluation design.

CASE STUDIES: ILLUSTRATIONS OF PROGRAM EVALUATIONS

The chapter on helping homeless and runaway youth with drug problems (Chapter 3) and the chapter on codependency (Chapter 5) have been used to provide concrete examples of evaluation questions, possible approaches, measures, and outcomes of family-focused program evaluations. The case studies illustrate a number of the points raised in the preceding discussion. One of the suggested programmatic interventions for each topic will be selected, and some of the key evaluation issues will be discussed.

Helping Homeless and Runaway Youth With Drug Abuse Problems

Synopsis. Chapter 3 describes the incidence and process leading youth to run away and develop alcohol and other drug problems. It further details the connection between developmental issues and running away. In addition, the chapter suggests a number of policy and programmatic strategies that can be implemented to achieve the goal of effective independent living for runaway youth and the elimination of societal conditions that hamper the achievement of the goal. One of the potentially effective strategies suggested is the use of small group homes. This approach is used as the basis to illustrate a number of potential evaluation questions, issues, and strategies.

Program Components. The proposed program was designed to provide alternative family structures to achieve the above goals. The task-centered family systems program components included the following:

AOD counseling and treatment
Educational and/or vocational services
Independent living workshops
Self-assessment and monitoring of independent living skills
Task groups
Family meetings
Mentoring

Evaluation Plan. As a new and innovative program, major emphasis should be on identifying needs and resources, specifying and quantifying the goals and objectives, and assessing the implementation of the program process (the first three steps/levels of the author's evaluation model). The program evaluation will use a staged implementation approach whereby initially the formative evaluation tasks will be conducted to document and monitor program implementation and to provide information for guiding further program development and improvement. These tasks could be followed by the collection of summative data through the use of an outcome evaluation. The outcome evaluation can provide information on the effectiveness of the program at achieving the stated objectives. Impact evaluation is not recommended at this time because the proposed program is too new and its potential effectiveness has not been documented.

Although a generalized need for the program may have been indicated, it is vitally important that a thorough *needs assessment* be implemented. This needs assessment will identify the following:

The number of youth who are running away
Where they are going
The activities they engage in
The number who return home

The extent and type of drugs used
The gender, ethnic, and socioeconomic makeup of the runaways
Current resources available
How the resources are organized
How effective they are
What provisions/resources are missing from the current services
How the community perceives the problem
How the youth perceive the problem
What needs the runaways themselves see
How receptive the community is to group homes or other forms of service
What types of needs, issues, and problems are being experienced by the runaways

The needs assessment will provide the necessary information to ascertain whether an approach using a family systems theoretical framework that emphasizes building and enhancing strengths is needed. It also will help predict whether such an approach is likely to be successfully implemented and effective in reducing AOD problems and family losses of runaways.

The *specification of the program goals and objectives* is extremely crucial, particularly for this program. The issues are so complex: drug use, runaways, criminal acts, family dysfunction, arrested human development, educational and vocational skills, sexual issues, child care and parenting, independent living skills, and racial discrimination. It is vital that the objectives ultimately specified are realistic and achievable, based on the needs of the youth, resources available, and services to be provided.

Another key feature of the objectives for this program is the importance of specifying objectives focused on the linkages and interactions between the various components of the program. In addition, the objectives should address the crosscutting issues of ethnicity, culture, and discrimination. Finally the objectives should be structured to allow for differential program effectiveness and the recognition that there will be a number of possible positive outcomes for participants in the program, depending on their individual needs and situations, rather than a standardized set of what constitutes a positive outcome.

The *process evaluation* will document how the program implemented the family systems group home approach. The issues to be addressed include the following:

Staff selection and performance
Community relations
Securing a facility
Linking with other resources in the community
What services were implemented
How successful they were at implementing the services
What barriers existed that had to be overcome
What support they received
How successful the program was at reaching and serving the youth
What unplanned steps or services were implemented
The quality of the services

The key use for this information is to feed it back continually into the program development process. Therefore process evaluation information should be collected and analyzed on a frequent basis. Formal systems should be established to ensure that the information is incorporated into ongoing program improvement processes.

A crucial consideration is to maximize the involvement and understanding of the process evaluation among all of the program staff. Conversely the evaluation staff must have a sound understanding of the theoretical and programmatic basis for the program. The data must be presented in a manner and format to ensure that they are both useful and usable.

The *outcome evaluation* will assess the success of the program at achieving the stated objectives. The goals of the program are to build an alternative family structure and to develop skills of independent living. The outcome evaluation will assess changes in the specific objectives selected by the program to affect the above-mentioned goals. In addition to measuring the effectiveness of the specific components, the evaluation should be capable of assessing the differential effectiveness of a variety of mixes of services based on the individualized needs of program participants. The program design emphasizes self-assessment of independent living skills and psychosocial functioning. Therefore the outcome evaluation must employ measures and use instruments that are both technically sound and capable of being effectively administered by youth at varying degrees of reading proficiency. The use of task groups and family meetings necessitates developing measures that assess outcomes based on the objectives of the task groups and the problems or needs to be addressed or resolved in the family meeting. Because the power of the program lies in its comprehensiveness, the outcome evaluation should focus on the effectiveness of the integration of the components, as opposed to focusing on the effectiveness of the separate services provided.

Summary

By implementing a carefully staged evaluation design, a rich and powerful evaluation of a runaway group home program can be implemented. The evaluation can provide substantial data that can assist in program development and continued enhancement. It can lay the groundwork for further evaluations to determine the impact of the approach on reducing AOD problems and improving the opportunities for successful independent living among runaways.

Codependency: Helping Clients Move From Enabling to Autonomous Relationships

Synopsis. Chapter 5 provides a foundation for defining *codependency* and its implications for effective treatment and prevention. The chapter presents a problem-solving family systems treatment approach that is consistent with the codependency perspective of the authors. This perspective views codependency as a process and from a strength rather than a pathological perspective. It involves ineffective problem solving and the assumption of role responsibilities for the chemically dependent partner in order to maintain the family system. The approach involves the use of a variety of methods for:

Developing a knowledge base about addictions and codependency
Assessing the personal and systems goals of members of the family unit
Identifying the source of blocks to goal attainment
Relating these obstacles to chemical abuse
Evaluating the effectiveness of current problem-solving strategies
Developing new strategies for problem solving and goal attainment

Program Components. The treatment process as suggested above serves as the basis for a proposed program consisting of the following components to be evaluated:

Community outreach
Client intake

Ancillary and support services
Information and referral
Client assessment
AOD education
Group counseling
Self-help group referral
Individual and family counseling

Evaluation Plan. The evaluation plan is designed to assess the program's ability to implement successfully the treatment process and the effectiveness of the program in facilitating the use of new strategies for problem solving and goal attainment. The evaluation plan will emphasize clarity of objectives to ensure that they are attainable and consistent with the perspective on codependency proposed by the authors. The plan also will be focused on providing information needed to manage the program effectively. The strategies will be assessed to determine the success of their implementation and the effectiveness of each phase of treatment on meeting the needs of participants at that level. Impact evaluation is not indicated at this time due to the early stage of development this program is in.

Prior to program implementation, a *needs assessment* is necessary to determine the potential number of families affected by alcohol and other drug problems. The potential sources of the clients should be identified and assessed to determine the possible number of codependent individuals in the community. The potential resources for treatment and self-help must be identified. Also, because clients will experience immediate needs such as medical and child care, financial assistance, and legal help, community resources must be identified and secured. In addition, referral sources must be interviewed to determine their perceptions about the need for services and the type of problems encountered by the potential clients.

The *goals and objectives* must be tied directly to the implementation of the problem-solving approach to codependency. Objectives should be specified for each phase of the program. Because the effectiveness of the program is based to a large degree on the identification and use of external resources, objectives also should focus on the linkages and interactions between the program, resources, and clients. Also, because the clients will determine what their needs are and the problems they choose to address, the objectives should be framed to provide for the use of a number of different indicators of effectiveness.

The *process evaluation* will take each phase of treatment and determine the implementation tasks and objectives necessary for that phase. It then will assess the degree of success experienced by the program in completing the task. For the initial client contact, the effectiveness of identifying, establishing, and using referral networks will be important. Questions such as "How many participants came from each source?" and "What types of relationships with chemically dependent individuals are experienced by clients in the program?" should be addressed. For ongoing treatment, the evaluation will document the types of problems encountered by the clients, what services were provided, whom they were referred to, and the problems they encountered with establishing referral linkages. In addition, documentation of how many clients followed up on the referrals, what support materials such as books were provided, and how many discontinued treatment at this stage and for what reasons are important.

As clients enter the second phase, the process evaluation will document the number and types of clients who continue in the program. It will identify also the usage rates of the codependency assessment tools and which ones were well received. The number of interventions with the codependent individuals would be documented, as well as referrals and participation in self-help and other therapeutic encounters. If peer or family groups are used, the quantity, type, and frequency of the groups is documented, as well as the number of participants in each of them and the issues addressed. Finally the process evaluation will assess participation in ongoing growth and development classes and other educational activities, the type of resources used, and the skills identified to be addressed.

The evaluation plan also will assess the ability of the program and the strategies employed to reach and effectively address the problems and needs of different ethnic and cultural groups. It will explore which methods worked for which ethnic groups and what culturally competent strategies were necessary to effectively serve multiethnic populations.

The *outcome evaluation* will assess the achievement of the objectives identified for each phase of treatment. For the initial contact, the evaluation will measure the program effectiveness in identifying and involving clients, in identifying and effectively addressing the presenting problems, and in examining and addressing clients' current goals. For the second phase, the evaluation will determine the number of clients who effectively assess their degree of codependency and the effectiveness of the program in educating the clients on the impact of alcoholism and other drug dependence. At the third phase, the evaluation will assess the effectiveness of the groups in developing or increasing the interpersonal relationship building, problem solving, and communication and listening skills. In addition, the relative effectiveness of individual versus group processes will be assessed. The outcome evaluation for the final phase will measure the number of clients who strengthened their ability to function more effectively and autonomously in achieving personal goals.

Summary

The implementation of an evaluation plan that places equal emphasis on the formative processes of needs assessments, goal and objective specification, and program implementation, as well as the summative process of measuring program effectiveness, yields information that will provide ongoing guidance for program improvement. This plan allows the family codependency program to identify what phases and activities worked for whom. It also lays the foundation for both single system evaluation and impact evaluation at a later time.

CONCLUSION

This chapter has provided an overview of a number of the issues involved in developing, implementing, and using evaluations of family-focused AOD programs. A number of points have been highlighted in the discussion. Among them are the following:

- A primary emphasis of evaluation should be on developing methodologies that support program development and improvement and that are designed to meet the needs of policy and programmatic decision makers.
- The evaluations should be sensitive to, based on, and designed with the ethnic population(s) being served by the program.
- Equal attention should be devoted to both process and outcome evaluation. The evaluation steps should include needs assessment, goal and objective specification, interpretation and implications of findings, dissemination, and technology transfer.

Finally the chapter advocates designing evaluations that focus on looking at the interdependence, interrelatedness, and interaction of family systems and the AOD-related programs developed to serve them. Only with this type of comprehensive and systemic approach can program evaluations of AOD family-focused services become an expected and valued part of such services.

REFERENCES

Cronbach, L. J. (1982). *Designing evaluations of education and social programs.* San Francisco: Jossey-Bass.

Cunningham, M. S. (1992). Multiethnic community empowerment: Affirming diversity, respecting differences, and building common-unity. In State of Washington Division of Substance Abuse, *Planning the future of prevention II in Washington State* (pp. B1-10). Olympia, WA: Developmental Research and Programs.

Dunst, C., Trivette, C., & Deal, A. (1988). *Enabling and empowering families.* Cambridge, MA: Brookline Books.

Hawkins, J. D., Catalano, R. F., & Miller, J. Y. (1992). Risk and protective factors for alcohol and other drug problems in adolescence and early adulthood: Implications for substance abuse prevention. In State of Washington Division of Substance Abuse, *Planning the future of prevention in Washington State* (Vol. II pp. A1-11). Olympia, WA: Developmental Research and Programs.

Jacobs, F. (1984). The state-of-the-art in family program evaluation. In H. Weiss & F. Jacobs (Eds.), *Final report to the Mott Foundation: The effectiveness and evaluation of family support and education programs* (pp. 64-98). Cambridge, MA: Harvard Family Research Project.

Jacobs, F. H. (1988). The five-tiered approach to evaluation: Context and implementation. In H. B. Weiss & F. H. Jacobs (Eds.), *Evaluating family programs* (pp. 37-68). Hawthorne, NY: Aldine.

Littell, J. H. (1986). *Building strong foundations: Evaluating strategies for family resource programs.* Chicago: Family Resource Coalition.

National Institute on Drug Abuse (NIDA). (1991). *Drug abuse and drug abuse research: The third triennial report to Congress from the Secretary, Department of Health and Human Services* (DHHS Publication No. ADM 91-1704). Washington, DC: Government Printing Office.

Office of Substance Abuse Prevention (OSAP). (1990). *Prevention research findings: 1988* (DHHS Publication No. ADM 89-1615). Washington, DC: Government Printing Office.

Office of Substance Abuse Prevention (OSAP). (1991). *Prevention plus III* (DHHS Publication No. ADM 91-1817). Washington, DC: Government Printing Office.

Schorr, L., & Schorr, D. (1988). *Within our reach.* New York: Anchor.

Sigafoos, A., Reiss, D., Rich, J., & Douglas, E. (1985). Pragmatics in the measurement of family functioning: An interpretive framework for methodology. *Family Process, 24,* 189-203.

Slaughter, D. T. (1988). Programs for racially and ethnically diverse American families: Some critical issues. In H. B. Weiss & F. H. Jacobs (Eds.), *Evaluating family programs* (pp. 461-476). Hawthorne, NY: Aldine.

Springer, J. F. (1990). Learning from prevention policy: A management-focused approach. In *Prevention research findings: 1988* (pp. 231-242). DHHS Publication No. (ADM) 89-1615. Washington, DC: Government Printing Office.

Walker, D. K., & Crocker, R. W. (1988). Measuring family system outcomes. In H. B. Weiss & F. H. Jacobs (Eds.), *Evaluating family programs* (pp. 153-176). Hawthorne, NY: Aldine.

Weiss, C. H. (1983). The stakeholder approach to evaluation: Origins and promise. In A. S. Bryk (Ed.), *Stakeholder-based evaluation* (pp. 3-14). San Francisco: Jossey-Bass.

Weiss, H. B., & Jacobs, F. H. (1988). *Evaluating family programs.* Hawthorne, NY: Aldine.

Epilogue

THE FAMILY SYSTEM RECOVERY PROCESS
What Is Lasting Change?

EDITH M. FREEMAN

The life span developmental framework of this book has provided numerous opportunities throughout these pages to emphasize the importance of acknowledging and building on individual and family strengths. As noted in the African proverb in the epigraph, each member of a family can contribute to the overall unit's strengths to resolve the problem of addiction. In circumstances in which hope for recovery and other positive changes has been lost, the responsibility for building on existing strengths and helping families develop new strengths assumes even more importance. Both the initiative for change and an effective family treatment process are greatly dependent on the family's and practitioner's skills in using their individual and system strengths.

THE FAMILY SYSTEMS PERSPECTIVE

Although an emphasis on strengths has been the cornerstone of this book, the focus also has been on a broad range of issues related to substance abuse treatment from a family systems perspective. However, a comprehensive approach has required attention to the other two areas on the substance abuse continuum of care during many of the discussions: intervention and prevention, as well as treatment. The advantages of using a family systems perspective throughout the book has been the guidelines it provides for maintaining a focus on all factors relevant to addiction development and recovery at key points during the life cycle of individuals and families. Substance abuse problems at various developmental stages often combine with other issues in the lives of families—for example, with issues related to cultural identity, sexual dysfunctioning, or mental illness. Moreover, life cycle issues themselves (such as separation from the family of origin and the aging process) have become more complex in recent years due to the changing nature of families and the shifting social context described in this book's preface. These complexities can result automatically in a more complicated, and often less effective, treatment process.

SUBSTANCE ABUSE TREATMENT EFFECTIVENESS

Treatment effectiveness with addicted families is both a short-term and a long-term issue, as noted in the research and evaluation section of this book (the first year of recovery vs. a lifetime of recovery). The first goal in substance abuse treatment is to facilitate recovery by using the family system's initial disequilibrium to keep the unit open and vulnerable to change. The unit's initiative for change is always counterbalanced by its attempts to maintain the status quo (the addictive cycle and other related problems of the system). Short-term recovery involves helping the system understand how it can survive and yet change by building on and enhancing strengths that move the unit toward recovery while preserving other aspects of the system that it needs to maintain (the system's desire to eliminate the substance abuse, the members' commitment to each other, or a member's insight about the family dynamics related to the addiction). Regression during treatment and aftercare, rather than being viewed as a threat to long-term recovery, can be reframed on systems concepts as an opportunity to strengthen short-term recovery (Watzlawick, Weakland, & Fisch, 1974).

The family may learn additional information about the addicted individual and the system that clarifies the triggers for relapse and the unit's pattern of dysfunctional responses to critical incidences. Such information can strengthen the family's ability to maintain the recovery process. In addition, strengths within the extended family, neighborhood or community organizations, and informal role models (e.g., peer counselors or natural leaders in the community) can be used to maintain the recovery process as well. Other aspects of effective treatment, as noted throughout this book, include the analysis of life cycle issues; the use of approaches that can address the diversity in family forms, structure, and functions that are encountered in substance abuse treatment; the focus on the family internally and in terms of its larger environment; and the various roles that the range of practitioners from various professional disciplines must use to serve families effectively. All of these factors can contribute to effective recovery in the short term.

WHAT IS LASTING CHANGE?

What about the long-term recovery process and lasting change? Watzlawick et al. (1974) indicated that change can occur on two distinct levels in terms of strategic family systems theory. In *first-order change,* a system (society) can change within its given way of behaving. The result does not change the system itself but does bring about changes in the members of the system within its limited repertoire of changes (Papp, 1983; Watzlawick et al., 1974). Presently substance abuse treatment, intervention, and prevention efforts are aimed at the individual family or community; the result is short-term changes for those targets, but the system itself (society) does not change. The underlying problem of addiction does not go away for society at large, although individual families and communities are benefitted in recovery and prevention in the short term.

They may benefit also in the long term if they are able to achieve second-order change on their own. *Second-order change* occurs when there is a change in the premises that govern a system so that the system itself is changed (Watzlawick et al., 1974). In the individual family or community, second-order change may occur during treatment or prevention services based on a change in the family's or community's beliefs about the problem. Second-order change may be achieved from a reframe by the practitioner that the addicted person's problem is really a family problem. The reframe changes beliefs of the family about the problem that may have helped maintain the problem in the past. This type of change in the family's beliefs about the addiction and related problems can help mobilize resources for change that the members were unaware of due to their previous views (e.g., by no longer pretending the addiction does not exist, they can ask for support and problem-solving resources from extended family members). This type of strategic family systems intervention also reduces the family's ability to continue their collusion in blaming the addicted member for all of the problems.

Another example is an empowerment prescription by a preventionist; he or she might say that other parts of a city have given up on a community's chances of surviving an increasing addiction rate, so it would be easy to see why the community itself might give up on resolving its problem. This type of second-order change prescription is paradoxical because it prescribes the very behavior that is maintaining the problem (Watzlawick et al., 1974), and once it is acknowledged by the community, it allows them to see the problem as resolvable rather than insurmountable. It is the community's belief that the problem cannot be resolved that helps to maintain it.

Given the distinctions between first- and second-order change, it is clear that to strengthen the family recovery process and to eliminate the problem of addiction, second-order change is needed at a societal level. This type of lasting change can be accomplished only through the following tasks related to society (Freeman, 1992; Kerr, 1982; Watzlawick et al., 1974; Wyers, 1991):

- A closer collaboration between policy and practice in the substance abuse treatment field, leading to policy-practice advocates for and participants in policy formulation, implementation, and change (policies that reduce the stresses that support and contribute to addiction on a large scale, such as liquor advertising)
- An increase in the collaboration between the helping professions that work in substance abuse treatment: the practice/policy/research area to address large-scale policy, funding, and practice issues (social work, psychiatry, psychology, nursing, gerontology, family therapy, occupational therapy, physical therapy, sex therapy, and education)
- The application of second-order change techniques to policy-making organizations (e.g., private funders and legislators) and treatment and prevention programs in order to change their beliefs and values that may help maintain the problem of large-scale addiction (e.g., a belief that substance abuse is only a problem in particular ethnic, age, and socioeconomic segments of the population and that the behavior within those groups alone has contributed to what is viewed as an individual problem)

CONCLUSION

These and other recommendations are necessary to achieve lasting changes in this society related to the elimination of substance abuse as a problem. In the same way that systems theory has been useful throughout this book in addressing issues of treatment with families, it is equally useful in addressing aspects of the problem at the level of organizations, communities, and society. The distinctions between first- and second-order change based on strategic family systems theory provide a practical framework for clarifying how important changes can occur within individual families and communities without society at large changing as needed. For those individual changes to be supported in the family recovery process, practitioners, policy makers, and researchers must turn their attention to methods for ensuring that second-order changes will occur in society itself.

REFERENCES

Freeman, E. M. (1992, April). *The role of developmental research in training substance abuse professionals to apply a multicultural perspective.* Paper presented at the Faculty Seminar Series on Alcohol and Other Abuse, University of Kansas, Lawrence, KS.

Kerr, M. E. (1982). Application of family systems theory to a work system. In R. Sagar & K. Wiseman (Eds.), *Understanding organizations* (pp. 121-129). Washington, DC: Georgetown University Family Center.

Papp, P. (1983). *The process of change.* New York: Guilford.

Watzlawick, P., Weakland, J., & Fisch, R. (1974). *Change: The principles of problem formulation and problem resolution.* New York: Free Press.

Wyers, N. L. (1991). Policy-practice in social work: Models and issues. *Journal of Social Work Education, 27,* 241-250.

AUTHOR INDEX

SUBJECT INDEX

ABOUT THE AUTHORS

MARIAN A. AGUILAR is an Assistant Professor at The University of Texas at Austin, School of Social Work. She received her PhD in Social Work and the Sociology of Medicine from the University of Illinois at Champaign-Urbana in 1983. Her publications and scholarly activities range from social issues that adversely impact on minorities, Mexican Americans, minority women, and minority aged to issues related to health care, education, and progress of minorities and social work practice and education in general.

STEPHANIE COVINGTON is a clinician, author, organizational consultant, and lecturer. She is recognized for her pioneering work on women's issues and specializes in programs on addiction, sexuality, families, and relationships. She has a PhD in Psychology and is a licensed clinical social worker and marriage and family therapist. At the Betty Ford Center she is Program Designer and Clinical Consultant for Women's Treatment. Her work in organizations focuses on the development of caring, compassionate, and empowering environments. She has served on the faculties of the University of Southern California, San Diego State University, and the California School of Professional Psychology. She has conducted seminars for health professionals, business and community organizations, and recovery groups in the United States and other countries. She has published numerous articles and co-authored the book *Leaving the Enchanted Forest: The Path from*

Relationship Addiction to Intimacy. Her newest book is *Awakening Your Sexuality: A Guide for Recovering Women and Their Partners.*

BRENDA CRAWLEY, PhD, is Associate Professor at the University of Kansas. Her research and numerous publications have focused on the elderly, African-American families, and social policy analysis in such areas as employment and entitlement programs. She has worked in the area of gerontology in direct practice and program development. She was a Fulbright Scholar in the country of Lesotho in Africa for the 1991-1992 academic year.

MICHAEL S. CUNNINGHAM has been Vice President and Director of Operations of Sacramento Office, The Circle, Inc., since 1989. He has expertise in acquiring and using current health-related prevention technology for agencies and organizations to use. He is also skilled in designing, implementing, and evaluating alcohol and other drug abuse prevention systems. He has an MA in Government from the Claremont Graduate School, and has done doctoral work at the Claremont Graduate School from 1974-1975.

ROBERT FAHNESTOCK is Team Leader at the Maui County Vet Center in Hawaii. He is a member of the DVA's Readjustment Counseling Service National Joint Committee on Post-Traumatic Stress and Psychoactive Substance Disorders. He earned an MSW from the University of Kansas in 1988. Prior to completing college, he served on active duty in the Navy for 20 years, the latter 5 as an alcohol and drug counselor, counseling and assistance center director, and drug abuse program advisor.

EDITH M. FREEMAN, is a Professor in the School of Social Welfare and has an adjunct appointment in the Department of African and African-American Studies at the University of Kansas. She earned a PhD in Developmental Psychology from the University of Kansas (Departments of Psychology and Human Development and Family Life) after receiving an MSW from the University of Kansas. Her scholarship efforts have resulted in four books on alcohol problems, the addiction process across substances, practice with African-American families, and practice with children in the school and community. She also has published numerous articles and chapters on the topics of substance abuse, cultural and gender-related issues in practice with families, teenage pregnancy, and effective consultation to community agencies. As a consultant, she is highly involved with substance abuse prevention and treatment programs, community organizations, hospitals, public schools, and child welfare agencies.

JACOB U. GORDON, PhD, is Professor of African and African-American Studies, Research Fellow in the Institute for Life Span Studies, and Executive Director of the Institute for Black Leadership Development and Research at the University of Kansas. Among his scholarly publications are books, monographs, research reports, more than 100 articles in professional journals, several book reviews and chapters, editorial works, and more than 200 presentations within the past 5 years. His latest book is *History of the National Bar Association: Black Lawyers in the United States.* For several years, he has been engaged in alcohol and other drug abuse prevention, intervention, and treatment research and activities, especially from multicultural perspectives.

MAN KEUNG HO was Professor of Social Work at the University of Oklahoma when he died in August, 1992. He was an approved supervisor and a clinical member or the American Association for Marriage and Family Therapy. His most recent books were *Building a Successful Intermarriage* (1984), *Family Therapy With Ethnic Minorities* (1987), and *Intermarried Couples in Therapy* (1990).

RUTH G. McROY, PhD, MSW, CSW-ACP, is the Ruby Lee Piester Centennial Professor in Services to Children and Families of the University of Texas at Austin School of Social Work. She has co-authored several articles on treatment strategies and issues for culturally diverse clients with substance abuse problems and is a co-editor of *Social Work Practice With Black Families.*

ELIZABETH J. NICKEL is a Senior Research Coordinator with the University of Kansas Medical Center. She received her BA in 1975 from Rockhurst College with a major in Psychology. In 1983 she received an MA in Psychology from the University of Missouri in Kansas City. She has coordinated three major alcoholism research grants at the Kansas City VA Medical Center, where she has guided many graduate students and her colleagues through the mazes of data analysis and manuscript preparation.

ELIZABETH C. PENICK, PhD, is Professor of Psychiatry and Director of the Division of Psychology at the University of Kansas Medical Center. She received her BA from Sophie Newcomb College in 1957, her MS in Experimental Psychology from Tulane University in 1960, and, after 2 years of postgraduate work in London, England, she received her PhD in 1975 in Clinical Psychology from Washington University in St. Louis. She has been active in the field of alcoholism treatment and alcoholism research for the past 17 years and is currently an investigator in an NIAAA follow-up study in Denmark of adult sons of alcoholics.

MARSHA R. READ, PhD, ACSW, is Clinical Associate Professor of Psychiatry at the University of Kansas Medical Center. She teaches a course in psychotherapy and provides psychotherapy supervision to psychiatry residents. In addition, she has an adjunct appointment in the University of Kansas School of Social Welfare, where she periodically teaches a seminar in psychopathology to MSW students. Her research background is in the area of alcoholism, family history, and subgroups of persons with drinking disorders. She is a co-author of a clinical diagnostic interview and co-developer of diagnosis-specific psychotherapy. Direct service includes psychotherapy with individuals, couples, and groups. She received her AB in 1964 from Milligan College in Tennessee, her MSW in 1968 from the Washington University George Warren Brown School of Social Work, and her PhD in 1981 in Medical Sociology with a minor in Social Work from the University of Kentucky.

WILLA ROSEN, MSSW, CSW, LCDC, is a clinical social worker at Dayglo Family Treatment Program in Austin, Texas. She works with chemically dependent adults, children of chemically dependent parents, and their families.

CLAYTON T. SHORKEY, MSW, CSW, ACP, PhD, is the Cullen Trust Centennial Professor of Alcohol Studies and Education of the University of Texas at Austin. He is Chair of the Mental Health and Chemical Dependence Concentration at the School of Social Work and is involved in teaching, research, and clinical practice.